Inherited Retinal Disease

Hyeong-Gon Yu
Editor

Inherited Retinal Disease

Springer

Editor
Hyeong-Gon Yu
Department of Ophthalmology
Seoul National University Hospital
Seoul, Korea (Republic of)

ISBN 978-981-16-7336-8 ISBN 978-981-16-7337-5 (eBook)
https://doi.org/10.1007/978-981-16-7337-5

This Springer imprint is published by the registered company Springer Nature Singapore Pte Ltd.
The registered company address is: 152 Beach Road, #21-01/04 Gateway East, Singapore 189721, Singapore

Preface

Inherited retinal diseases are hereditary diseases causing bilateral irreversible retinal degeneration and subsequent visual impairment. They are a large group of genetically and clinically heterogenous disorders which constitute the leading cause of vision loss in working-age adults or children. They can be stationary in some diseases, but most vision-threatening inherited retinal diseases are progressive. Retinitis pigmentosa, the most well-known inherited retinal disease, usually progresses slowly over decades, leading to visual impairment as the result of diffuse retinal degeneration. However, some inherited retinal diseases are congenital or early-infantile onset and affected individuals are legally blind from birth or early infancy.

Diagnosis of inherited retinal disease is often challenging, and reliable guidance to precise diagnosis is essential for proper management. Although currently no curative treatment is known for most disorders, patients with inherited retinal diseases can benefit from genetic counseling, supportive medication, correction of refractive error, and treatment of associated complications. In recent years, there has been great improvement in our knowledge of the genetic and cytological background of inherited retinal diseases. Genetic analysis methods such as next generation sequencing have remarkably reduced the time and cost required for large-scale analysis of patients' samples. In addition, molecular genetic testing is crucial for the treatment prospects of targeted therapeutics as well as for accurate diagnosis and prognostication. Studies on gene therapy and stem cell therapy have been successfully carried out in animal models of inherited retinal diseases. In particular, gene therapy for Leber congenital amaurosis by *RPE65* mutation is now available.

In this book, we first provide an overview of inherited retinal diseases, including molecular genetics, general principle of treatment, genetic counseling, and novel treatment methods under research. For each individual disorder, essential information regarding the genetics, diagnosis, clinical features, and possible management are discussed based on up-to-date knowledge. Experts for each inherited retinal disease were recruited as authors of this treatise, and they tried to include as many images as possible which they encountered during clinical practice. Undoubtedly, this treatise will guide the practice of not only ophthalmologists but also medical students who are seeing patients with inherited retinal diseases. I would like to thank all of the authors and the project coordinators for their special contribution to this work.

Seoul, Korea Hyeong Gon Yu

Contents

1 Molecular Genetics of Inherited Retinal Diseases

Dae Joong Ma

Abstract

In the last decade, our understanding of inherited retinal diseases (IRDs) has undergone significant advances owing to major achievements in molecular biology and genetic technologies. The study of molecular genetics of the IRDs provides not only a better understanding of the underlying pathogenesis but also the development of new therapeutic alternatives. In this chapter, we review the molecular genetic characteristics and techniques of genetic analysis associated with IRDs. We also discuss the molecular biology of the common mutations causing IRDs.

Keywords

Inherited retinal disease · Genetic analysis
Molecular genetics · Next-generation sequencing

1.1 Introduction

Inherited retinal diseases (IRDs) are a clinically and genetically heterogeneous group of inherited eye disorders characterized by rod and/or cone photoreceptor degeneration, such as retinitis pigmentosa (RP), Leber congenital amaurosis (LCA), Stargardt disease (STGD), Best vitelliform macular dystrophy (BVMD), and Usher syndrome (USH). Their estimated prevalence varies with the IRD subtype: 1/3000–1/50,000 for RP, 1/50,000–1/33,000 for LCA, 1/8000–1/10,000 for STGD, 1/5000–1/67,000 for BVMD, and 1/30,000 for USH (http://www.orpha.net).

IRDs can be classified clinically based on the following features: (1) which cell type or anatomical location is mainly affected among rod photoreceptors (RP, rod-cone dystrophy), cone photoreceptors (cone and cone-rod dystrophy and achromatopsia), macular dystrophy (STGD, BVMD, Pattern dystrophy, and Sorsby's fundus dystrophy), and choroidal dystrophy (choroideremia, central areolar choroidal atrophy, and gyrate atrophy); (2) whether or not the ocular phenotypes are associated with other organ pathologies (syndromic and non-syndromic forms); (3) whether the disease is stationary or progressive over time; and (4) the mode of inheritance (autosomal dominant, autosomal recessive, X-linked, mitochondrial, and simplex) [1, 2].

Presently, the diagnosis of IRDs is mostly based on clinical findings. However, the variable age of onset, genotypic heterogeneity (one phenotype caused by multiple genes), phenotypic heterogeneity (various mutations in a single gene resulting in various phenotypes), incomplete penetrance, unclear inheritance, and progressive

D. J. Ma (✉)
Hallym University Kangnam Sacred Heart Hospital, Seoul, South Korea

H.-G. Yu (ed.), *Inherited Retinal Disease*, https://doi.org/10.1007/978-981-16-7337-5_1

nature of IRDs impede the definitive diagnosis, and therefore, molecular genetic testing is imperative for the definitive diagnosis of IRDs.

1.2 Importance of Molecular Genetic Diagnostics in IRD

Obtaining the molecular genetic diagnosis in IRDs remains challenging because of the large number of causative genes. To date, more than 270 causative genes have been identified for IRDs (http://www.sph.uth.tmc.edu/retnet/). Frequent genetic overlaps also complicate the molecular genetic diagnosis of IRDs (Fig. 1.1). For example, some genes responsible for RP have also been associated with other IRDs, such as STGD, congenital stationary night blindness (CSNB), and LCA. Likewise, genes responsible for syndromic IRDs, such as Bardet–Biedl syndrome (BBS), have also been associated with non-syndromic IRDs, such as RP [1]. However, this genetic overlap among IRDs with different phenotypes suggests the common genetic pathways with similar underlying mechanisms, which emphasize the importance of a molecular genetic approach in IRDs for understanding the pathophysiology and developing the novel therapeutic

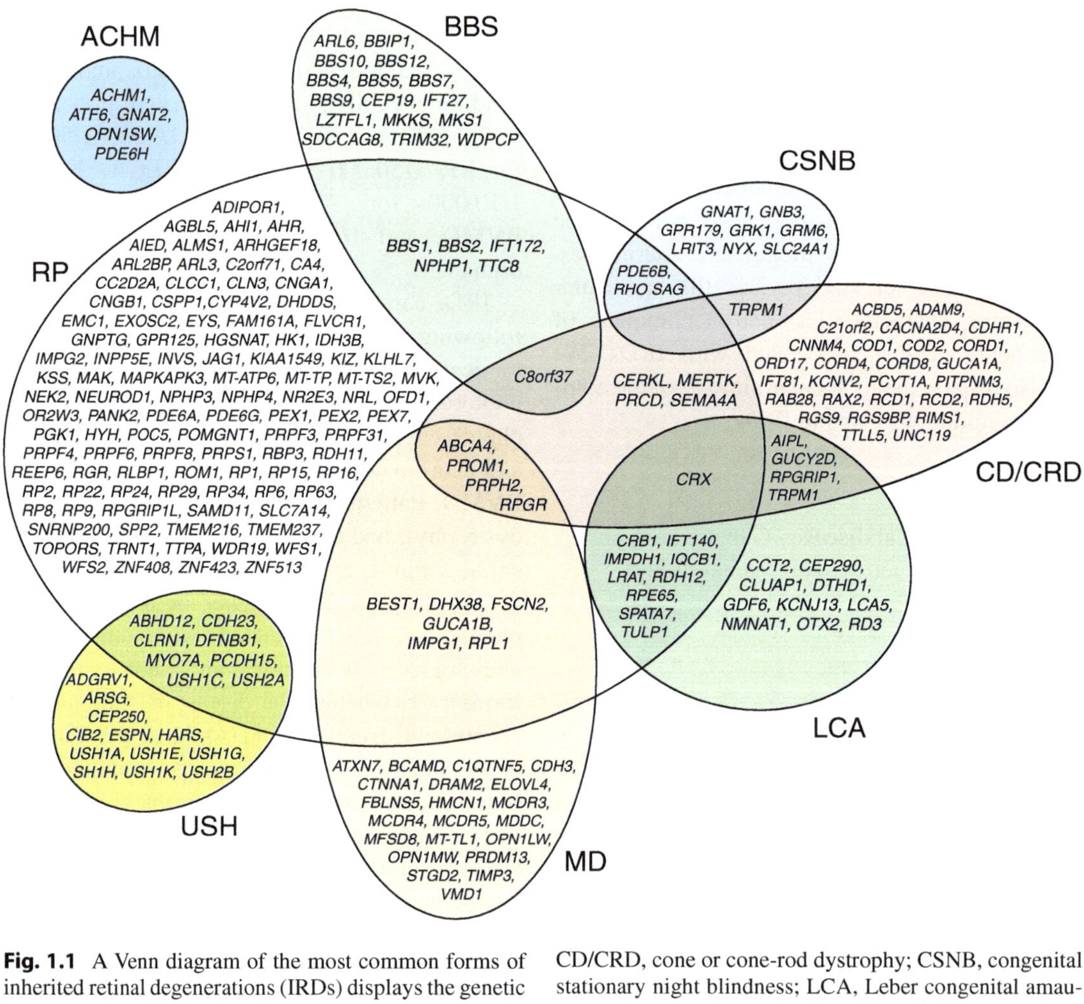

Fig. 1.1 A Venn diagram of the most common forms of inherited retinal degenerations (IRDs) displays the genetic heterogeneity of IRDs. Overlapping regions represent the same gene that is responsible for different disorders. ACHM, achromatopsia; BBS, Bardet–Biedl syndrome; CD/CRD, cone or cone-rod dystrophy; CSNB, congenital stationary night blindness; LCA, Leber congenital amaurosis; MD, macular dystrophy; RP, retinitis pigmentosa, USH, Usher syndrome (http://www.sph.uth.tmc.edu/retnet/, accessed March 2020)

choice. In addition, the variable expression, oligogenic inheritance, and incomplete penetrance also complicate the molecular genetic diagnosis of IRDs [3].

Nevertheless, the molecular genetic diagnosis of IRDs has several clinical values. First, the detection of pathogenic genes and mutations helps obtain the definitive diagnosis of the retinal condition, which can yield information about the prognosis. Second, early identification of syndromic IRDs allows the prediction of the systemic complications that may arise. Some extraocular features, such as hearing loss and vestibular dysfunction in USH, obesity in BBS, and cardiomyopathy in Alström syndrome, may not be seen until late childhood [4]. Molecular genetic testing can identify the risk of systemic involvement and offer the opportunity to prepare [5]. Third, based on the molecular genetic findings, treating physicians can provide genetic counseling to family members, identify carriers, make the diagnosis prenatally, and reduce the risk of transmission.

Fourth, the molecular genetic diagnosis can provide an opportunity for the optimal treatment for patients. Voretigene neparvovec-rzyl (Luxturna™) was approved by the US Food and Drug Administration (FDA) in December 2017 and indicated for biallelic *RPE65* mutation-associated retinal dystrophy. Currently, more than 30 clinical trials in relation to gene therapy for IRDs are registered at ClinicalTrials.gov, RP with *LRAT*, *MERTK*, *PDE6B*, *RLBP1*, *RPE65*, or *RPGR* mutation, LCA with *RPE65* or *LRAT* mutation, X-linked juvenile retinoschisis with *RS1* mutation, achromatopsia with *CNGA3* or *CNGB3* mutation, choroideremia with *CHM* mutation, and USH with *MYOA7A* mutation (https://clinicaltrials.gov/). Thus, identification of the applicable mutation is a prerequisite for enrollment in these ongoing gene therapy trials.

Last, knowledge of the molecular genetic basis of IRDs can lead to a better understanding of the retinal physiology and pathophysiology, which can aid in the development of a novel treatment strategy [6–8]. The latest development in gene therapy is primarily based on the recent achievement of genetic analysis in IRDs. The design of other therapeutic interventions also depends on the molecular biology and genetic characteristics of inherited diseases. For example, approximately 10% of cases of cystic fibrosis are caused by the nonsense mutations that cause protein truncation, leading to function loss of cystic fibrosis transmembrane conductance regulator (CFTR) and consequent disease [9, 10]. Certain aminoglycoside antibiotics (e.g., gentamicin) can induce ribosomes to read through a premature stop codon in mRNA, continue the translation, and produce a complete protein [11]. Topical application of gentamicin drops to the nasal mucosa cause a local increase in CFTR-mediated chloride transport [12].

1.3 Techniques of Genetic Analysis

After the *OAT* gene was found to cause gyrate atrophy in 1988, the methods and tools available for the molecular genetic diagnosis of IRDs continuously evolved [13]. Currently, more than 270 genes have been found to be associated with IRDs (http://www.sph.uth.tmc.edu/retnet/).

In general, the aim of genetic analyses is to determine genomic variations, such as single nucleotide variants (SNVs), small DNA insertions or deletions (inDels), copy number variations (CNVs), or other structural variants (SVs) and relates these variations to human phenotypes. The molecular genetic diagnosis can be made through a direct analysis of the targeted gene mutation, direct sequence analysis, or linkage study [14]. A direct mutation analysis is possible when the related gene has been identified. However, this approach has less value for IRDs because of more than 270 disease-associated genes, heterogeneity of the genotype and phenotype, and unclear inheritance patterns, making it difficult to select genes for direct mutation analysis.

Given the extreme heterogeneity of IRDs, next-generation sequencing (NGS), also known as massively parallel sequencing, has been suggested as a cost-effective approach for the identification of mutations [15, 16]. The introduction of

Table 1.1 Comparison of next-generation sequencing methods in terms of inherited retinal degenerations [19–21]

	TES	WES	WGS
Depth	>500X	>50–100 X	>30 X
Size of capture	Variable (2–200)	4,000–20,000 genes	20,000 genes and non-coding area
Number of variants	~1000	~20,000	~4,000,000
Cost per sample ($)[a]	200–1000	500–1000	Short read: 1000–2500 Long read: 2750–20,000
Turnaround time [a]	3–6 weeks	8–12 weeks	8–12 weeks
Advantages	Customizable Lowest cost and time	Applicable in the case without certain clinical diagnosis Cheaper than WGS and multiple panels	Detect all variants in the genome No bias in target selection
Identify new variants	Yes	Yes	Yes
Identify new genes	No	Yes	Yes
Exonic Variants	Yes	Yes	Yes
Intergenic regions	No	No	Yes
Variant in regulatory regions	No	No	Yes
Deep intronic variants	No	No	Yes
Structural variations	No	No	Yes
Copy number variations	Mostly undetected	Mostly undetected	Yes
InDels	Yes	Yes	Yes
Large InDels	Mostly undetected	Mostly undetected	Yes
microRNAs	No	No	Yes

TES, targeted exome sequencing; WES, whole exome sequencing; WGS, whole genome sequencing
[a]May vary depending on the laboratory

NGS allows the analysis of all genes in a defined linkage interval (targeted NGS), all exons in the genome (whole exome sequencing [WES]), and even the entire genomic sequence (whole genome sequencing [WGS]). Table 1.1 displays the characteristics of common NGS methods [17, 18].

1.3.1 Linkage Analysis

The linkage analysis can be utilized when there are available polymorphic markers closely linked to a target gene but without the identification of the gene itself or when detection of mutations in the gene is difficult [22]. Traditionally, the linkage analysis evaluated trait segregation within a family. When particular traits were co-inherited, it was suggested that genes associated with the co-inherited traits were closely linked within the genome.

Polymorphic markers are now used to determine whether or not certain genetic polymorphisms are co-inherited with the certain phenotype and help locate the genome associated with the trait of interest [23]. Polymorphic markers can be single nucleotide polymorphisms, simple sequence length polymorphisms, and restriction fragment length polymorphisms.

The linkage analysis cannot be used to confirm the proband's diagnosis but can be used to determine whether or not other family members are likely to have inherited the mutated gene. This approach relies heavily on making the correct diagnosis in the proband and knowing the exact family relationships. However, this technique has gradually phased out as the techniques for identifying genetic mutations have advanced.

1.3.2 Sanger Sequencing

Sanger sequencing is the most widely adopted sequencing technique for a limited number of exons or amplicons and is still regarded as the gold standard DNA sequencing technique. Speed, flexibility, and accuracy are the advantages of Sanger sequencing. It is relatively cheap for a limited number of exons or amplicons. For genes with more exons or amplicons, it is better to use the NSG-based approach. In addition, the costs of Sanger sequencing for large genes, such as *ABCA4* and *USH2A*, are not cheaper than those of NGS [19].

The value of Sanger sequencing is limited for detecting mutations in diseases with high genetic heterogeneity, such as IRDs, because of the long time, high cost, and a lot of effort required to sequence many genes. However, Sanger sequencing is preferred for the segregation analysis of IRDs.

1.3.3 Next-Generation Sequencing

In the last decade, NGS has evolved in accuracy and throughput. IRDs are excellent candidates for screening NGS because of their wide genetic and phenotypic heterogeneity.

The most significant obstacle for the clinical application of NGS is the huge volume of data to analyze. For example, the number of variants detected is approximately 20,000–50,000 for each exome [17]. At least 150–500 variants remain as "probable pathogenic" after the application of various bioinformatics filters. Interpreting these variants is a challenging task in the clinical setting [18]. The higher error rate compared to that of Sanger sequencing can be another obstacle in NGS. The false-positive rate of NGS is approximately 14–27% [18]. False-positive results can be obtained from the artificial mutations generated during template amplification or sequencing. Therefore, each type of variant detected in NGS must be validated by Sanger sequencing, which increases the cost and turnaround time [7].

1.3.3.1 Targeted Exome Sequencing

In targeted exome sequencing (TES), also known as panel-based sequencing or targeted NGS, targeted genomic regions are selectively enriched and sequenced using NGS. TES can evaluate exons, introns, and intergenic regions of genes [20]. TES usually evaluates genes with a prior knowledge, which are known to be associated with a specific disease or group of related diseases; therefore, it is not suitable for discovering a new disease-related gene. TES can sequence more samples per run with increased reading depth and coverage and results in being much more sensitive than the holistic approach of NGS, including WES and WGS. Several researchers reported that TES discovered causal variants in IRDs in 50–76% of cases [24–28]. However, the sensitivity of a specific gene panel may vary among ethnic groups [29].

TES is suitable for diagnostic screenings because of its low costs, short turnaround time, and less computational burden compared to the holistic approach of NGS [30]. In IRDs, TES can be utilized as a first-tier test. If this test is negative, the holistic approach of NGS, including WES and WGS, can be considered as the second-tier test.

However, there are several limitations to TES. First, researchers need to redesign the panel to incorporate new genomic regions at an additional expense. Second, the role of gene modifiers and structural genomic rearrangements cannot be adequately analyzed with TES [6, 15]. Furthermore, because of the limitations inherent to polymerase chain reaction (PCR) amplification, low coverage of regions, such as GC- and AG-rich regions, can occur [6].

1.3.3.2 Whole Exome Sequencing

In WES, all protein-coding genes within a genome containing approximately 180,000 exons are enriched and sequenced. Protein-coding genes constitute ~1% of the whole genome but harbor 85% of the disease-causing mutations [31]. The intergenic and intronic regions constitute the remaining 99%, which might cause ~15% of cases. Compared to WGS, WES sequences exons with higher coverage but generate fewer data and require fewer data storage resources, making the analysis easier [32]. WES capture kits are expensive, but WES is more cost-effective than WGS in clinical applications.

WES is commonly used for the genetic analysis of a large number of samples in a short time period. Because most causative mutations can occur in different coding regions, WES is the best approach for detecting mutations in heterogeneous Mendelian disorders. Patients who have probable genetic causes but with a nonspecific or an unusual disease manifestation and those with clinical diagnoses of genetic heterogeneity were also good candidates for WES [33, 34]. In a study comparing WES and three commercial gene panels, WES discovered causative mutations of genes in 42% of cases, which were not included in at least one commercial panel [35]. Several researchers reported success rates of genetic diagnosis in IRDs with WES ranging from 55 to 72% [36–38].

There are some clear limitations to WES. First, WES often misses deep intronic variants, large chromosomal SVs, and CNVs [39]. Second, the enrichment methods based on PCR may result in low coverage of regions, such as GC- and AG-rich regions, similar to TES [40]. Last, this method captures 92–95% of the exons, so even if that region is included in the capture probe design, some mutations may be missed [20].

1.3.3.3 Whole Genome Sequencing

WGS sequences the whole genome containing coding (exons) and non-coding regions (introns, regulatory, and intergenic sequences). This allows the detection of CNVs, intergenic variants, and other structural rearrangements as well as exonic sequences, which can cover more than 95% of the entire human genome [41]. WGS offers extraordinary power, particularly for discovering three groups of pathogenic variants: SVs, variants in GC-rich regions, and variants in non-coding regulatory regions, of which coverage is significantly improved compared to WES [42]. Furthermore, recent studies showed that variants located in microRNA regions and deep intronic regions could be responsible for IRDs [43, 44].

As the cost of WGS is continually declining, more laboratories have access to technology. However, analyzing vast amounts of genomic variant data remains challenging.

1.4 Molecular Genetics of Inherited Retinal Disease

Molecular biological mechanisms associated with IRD genes are very complex and heterogeneous (Fig. 1.2). They include photoreceptor development defect (*CRX*, *NR2E3*, and *NRL*), defects in intracellular trafficking and cilia function (*BBSs*, *CEP290*, *MYO7A*, RAB28, *ROM1*, *RPGR*, *TULP1*, and USH2A), phototransduction and outer segment (OS) structure formation defects (*AIPL1*, *CNGAs*, *CNGBs* GNATs, *GRK1*, *PDE6s*, *PRPH2*, *RHO*, and SAG), synaptic transmission defects (CACNA1F, CACNA2D4, UNC119, and *RIMS1*), and defects in RPE integrity and function (*LRAT, MERTK, and RPE65*) [2, 45].

1.4.1 Genes Affecting Photoreceptor Development

1.4.1.1 *CRX*

The cone-rod homeobox (*CRX*) gene encodes a transcription factor that is preferentially expressed in the photoreceptor of vertebrates. It regulates gene expression, development, and maintenance of photoreceptors [46]. Mutations in *CRX* cause autosomal dominant RP, autosomal dominant cone-rod dystrophy, and autosomal dominant as well as recessive LCA [47–51].

1.4.2 Genes Affecting Intracellular Trafficking and Cilia Function

Primary cilia consist of nine microtubule triplets arranged in a circle with an outer membrane ("9+0" structure) [52]. Intraflagellar transport (IFT) and active protein transport along the microtubules are necessary for the formation and maintenance of cilia. IFT plays an important role in cell mobility, fluid transport over epithelial cells, and sensory perception.

Photoreceptor-connecting cilia (CC) is very similar in structure to the standard primary cilia. It acts as a conduit for uni- or bi-directional

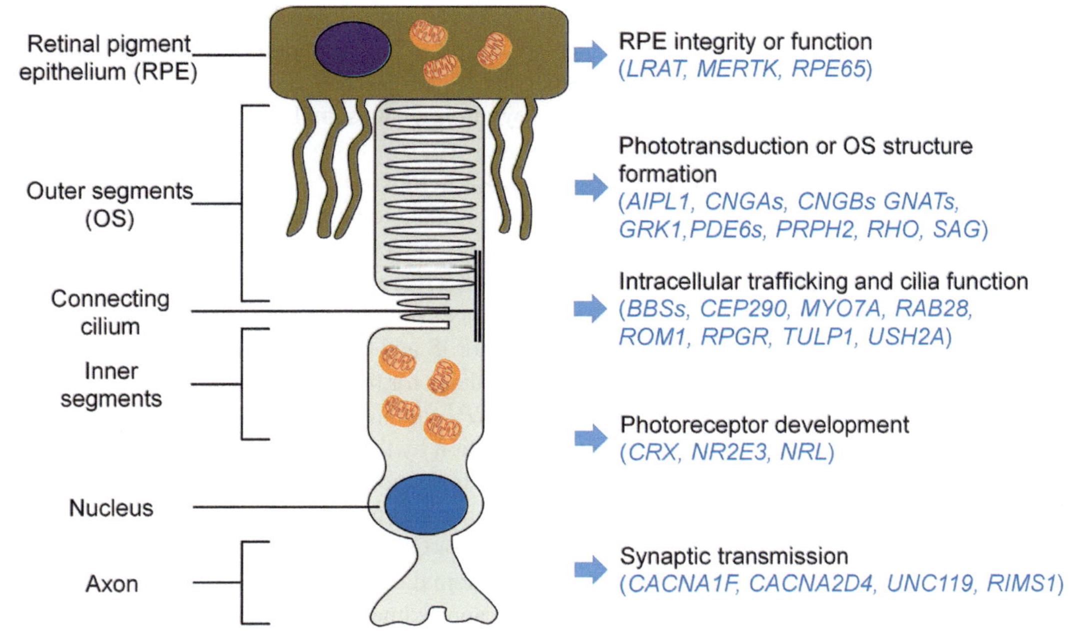

Fig. 1.2 Cellular functions and associated genes in photoreceptors and retinal pigment epithelium

cargo transition compartment between the inner segments (IS) and OS. Approximately 10% of OS renews daily, which depends on the synthesis and transport from the IS across the CC. Therefore, precise control of ciliary transport is crucial. For example, rhodopsin is synthesized in the IS and transported to the disk-forming region within the OS across the CC using vesicle trafficking [53].

1.4.2.1 *CEP290*

Centrosomal protein 290 (CEP290) is a centrosomal-cilia protein that is highly expressed in the nasal epithelium and neural retina and plays an important role in centrosome and cilia function [54, 55]. Mutations in *CEP290* cause ciliogenesis defects, i.e., ciliopathies. *CEP290* mutations account for up to 20% of LCA cases in the Caucasian population as the most common genetic cause.

Mutations in *CEP290* are also associated with the Senior-Løken syndrome, Joubert syndrome, BBS, and Meckel syndrome [56–59].

1.4.2.2 *BBSs*

BBS is a clinically and genetically heterogeneous syndromic ciliopathy with autosomal recessive inheritance. It is characterized by six major defects, including retinal degeneration, renal abnormalities, mental retardation, truncal obesity, hypogenitalism, and postaxial polydactyly [60].

At least 19 genes are associated with BBS, but mutations in *BBS1* to *BBS18* gene account for approximately 70–80% [61]. The BBS (1, 2, 4, 5, 7, 8, 9, and 18) proteins form a BBSome complex, which acts as cargo for the antero- and retrograde transport at the ciliary transition zone [61]. This complex formation is facilitated by the BBS-chaperonin complex formed by BBS-6, 10, and 12 with BBS7. The other BBS proteins work independently for recruiting the BBSome at the base of the cilium or in the centrosome. It has been hypothesized that ciliary trafficking of the rhodopsin is mediated by the BBSome complex along with Rab8, and they interact during IFT [53].

Mutations in *BBS* genes express both cone-rod and rod-cone phenotypes of IRDs [53].

1.4.2.3 *RPGR*

The retinitis pigmentosa GTPase regulator (RPGR) protein is predominantly localized to the CC [62]. It is presumed to play a role in nucleo-cytoplasmic transport, intracellular transport of opsins from the IS to OS, and regulation of disk morphogenesis.

The *RPGR* gene is located on the X chromosome, and approximately 70% of X-linked RP accounts for the *RPGR* gene mutations [63–65]. In addition, mutations of *RPGR* are also detected in male simplex RP patients, RP families with provisional autosomal dominant inheritance, CRD patients, and MD patients [66–70].

1.4.2.4 *MYO7A*

Myosin VIIA (MYO7A) is primarily expressed in the RPE, photoreceptors, and cochlear and vestibular neuroepithelia of the inner ear [71]. It plays a role in the transport of opsin to the OS through the ciliary plasma membrane in the photoreceptors [72] and the movement of melanosomes and phagosomes in the RPE [73]. Without MYO7A, melanosomes are unable to move along actin filaments and are therefore absent from the apical RPE [73]. Mutations in *MYO7A* result in an abnormally high opsin level in the CC, slowed distal migration of the disk membranes, and delayed digestion of phagocytosed photoreceptor disk membranes [72].

MYO7A mutations cause USH type I, the most severe subtype with profound congenital deafness and vestibular dysfunction [74, 75].

1.4.2.5 *USH2A*

The *USH2A* gene encodes two alternatively spliced isoforms, 170 kDa USH2A isoform a and 580 kDa USH2A isoform b [76]. USH2A isoform a is a basement membrane protein [77, 78]. USH2A isoform b encodes usherin, which is the major isoform in the retina and inner ear [79]. In photoreceptors, usherin is expressed particularly in the CC and involved in the cargo delivery from the IS to the OS [76, 79]. However, the exact function of USH2A in the retina has not been fully elucidated.

Mutations in *USH2A* are the most common cause of USH, accounting for up to 85% of USH type II cases and causing up to 23% of non-syndromic autosomal recessive RP [73].

1.4.2.6 *RP1*

RP1 is a photoreceptor-specific protein expressed in both rod and cone photoreceptors, localized at the CC. It is responsible for cilia structure maintenance, protein transport between the photoreceptor IS and OS, and capturing and stacking the OS disks for the correct orientation [80].

RP1 mutations may cause photoreceptor dysfunction by the misalignment of the OS disk and disk formation disruption. In addition, *RP1* may also account for rhodopsin transport to the photoreceptor OS [81]. *RP1* mutations can cause either autosomal dominant or recessive RP, accounting for approximately 5.5% and 1% of cases, respectively [82]. In addition, some recent works suggested that the phenotypic spectrum associated with *RP1* mutations should be expanded to MD and cone-rod dystrophy [83, 84]. Although the exact mechanism underlying the autosomal dominant or recessive mutation effect of *RP1* is still unclear, different classes of the truncated protein can cause various effects on the etiology of RP [85, 86].

1.4.3 Genes Affecting Phototransduction and Structure Formation

The phototransduction cascades are basically the same in both rod and cone photoreceptors [45]. During phototransduction, the captured photons activate rhodopsin, which leads to dissociation of transducin subunits βγ from Gα, followed by activation of cGMP-phosphodiesterase (PDE). PDE hydrolyzes cGMP to GMP [87, 88], which leads to the cyclic-nucleotide-gated (CNG) channel closure in the OS membrane of the photoreceptor. The CNG channels closure results in hyperpolarization of the photoreceptor and electrochemical signal transmission to the second-order neurons.

1.4.3.1 *PRPH2*

The *PRPH2* gene, also known as the Retinal Degeneration Slow (*RDS*) gene, encoded a photoreceptor-specific transmembrane glycoprotein, peripherin-2 [89, 90]. Peripherin-2 may account for disk morphogenesis and maintenance [91]. In addition, peripherin-2 is predicted to play a role in regulating disk alignment and size as a complex with rod OS membrane protein-1 (ROM1) [92, 93].

Mutations in *PRPH2* account for 5–10% of autosomal dominant RP, with primary loss of the rod photoreceptors and secondary delayed loss of the cone photoreceptors [94]. However, *PRPH2* mutations can also cause autosomal dominant MD, with cone photoreceptors and central-vision defects [90]. The different mutation loci caused the difference in *PRPH2* mRNA splicing efficiencies, which may result in the phenotypic heterogeneity of *PRPH2* mutations.

The PRPH2 upregulation and function defects may lead to cone photoreceptor degeneration. In contrast, the *PRPH2* mutations specific to rod photoreceptors can cause PRPH2 downregulation and protein localization impairment [95]. These results suggest that the different penetrance of *PRPH2* mutants between rod and cone photoreceptors may result from mRNA splicing.

1.4.3.2 *RHO*

The *RHO* gene encodes rhodopsin, which is a photo-excitable G protein-coupled receptor located on the disk membrane of the OS in the rod photoreceptor. As rhodopsin plays a crucial role in phototransduction, mutations in rhodopsin can cause dysfunction of the photoreceptor with or without degeneration. Mutations of *RHO* account for 20–30% of autosomal dominant RP. Currently, there are more than 200 disease-causing *RHO* mutations, which can be divided into seven classes [96, 97]. Class I mutations result in the impairment of post-Golgi trafficking and OS targeting. Class II mutations cause misfolding and endoplasmic reticulum retention and instability. Class III mutations result in vesicular trafficking and endocytosis disruption. Class IV mutations are responsible for alterations in the post-translational modifications and reduced stability. Class V mutations alter transducin activation. Class VI mutations affect constitutive activation. Class VII mutations result in dimerization deficiency. These classifications are not mutually exclusive. In addition, there are more mutations that cannot be placed in these categories.

There is a clinical classification based on their broad phenotype-genotype correlation, consisting of two classes [96]. Class A shows severe rod photoreceptor dysfunction with early onset. Class B shows a milder phenotype with later onset and slower progression. This different presentation is probably the underlying molecular biology associated with the mutation and genetic modifiers and environment.

1.4.3.3 *PDE6s*

Rod cGMP-specific phosphodiesterase 6 (PDE6) is a protein complex composed of α, β, and two γ subunits, which are encoded by *PDE6A, PDE6B, and PDE6G* genes. The PDE6 complex is located on the photoreceptor OS and hydrolyses cGMP in response to light stimulations, regulates the cGMP-gated cation (Na^+, Ca^{2+}) channels opening in rod and cone photoreceptors [98].

Mutations in *PDE6A* and *PDE6B* cause a calcium influx into rod photoreceptors and subsequent apoptosis, which results in autosomal recessive RP [99–104]. However, there was a report of a large consanguineous family with *PDE6G* mutation, manifesting with an early-onset RP phenotype [105].

1.4.3.4 *CNGAs* and *CNGBs*

The CNG channel is a protein complex composed of α-(CNGA) and β-(CNGB) subunits in rod and cone photoreceptors [106]. The opening of CNG channels in the dark-adapted state results in sodium and calcium influx, leading to inward negative current flow. In contrast, the closure of CNG channels during phototransduction generates a hyperpolarization wave in the photoreceptors [107].

Mutations in *CNGA1* and *CNGB1*, which encode the CNG channel subunits of the rod photoreceptor, cause autosomal recessive RP [108, 109]. Mutations in the *CNGA3* and *CNGB3* genes, which encode the CNG channel subunits of the cone photoreceptor, are responsible for complete and incomplete achromatopsia [106, 110, 111].

1.4.4 Genes Affecting Synaptic Transmission

Photons are converted into electrochemical signals at photoreceptor ribbon synapses with bipolar cells. In the dark, an opening of the L-type calcium channels in the photoreceptor results in calcium influx into the cytoplasm, leading to glutamate release. When activated by light, the glutamate release gradually decreases at the ribbon synapses, which mediates signal transmission from the photoreceptor to the bipolar cell [112].

1.4.4.1 *CACNA1F*

CACNA1F encodes a subunit of the voltage-gated L-type calcium channels. Mutations in *CACNA1F* account for X-linked CSNB, X-linked cone-rod dystrophy, and Åland island eye disease [113–115].

1.4.5 Genes Affecting RPE Integrity or Function

1.4.5.1 *RPE65*

The *RPE65* gene encodes retinal pigment epithelium 65 kDa protein (RPE65), also known as retinoid isomerohydrolase, is responsible for the visual pigment restoration [116]. In the initial step of the phototransduction cascade, 11-*cis*-retinal is photoisomerized to all-*trans*-retinal. The reconversion of all-*trans* to 11-*cis*-retinal is catalyzed by RPE65 in the RPE, which is crucial for recombination with opsin and active visual pigment formation.

The absence of RPE65 activity results in the 11-*cis*-retinal level reduction and retinal esters accumulation in RPE cells, severe rod and cone photoreceptor response attenuation, and progressive retinal degeneration because of the block in the regeneration of 11-*cis*-retinal [116]. Biallelic mutations in the *RPE65 gene*, which disrupt the visual cycle, are responsible for approximately 6% of LCA and 2% of autosomal recessive RP [117–119].

Using a viral vector, the healthy *RPE65* gene can be delivered to the retina. Adeno-associated virus (AAV) has become the best vector for most gene therapy applications. It can be manufactured to contain only genetic information, which is intended to be transferred for gene therapy [120]. AAV has proven to have a favorable safety profile for many types of gene therapy, no known associations of diseases, no reproducibility without helper viruses, and less immunogenicity than other viruses. AAV serotype 2 (AAV2) is used for the treatment of *RPE65*-associated IRDs. It has a natural predilection for retinal cell types and can induce prolonged levels of gene expression, which can maximize the intended therapeutic effects [121]. Instead of eliminating or repairing defective genes, gene therapy with AAV2 introduces a normal copy of the gene into the cells as free-floating DNA outside the chromosome [122].

Voretigene neparvovec (AAV2-hRPE65v2), the first FDA-approved gene replacement therapy, consists of an AAV2 viral vector containing the human *RPE65* cDNA. Voretigene neparvovec also includes a modified Kozak sequence and utilizes a hybrid chicken β-actin promoter using a cytomegalovirus enhancer [123]. Voretigene neparvovec introduces normal copies of the *RPE65* gene in the RPE cells and causes the production of a functional enzyme. For the first intervention participants in the phase 3 trial, average multi-luminance mobility test, full-field light sensitivity test, visual field, and visual acuity measures have been maintained for 3 years, and the follow-up is ongoing [123, 124].

1.4.5.2 *MERTK*

The MER proto-oncogene tyrosine kinase (*MERTK*) gene encodes a receptor tyrosine kinase that is a member of the MER/AXL/TYRO3 receptor kinase family. It is expressed in several tissues but strongly in the RPE and macrophages, which are capable of phagocytosis. It plays a critical role in regulating cytoskeleton rearrangement during phagocytosis, an essential circadian process for homeostasis in photoreceptors [125]. In the RPE, MERTK is essential in the shed photoreceptor OS engulfment before phagocytosis [126].

Mutations in *MERTK* were identified in autosomal recessive RP patients, resulting from defective OS phagocytosis by the RPE [127]. The associated phenotype is characterized by an early onset with rapid macular involvement.

1.4.6 Others

1.4.6.1 *ABCA4*

ATP-binding cassette sub-family A (ABC1) member 4 (*ABCA4*) encodes the photoreceptor-specific ABCR protein. It is an ATP-binding transporter protein that is localized at the OS disk membranes [128]. It functions as a flippase for N-retinylidene-phosphatidylethanolamine that facilitates the transport from the disk lumen to the cytoplasm [129]. This transport activity makes retinoids not be accumulated in disk membranes.

Mutations in the *ABCA4* gene result in the accumulation of the toxic bisretinoid A2E and yellow fundus flecking, leading to RPE atrophy and photoreceptor cell death [130]. Mutations in the *ABCA4* gene cause autosomal recessive IRDs, including STGD, RP, cone-rod dystrophy, and increased susceptibility to age-related macular degeneration [130].

1.4.6.2 *EYS*

The eyes shut homolog (*EYS*) gene encodes the EYS protein that is expressed predominantly in the retina [131, 132]. It is an ortholog of the Drosophila spacemaker (spam) protein, which plays a key role in maintaining the photoreceptor morphology [133]. However, little is known about the exact function of EYS and the underlying pathogenic mechanism of RP associated with *EYS*.

Studies on *EYS*-knockout zebrafish suggest that EYS is required for maintaining the integrity of the ciliary pocket lumen in cone photoreceptors, photoreceptor OS protein localization, and maintaining photoreceptor actin filaments [134, 135]. *EYS* mutations are the commonest cause of non-syndromic autosomal recessive RP, accounting for 5–23.5% of cases [136, 137], and are also associated with autosomal recessive cone-rod dystrophy [138].

1.4.6.3 *CHM*

Choroideremia is an X-linked recessive IRD caused by hemizygous duplication mutations or nullizygous deletion in the *CHM* gene, which encodes the major transporter REP-1 [139]. REP-1 is involved in the isoprenylation of monomeric Rab GTPases (Rabs), which plays a key role in the regulation of vesicular trafficking, phagosome fusion, and maturation [140].

CHM mutations cause underprenylation of Rabs, vesicle trafficking deficiency, and defect in OS dick phagocytosis by RPE cells [140], which results in progressive degeneration of choriocapillaris, RPE, and photoreceptors.

1.4.6.4 *BEST1*

The *BEST1* gene encodes Bestrophin 1 (Best1), an RPE-specific transmembrane channel [141]. It acts as a pentameric anion channel and regulator of intracellular calcium signaling and cell volume [142, 143].

BEST1 mutations cause various RPE-photoreceptor abnormalities, including an imbalance between the photoreceptor OS turnover and RPE phagocytosis [144]. This results in an excessive lipofuscin accumulation expressed as the formation of vitelliform lesions, a consistent pathological finding among *BEST1*-associated maculopathies.

Mutations in *BEST1* are associated with several clinically heterogeneous IRDs, termed as bestrophinopathies, including Best vitelliform macular dystrophy, adult-onset vitelliform macular dystrophy, RP, autosomal recessive bestrophinopathy, and autosomal dominant vitreoretinochoroidopathy [145].

1.5 Conclusion

IRDs have long been proven to be a clinical diagnostic challenge because of the overlapping phenotypes, variable onset ages, and unclear inheritance patterns. Advances in molecular biology and NGS technology have greatly revolutionized the molecular genetic diagnosis of IRDs. To increase our knowledge of IRDs, molecular genetics may play a key role in identifying the underlying mechanism, which is yet to be fully identified, and is an essential element in the development of the novel treatment modalities for this near-incurable devastating disease.

References

1. Berger W, Kloeckener-Gruissem B, Neidhardt J. The molecular basis of human retinal and vitreoretinal diseases. Prog Retin Eye Res. 2010;29(5):335–75. https://doi.org/10.1016/j.preteyeres.2010.03.004.
2. Dias MF, Joo K, Kemp JA, Fialho SL, da Silva Cunha A Jr, Woo SJ, Kwon YJ. Molecular genetics and emerging therapies for retinitis pigmentosa: basic research and clinical perspectives. Prog Retin Eye Res. 2018;63:107–31. https://doi.org/10.1016/j.preteyeres.2017.10.004.
3. Nash BM, Wright DC, Grigg JR, Bennetts B, Jamieson RV. Retinal dystrophies, genomic applications in diagnosis and prospects for therapy. Transl Pediatr. 2015;4(2):139–63. https://doi.org/10.3978/j.issn.2224-4336.2015.04.03.
4. Sadagopan KA. Practical approach to syndromic pediatric retinal dystrophies. Curr Opin Ophthalmol. 2017;28(5):416–29. https://doi.org/10.1097/icu.0000000000000404.
5. Werdich XQ, Place EM, Pierce EA. Systemic diseases associated with retinal dystrophies. Semin Ophthalmol. 2014;29(5-6):319–28. https://doi.org/10.3109/08820538.2014.959202.
6. Chacon-Camacho OF, Garcia-Montano LA, Zenteno JC. The clinical implications of molecular monitoring and analyses of inherited retinal diseases. Expert Rev Mol Diagn. 2017;17(11):1009–21. https://doi.org/10.1080/14737159.2017.1384314.
7. Efthymiou S, Manole A, Houlden H. Next-generation sequencing in neuromuscular diseases. Curr Opin Neurol. 2016;29(5):527–36. https://doi.org/10.1097/wco.0000000000000374.
8. Gillespie RL, Hall G, Black GC. Genetic testing for inherited ocular disease: delivering on the promise at last? Clin Experiment Ophthalmol. 2014;42(1):65–77. https://doi.org/10.1111/ceo.12159.
9. Bobadilla JL, Macek M Jr, Fine JP, Farrell PM. Cystic fibrosis: a worldwide analysis of CFTR mutations—correlation with incidence data and application to screening. Hum Mutat. 2002;19(6):575–606. https://doi.org/10.1002/humu.10041.
10. Hanrahan JW, Sato Y, Carlile GW, Jansen G, Young JC, Thomas DY. Cystic fibrosis: proteostatic correctors of CFTR trafficking and alternative therapeutic targets. Expert Opin Ther Targets. 2019;23(8):711–24. https://doi.org/10.1080/14728222.2019.1628948
.
11. Du M, Jones JR, Lanier J, Keeling KM, Lindsey JR, Tousson A, Bebok Z, Whitsett JA, Dey CR, Colledge WH, Evans MJ, Sorscher EJ, Bedwell DM. Aminoglycoside suppression of a premature stop mutation in a Cftr-/- mouse carrying a human CFTR-G542X transgene. J Mol Med (Berl). 2002;80(9):595–604. https://doi.org/10.1007/s00109-002-0363-1.
12. Wilschanski M, Yahav Y, Yaacov Y, Blau H, Bentur L, Rivlin J, Aviram M, Bdolah-Abram T, Bebok Z, Shushi L, Kerem B, Kerem E. Gentamicin-induced correction of CFTR function in patients with cystic fibrosis and CFTR stop mutations. N Engl J Med. 2003;349(15):1433–41. https://doi.org/10.1056/NEJMoa022170.
13. Mitchell GA, Brody LC, Looney J, Steel G, Suchanek M, Dowling C, Der Kaloustian V, Kaiser-Kupfer M, Valle D. An initiator codon mutation in ornithine-delta-aminotransferase causing gyrate atrophy of the choroid and retina. J Clin Invest. 1988;81(2):630–3. https://doi.org/10.1172/jci113365.
14. Harada S, Korf BR. Overview of molecular genetic diagnosis. Curr Protoc Hum Genet. 2013;Chapter 9:Unit 9.1. https://doi.org/10.1002/0471142905.hg0901s76.
15. Bernardis I, Chiesi L. Unravelling the complexity of inherited retinal dystrophies molecular testing: added value of targeted next-generation sequencing. Biomed Res Int. 2016;2016:6341870. https://doi.org/10.1155/2016/6341870.
16. Chiang JP, Lamey T, McLaren T, Thompson JA, Montgomery H, De Roach J. Progress and prospects of next-generation sequencing testing for inherited retinal dystrophy. Expert Rev Mol Diagn. 2015;15(10):1269–75. https://doi.org/10.1586/14737159.2015.1081057.
17. Caspar SM, Dubacher N, Kopps AM, Meienberg J, Henggeler C, Matyas G. Clinical sequencing: from raw data to diagnosis with lifetime value. Clin Genet. 2018;93(3):508–19. https://doi.org/10.1111/cge.13190.
18. Xue Y, Ankala A, Wilcox WR, Hegde MR. Solving the molecular diagnostic testing conundrum for Mendelian disorders in the era of next-generation sequencing: single-gene, gene panel, or exome/genome sequencing. Genet Med. 2015;17(6):444–51. https://doi.org/10.1038/gim.2014.122.
19. Jin Z-B. Whole genome sequencing in genetic eye diseases. In: Prakash G, Iwata T, editors. Advances

in vision research, Volume I: Genetic eye research in Asia and the Pacific. Tokyo: Springer; 2017. p. 21–9. https://doi.org/10.1007/978-4-431-56511-6_3.
20. Salmaninejad A, Motaee J, Farjami M, Alimardani M, Esmaeilie A, Pasdar A. Next-generation sequencing and its application in diagnosis of retinitis pigmentosa. Ophthalmic Genet. 2019;40(5):393–402. https://doi.org/10.1080/13816810.2019.1675178.
21. Seleman M, Hoyos-Bachiloglu R, Geha RS, Chou J. Uses of next-generation sequencing technologies for the diagnosis of primary immunodeficiencies. Front Immunol. 2017;8:847. https://doi.org/10.3389/fimmu.2017.00847.
22. Korf BR. Overview of molecular genetic diagnosis. Curr Protoc Hum Genet. 2006;Chapter 9:Unit 9.1. https://doi.org/10.1002/0471142905.hg0901s48.
23. Teare MD, Santibanez Koref MF. Linkage analysis and the study of Mendelian disease in the era of whole exome and genome sequencing. Brief Funct Genomics. 2014;13(5):378–83. https://doi.org/10.1093/bfgp/elu024.
24. Audo I, Bujakowska KM, Leveillard T, Mohand-Said S, Lancelot ME, Germain A, Antonio A, Michiels C, Saraiva JP, Letexier M, Sahel JA, Bhattacharya SS, Zeitz C. Development and application of a next-generation-sequencing (NGS) approach to detect known and novel gene defects underlying retinal diseases. Orphanet J Rare Dis. 2012;7:8. https://doi.org/10.1186/1750-1172-7-8.
25. Consugar MB, Navarro-Gomez D, Place EM, Bujakowska KM, Sousa ME, Fonseca-Kelly ZD, Taub DG, Janessian M, Wang DY, Au ED, Sims KB, Sweetser DA, Fulton AB, Liu Q, Wiggs JL, Gai X, Pierce EA. Panel-based genetic diagnostic testing for inherited eye diseases is highly accurate and reproducible, and more sensitive for variant detection, than exome sequencing. Genet Med. 2015;17(4):253–61. https://doi.org/10.1038/gim.2014.172.
26. Glockle N, Kohl S, Mohr J, Scheurenbrand T, Sprecher A, Weisschuh N, Bernd A, Rudolph G, Schubach M, Poloschek C, Zrenner E, Biskup S, Berger W, Wissinger B, Neidhardt J. Panel-based next generation sequencing as a reliable and efficient technique to detect mutations in unselected patients with retinal dystrophies. Eur J Hum Genet. 2014;22(1):99–104. https://doi.org/10.1038/ejhg.2013.72.
27. Weisschuh N, Mayer AK, Strom TM, Kohl S, Glockle N, Schubach M, Andreasson S, Bernd A, Birch DG, Hamel CP, Heckenlively JR, Jacobson SG, Kamme C, Kellner U, Kunstmann E, Maffei P, Reiff CM, Rohrschneider K, Rosenberg T, Rudolph G, Vamos R, Varsanyi B, Weleber RG, Wissinger B. Mutation detection in patients with retinal dystrophies using targeted next generation sequencing. PLoS One. 2016;11(1):e0145951. https://doi.org/10.1371/journal.pone.0145951.
28. Yoon CK, Kim NK, Joung JG, Shin JY, Park JH, Eum HH, Lee HO, Park WY, Yu HG. The diagnostic application of targeted re-sequencing in Korean patients with retinitis pigmentosa. BMC Genomics. 2015;16:515. https://doi.org/10.1186/s12864-015-1723-x.
29. Vincent AL, Abeysekera N, van Bysterveldt KA, Oliver VF, Ellingford JM, Barton S, Black GC. Next-generation sequencing targeted disease panel in rod-cone retinal dystrophies in Maori and Polynesian reveals novel changes and a common founder mutation. Clin Experiment Ophthalmol. 2017;45(9):901–10. https://doi.org/10.1111/ceo.12983.
30. Dilliott AA, Farhan SMK, Ghani M, Sato C, Liang E, Zhang M, McIntyre AD, Cao H, Racacho L, Robinson JF, Strong MJ, Masellis M, Bulman DE, Rogaeva E, Lang A, Tartaglia C, Finger E, Zinman L, Turnbull J, Freedman M, Swartz R, Black SE, Hegele RA. Targeted next-generation sequencing and bioinformatics pipeline to evaluate genetic determinants of constitutional disease. J Vis Exp. 2018;134. https://doi.org/10.3791/57266.
31. Choi M, Scholl UI, Ji W, Liu T, Tikhonova IR, Zumbo P, Nayir A, Bakkaloglu A, Ozen S, Sanjad S, Nelson-Williams C, Farhi A, Mane S, Lifton RP. Genetic diagnosis by whole exome capture and massively parallel DNA sequencing. Proc Natl Acad Sci U S A. 2009;106(45):19096–101. https://doi.org/10.1073/pnas.0910672106.
32. Lek M, Karczewski KJ, Minikel EV, Samocha KE, Banks E, Fennell T, O'Donnell-Luria AH, Ware JS, Hill AJ, Cummings BB, Tukiainen T, Birnbaum DP, Kosmicki JA, Duncan LE, Estrada K, Zhao F, Zou J, Pierce-Hoffman E, Berghout J, Cooper DN, Deflaux N, DePristo M, Do R, Flannick J, Fromer M, Gauthier L, Goldstein J, Gupta N, Howrigan D, Kiezun A, Kurki MI, Moonshine AL, Natarajan P, Orozco L, Peloso GM, Poplin R, Rivas MA, Ruano-Rubio V, Rose SA, Ruderfer DM, Shakir K, Stenson PD, Stevens C, Thomas BP, Tiao G, Tusie-Luna MT, Weisburd B, Won HH, Yu D, Altshuler DM, Ardissino D, Boehnke M, Danesh J, Donnelly S, Elosua R, Florez JC, Gabriel SB, Getz G, Glatt SJ, Hultman CM, Kathiresan S, Laakso M, McCarroll S, McCarthy MI, McGovern D, McPherson R, Neale BM, Palotie A, Purcell SM, Saleheen D, Scharf JM, Sklar P, Sullivan PF, Tuomilehto J, Tsuang MT, Watkins HC, Wilson JG, Daly MJ, MacArthur DG. Analysis of protein-coding genetic variation in 60,706 humans. Nature. 2016;536(7616):285–91. https://doi.org/10.1038/nature19057.
33. de Ligt J, Willemsen MH, van Bon BW, Kleefstra T, Yntema HG, Kroes T, Vulto-van Silfhout AT, Koolen DA, de Vries P, Gilissen C, del Rosario M, Hoischen A, Scheffer H, de Vries BB, Brunner HG, Veltman JA, Vissers LE. Diagnostic exome sequencing in persons with severe intellectual disability. N Engl J Med. 2012;367(20):1921–9. https://doi.org/10.1056/NEJMoa1206524.
34. Yang Y, Muzny DM, Reid JG, Bainbridge MN, Willis A, Ward PA, Braxton A, Beuten J, Xia F, Niu Z, Hardison M, Person R, Bekheirnia MR, Leduc MS, Kirby A, Pham P, Scull J, Wang M, Ding Y,

Plon SE, Lupski JR, Beaudet AL, Gibbs RA, Eng CM. Clinical whole-exome sequencing for the diagnosis of Mendelian disorders. N Engl J Med. 2013;369(16):1502–11. https://doi.org/10.1056/NEJMoa1306555.
35. Dillon OJ, Lunke S. Exome sequencing has higher diagnostic yield compared to simulated disease-specific panels in children with suspected monogenic disorders. Eur J Hum Genet. 2018;26(5):644–51. https://doi.org/10.1038/s41431-018-0099-1.
36. de Castro-Miro M, Tonda R, Escudero-Ferruz P, Andres R, Mayor-Lorenzo A, Castro J, Ciccioli M, Hidalgo DA, Rodriguez-Ezcurra JJ, Farrando J, Perez-Santonja JJ, Cormand B, Marfany G, Gonzalez-Duarte R. Novel candidate genes and a wide spectrum of structural and point mutations responsible for inherited retinal dystrophies revealed by exome sequencing. PLoS One. 2016;11(12):e0168966. https://doi.org/10.1371/journal.pone.0168966.
37. Riera M, Navarro R, Ruiz-Nogales S, Mendez P, Bures-Jelstrup A, Corcostegui B, Pomares E. Whole exome sequencing using Ion Proton system enables reliable genetic diagnosis of inherited retinal dystrophies. Sci Rep. 2017;7:42078. https://doi.org/10.1038/srep42078.
38. Tiwari A, Bahr A, Bahr L, Fleischhauer J, Zinkernagel MS, Winkler N, Barthelmes D, Berger L, Gerth-Kahlert C, Neidhardt J, Berger W. Next generation sequencing based identification of disease-associated mutations in Swiss patients with retinal dystrophies. Sci Rep. 2016;6:28755. https://doi.org/10.1038/srep28755.
39. Nishiguchi KM. Whole genome sequencing in patients with retinitis pigmentosa. In: Prakash G, Iwata T, editors. Advances in vision research, Volume I: Genetic eye research in Asia and the Pacific. Tokyo: Springer; 2017. p. 83–91. https://doi.org/10.1007/978-4-431-56511-6_8.
40. Clark MJ, Chen R, Lam HY, Karczewski KJ, Chen R, Euskirchen G, Butte AJ, Snyder M. Performance comparison of exome DNA sequencing technologies. Nat Biotechnol. 2011;29(10):908–14. https://doi.org/10.1038/nbt.1975.
41. Nishiguchi KM, Tearle RG, Liu YP, Oh EC, Miyake N, Benaglio P, Harper S, Koskiniemi-Kuendig H, Venturini G, Sharon D, Koenekoop RK, Nakamura M, Kondo M, Ueno S, Yasuma TR, Beckmann JS, Ikegawa S, Matsumoto N, Terasaki H, Berson EL, Katsanis N, Rivolta C. Whole genome sequencing in patients with retinitis pigmentosa reveals pathogenic DNA structural changes and NEK2 as a new disease gene. Proc Natl Acad Sci U S A. 2013;110(40):16139–44. https://doi.org/10.1073/pnas.1308243110.
42. Carss KJ, Arno G, Erwood M, Stephens J, Sanchis-Juan A, Hull S, Megy K, Grozeva D, Dewhurst E, Malka S, Plagnol V, Penkett C, Stirrups K, Rizzo R, Wright G, Josifova D, Bitner-Glindzicz M, Scott RH, Clement E, Allen L, Armstrong R, Brady AF, Carmichael J, Chitre M, Henderson RHH, Hurst J, MacLaren RE, Murphy E, Paterson J, Rosser E, Thompson DA, Wakeling E, Ouwehand WH, Michaelides M, Moore AT, Webster AR, Raymond FL. Comprehensive rare variant analysis via whole-genome sequencing to determine the molecular pathology of inherited retinal disease. Am J Hum Genet. 2017;100(1):75–90. https://doi.org/10.1016/j.ajhg.2016.12.003.
43. Bax NM, Sangermano R, Roosing S, Thiadens AA, Hoefsloot LH, van den Born LI, Phan M, Klevering BJ, Westeneng-van Haaften C, Braun TA, Zonneveld-Vrieling MN, de Wijs I, Mutlu M, Stone EM, den Hollander AI, Klaver CC, Hoyng CB, Cremers FP. Heterozygous deep-intronic variants and deletions in ABCA4 in persons with retinal dystrophies and one exonic ABCA4 variant. Hum Mutat. 2015;36(1):43–7. https://doi.org/10.1002/humu.22717.
44. Conte I, Hadfield KD, Barbato S, Carrella S, Pizzo M, Bhat RS, Carissimo A, Karali M, Porter LF, Urquhart J, Hateley S, O'Sullivan J, Manson FD, Neuhauss SC, Banfi S, Black GC. MiR-204 is responsible for inherited retinal dystrophy associated with ocular coloboma. Proc Natl Acad Sci U S A. 2015;112(25):E3236–45. https://doi.org/10.1073/pnas.1401464112.
45. Veleri S, Lazar CH, Chang B, Sieving PA, Banin E, Swaroop A. Biology and therapy of inherited retinal degenerative disease: insights from mouse models. Dis Model Mech. 2015;8(2):109–29. https://doi.org/10.1242/dmm.017913.
46. Furukawa T, Morrow EM, Cepko CL. Crx, a novel otx-like homeobox gene, shows photoreceptor-specific expression and regulates photoreceptor differentiation. Cell. 1997;91(4):531–41. https://doi.org/10.1016/s0092-8674(00)80439-0.
47. Freund CL, Gregory-Evans CY, Furukawa T, Papaioannou M, Looser J, Ploder L, Bellingham J, Ng D, Herbrick JA, Duncan A, Scherer SW, Tsui LC, Loutradis-Anagnostou A, Jacobson SG, Cepko CL, Bhattacharya SS, McInnes RR. Cone-rod dystrophy due to mutations in a novel photoreceptor-specific homeobox gene (CRX) essential for maintenance of the photoreceptor. Cell. 1997;91(4):543–53. https://doi.org/10.1016/s0092-8674(00)80440-7.
48. Rivolta C, Berson EL, Dryja TP. Dominant Leber congenital amaurosis, cone-rod degeneration, and retinitis pigmentosa caused by mutant versions of the transcription factor CRX. Hum Mutat. 2001;18(6):488–98. https://doi.org/10.1002/humu.1226.
49. Sohocki MM, Sullivan LS, Mintz-Hittner HA, Birch D, Heckenlively JR, Freund CL, McInnes RR, Daiger SP. A range of clinical phenotypes associated with mutations in CRX, a photoreceptor transcription-factor gene. Am J Hum Genet. 1998;63(5):1307–15. https://doi.org/10.1086/302101.
50. Swain PK, Chen S, Wang QL, Affatigato LM, Coats CL, Brady KD, Fishman GA, Jacobson SG, Swaroop

A, Stone E, Sieving PA, Zack DJ. Mutations in the cone-rod homeobox gene are associated with the cone-rod dystrophy photoreceptor degeneration. Neuron. 1997;19(6):1329–36. https://doi.org/10.1016/s0896-6273(00)80423-7.
51. Swaroop A, Wang QL, Wu W, Cook J, Coats C, Xu S, Chen S, Zack DJ, Sieving PA. Leber congenital amaurosis caused by a homozygous mutation (R90W) in the homeodomain of the retinal transcription factor CRX: direct evidence for the involvement of CRX in the development of photoreceptor function. Hum Mol Genet. 1999;8(2):299–305. https://doi.org/10.1093/hmg/8.2.299.
52. Satir P, Pedersen LB, Christensen ST. The primary cilium at a glance. J Cell Sci. 2010;123(Pt 4):499–503. https://doi.org/10.1242/jcs.050377.
53. Mockel A, Perdomo Y, Stutzmann F, Letsch J, Marion V, Dollfus H. Retinal dystrophy in Bardet-Biedl syndrome and related syndromic ciliopathies. Prog Retin Eye Res. 2011;30(4):258–74. https://doi.org/10.1016/j.preteyeres.2011.03.001.
54. Chang B, Khanna H, Hawes N, Jimeno D, He S, Lillo C, Parapuram SK, Cheng H, Scott A, Hurd RE, Sayer JA, Otto EA, Attanasio M, O'Toole JF, Jin G, Shou C, Hildebrandt F, Williams DS, Heckenlively JR, Swaroop A. In-frame deletion in a novel centrosomal/ciliary protein CEP290/NPHP6 perturbs its interaction with RPGR and results in early-onset retinal degeneration in the rd16 mouse. Hum Mol Genet. 2006;15(11):1847–57. https://doi.org/10.1093/hmg/ddl107.
55. Papon JF, Perrault I, Coste A, Louis B, Gerard X, Hanein S, Fares-Taie L, Gerber S, Defoort-Dhellemmes S, Vojtek AM, Kaplan J, Rozet JM, Escudier E. Abnormal respiratory cilia in non-syndromic Leber congenital amaurosis with CEP290 mutations. J Med Genet. 2010;47(12):829–34. https://doi.org/10.1136/jmg.2010.077883.
56. Baala L, Audollent S, Martinovic J, Ozilou C, Babron MC, Sivanandamoorthy S, Saunier S, Salomon R, Gonzales M, Rattenberry E, Esculpavit C, Toutain A, Moraine C, Parent P, Marcorelles P, Dauge MC, Roume J, Le Merrer M, Meiner V, Meir K, Menez F, Beaufrere AM, Francannet C, Tantau J, Sinico M, Dumez Y, MacDonald F, Munnich A, Lyonnet S, Gubler MC, Genin E, Johnson CA, Vekemans M, Encha-Razavi F, Attie-Bitach T. Pleiotropic effects of CEP290 (NPHP6) mutations extend to Meckel syndrome. Am J Hum Genet. 2007;81(1):170–9. https://doi.org/10.1086/519494.
57. Leitch CC, Zaghloul NA, Davis EE, Stoetzel C, Diaz-Font A, Rix S, Alfadhel M, Lewis RA, Eyaid W, Banin E, Dollfus H, Beales PL, Badano JL, Katsanis N. Hypomorphic mutations in syndromic encephalocele genes are associated with Bardet-Biedl syndrome. Nat Genet. 2008;40(4):443–8. https://doi.org/10.1038/ng.97.
58. Sayer JA, Otto EA, O'Toole JF, Nurnberg G, Kennedy MA, Becker C, Hennies HC, Helou J, Attanasio M, Fausett BV, Utsch B, Khanna H, Liu Y, Drummond I, Kawakami I, Kusakabe T, Tsuda M, Ma L, Lee H, Larson RG, Allen SJ, Wilkinson CJ, Nigg EA, Shou C, Lillo C, Williams DS, Hoppe B, Kemper MJ, Neuhaus T, Parisi MA, Glass IA, Petry M, Kispert A, Gloy J, Ganner A, Walz G, Zhu X, Goldman D, Nurnberg P, Swaroop A, Leroux MR, Hildebrandt F. The centrosomal protein nephrocystin-6 is mutated in Joubert syndrome and activates transcription factor ATF4. Nat Genet. 2006;38(6):674–81. https://doi.org/10.1038/ng1786.
59. Valente EM, Silhavy JL, Brancati F, Barrano G, Krishnaswami SR, Castori M, Lancaster MA, Boltshauser E, Boccone L, Al-Gazali L, Fazzi E, Signorini S, Louie CM, Bellacchio E, Bertini E, Dallapiccola B, Gleeson JG. Mutations in CEP290, which encodes a centrosomal protein, cause pleiotropic forms of Joubert syndrome. Nat Genet. 2006;38(6):623–5. https://doi.org/10.1038/ng1805.
60. Khan SA, Muhammad N, Khan MA, Kamal A, Rehman ZU, Khan S. Genetics of human Bardet–Biedl syndrome, an updates. Clin Genet. 2016;90(1):3–15. https://doi.org/10.1111/cge.12737.
61. M'Hamdi O, Ouertani I, Chaabouni-Bouhamed H. Update on the genetics of Bardet-Biedl syndrome. Mol Syndromol. 2014;5(2):51–6. https://doi.org/10.1159/000357054.
62. Tee JJ, Smith AJ, Hardcastle AJ, Michaelides M. RPGR-associated retinopathy: clinical features, molecular genetics, animal models and therapeutic options. Br J Ophthalmol. 2016;100(8):1022–7. https://doi.org/10.1136/bjophthalmol-2015-307698.
63. Breuer DK, Yashar BM, Filippova E, Hiriyanna S, Lyons RH, Mears AJ, Asaye B, Acar C, Vervoort R, Wright AF, Musarella MA, Wheeler P, MacDonald I, Iannaccone A, Birch D, Hoffman DR, Fishman GA, Heckenlively JR, Jacobson SG, Sieving PA, Swaroop A. A comprehensive mutation analysis of RP2 and RPGR in a North American cohort of families with X-linked retinitis pigmentosa. Am J Hum Genet. 2002;70(6):1545–54. https://doi.org/10.1086/340848.
64. Vervoort R, Lennon A, Bird AC, Tulloch B, Axton R, Miano MG, Meindl A, Meitinger T, Ciccodicola A, Wright AF. Mutational hot spot within a new RPGR exon in X-linked retinitis pigmentosa. Nat Genet. 2000;25(4):462–6. https://doi.org/10.1038/78182.
65. Zito I, Gorin MB, Plant C, Bird AC, Bhattacharya SS, Hardcastle AJ. Novel mutations of the RPGR gene in RP3 families. Hum Mutat. 2000;15(4):386. https://doi.org/10.1002/(sici)1098-1004(200004)15:4<386::aid-humu23>3.0.co;2-4.
66. Ayyagari R, Demirci FY, Liu J, Bingham EL, Stringham H, Kakuk LE, Boehnke M, Gorin MB, Richards JE, Sieving PA. X-linked recessive atrophic macular degeneration from RPGR mutation. Genomics. 2002;80(2):166–71. https://doi.org/10.1006/geno.2002.6815.
67. Branham K, Othman M, Brumm M, Karoukis AJ, Atmaca-Sonmez P, Yashar BM, Schwartz SB, Stover

NB, Trzupek K, Wheaton D, Jennings B, Ciccarelli ML, Jayasundera KT, Lewis RA, Birch D, Bennett J, Sieving PA, Andreasson S, Duncan JL, Fishman GA, Iannaccone A, Weleber RG, Jacobson SG, Heckenlively JR, Swaroop A. Mutations in RPGR and RP2 account for 15% of males with simplex retinal degenerative disease. Invest Ophthalmol Vis Sci. 2012;53(13):8232–7. https://doi.org/10.1167/iovs.12-11025.
68. Churchill JD, Bowne SJ, Sullivan LS, Lewis RA, Wheaton DK, Birch DG, Branham KE, Heckenlively JR, Daiger SP. Mutations in the X-linked retinitis pigmentosa genes RPGR and RP2 found in 8.5% of families with a provisional diagnosis of autosomal dominant retinitis pigmentosa. Invest Ophthalmol Vis Sci. 2013;54(2):1411–6. https://doi.org/10.1167/iovs.12-11541.
69. Demirci FY, Rigatti BW, Wen G, Radak AL, Mah TS, Baic CL, Traboulsi EI, Alitalo T, Ramser J, Gorin MB. X-linked cone-rod dystrophy (locus COD1): identification of mutations in RPGR exon ORF15. Am J Hum Genet. 2002;70(4):1049–53. https://doi.org/10.1086/339620.
70. Sharon D, Sandberg MA, Rabe VW, Stillberger M, Dryja TP, Berson EL. RP2 and RPGR mutations and clinical correlations in patients with X-linked retinitis pigmentosa. Am J Hum Genet. 2003;73(5):1131–46. https://doi.org/10.1086/379379.
71. Weil D, Levy G, Sahly I, Levi-Acobas F, Blanchard S, El-Amraoui A, Crozet F, Philippe H, Abitbol M, Petit C. Human myosin VIIA responsible for the Usher 1B syndrome: a predicted membrane-associated motor protein expressed in developing sensory epithelia. Proc Natl Acad Sci U S A. 1996;93(8):3232–7. https://doi.org/10.1073/pnas.93.8.3232.
72. Liu X, Udovichenko IP, Brown SD, Steel KP, Williams DS. Myosin VIIa participates in opsin transport through the photoreceptor cilium. J Neurosci. 1999;19(15):6267–74. https://doi.org/10.1523/JNEUROSCI.19-15-06267.1999.
73. Gibbs D, Kitamoto J, Williams DS. Abnormal phagocytosis by retinal pigmented epithelium that lacks myosin VIIa, the Usher syndrome 1B protein. Proc Natl Acad Sci U S A. 2003;100(11):6481–6. https://doi.org/10.1073/pnas.1130432100.
74. Le Quesne Stabej P, Saihan Z, Rangesh N, Steele-Stallard HB, Ambrose J, Coffey A, Emmerson J, Haralambous E, Hughes Y, Steel KP, Luxon LM, Webster AR, Bitner-Glindzicz M. Comprehensive sequence analysis of nine Usher syndrome genes in the UK National Collaborative Usher Study. J Med Genet. 2012;49(1):27–36. https://doi.org/10.1136/jmedgenet-2011-100468.
75. Weil D, Blanchard S, Kaplan J, Guilford P, Gibson F, Walsh J, Mburu P, Varela A, Levilliers J, Weston MD, et al. Defective myosin VIIA gene responsible for Usher syndrome type 1B. Nature. 1995;374(6517):60–1. https://doi.org/10.1038/374060a0.
76. Reiners J, Nagel-Wolfrum K, Jurgens K, Marker T, Wolfrum U. Molecular basis of human Usher syndrome: deciphering the meshes of the Usher protein network provides insights into the pathomechanisms of the Usher disease. Exp Eye Res. 2006;83(1):97–119. https://doi.org/10.1016/j.exer.2005.11.010.
77. Huang D, Eudy JD, Uzvolgyi E, Davis JR, Talmadge CB, Pretto D, Weston MD, Lehman JE, Zhou M, Seemayer TAJG. Identification of the mouse and rat orthologs of the gene mutated in Usher syndrome type IIA and the cellular source of USH2A mRNA in retina, a target tissue of the disease. Genomics. 2002;80(2):195–203.
78. Weston M, Eudy JD, Fujita S, Yao S-F, Usami S, Cremers C, Greenberg J, Ramesar R, Martini A, Moller CJ, Smith RJ, Sumegi J, Kimberling WJ. Genomic structure and identification of novel mutations in usherin, the gene responsible for Usher syndrome type IIa. Am J Hum Genet. 2000;66(4):1199–210.
79. van Wijk E, Pennings RJE, te Brinke H, Claassen A, Yntema HG, Hoefsloot LH, Cremers FPM, Cremers CWRJ, Kremer H. Identification of 51 novel exons of the Usher syndrome type 2A (USH2A) gene that encode multiple conserved functional domains and that are mutated in patients with Usher syndrome type II. Am J Hum Genet. 2004;74(4):738–44. https://doi.org/10.1086/383096.
80. Liu Q, Zuo J, Pierce EA. The retinitis pigmentosa 1 protein is a photoreceptor microtubule-associated protein. J Neurosci. 2004;24(29):6427–36. https://doi.org/10.1523/jneurosci.1335-04.2004.
81. Gao J, Cheon K, Nusinowitz S, Liu Q, Bei D, Atkins K, Azimi A, Daiger SP, Farber DB, Heckenlively JR. Progressive photoreceptor degeneration, outer segment dysplasia, and rhodopsin mislocalization in mice with targeted disruption of the retinitis pigmentosa-1 (Rp1) gene. Proc Natl Acad Sci U S A. 2002;99(8):5698–703.
82. Hartong DT, Berson EL, Dryja TP. Retinitis pigmentosa. Lancet. 2006;368(9549):1795–809. https://doi.org/10.1016/s0140-6736(06)69740-7.
83. Riera M, Abad-Morales V, Navarro R, Ruiz-Nogales S, Mendez-Vendrell P, Corcostegui B, Pomares E. Expanding the retinal phenotype of RP1: from retinitis pigmentosa to a novel and singular macular dystrophy. Br J Ophthalmol. 2020;104(2):173–81. https://doi.org/10.1136/bjophthalmol-2018-313672.
84. Verbakel SK, van Huet RAC, den Hollander AI, Geerlings MJ, Kersten E, Klevering BJ, Klaver CCW, Plomp AS, Wesseling NL, Bergen AAB, Nikopoulos K, Rivolta C, Ikeda Y, Sonoda KH, Wada Y, Boon CJF, Nakazawa T, Hoyng CB, Nishiguchi KM. Macular dystrophy and cone-rod dystrophy caused by mutations in the RP1 gene: extending the RP1 disease spectrum. Invest Ophthalmol Vis Sci. 2019;60(4):1192–203. https://doi.org/10.1167/iovs.18-26084.
85. Berson EL, Grimsby JL, Adams SM, McGee TL, Sweklo E, Pierce EA, Sandberg MA, Dryja

TP. Clinical features and mutations in patients with dominant retinitis pigmentosa-1 (RP1). Invest Ophthalmol Vis Sci. 2001;42(10):2217–24.
86. Chen LJ, Lai TY, Tam PO, Chiang SW, Zhang X, Lam S, Lai RY, Lam DS, Pang CP. Compound heterozygosity of two novel truncation mutations in RP1 causing autosomal recessive retinitis pigmentosa. Invest Ophthalmol Vis Sci. 2010;51(4):2236–42. https://doi.org/10.1167/iovs.09-4437.
87. Hims M, Daiger S, Inglehearn C. Retinitis pigmentosa: genes, proteins and prospects. In: Genetics in ophthalmology, vol. 37. Basel: Karger; 2003. p. 109–25.
88. Palczewski K. G protein-coupled receptor rhodopsin. Annu Rev Biochem. 2006;75:743–67.
89. Boon CJ, den Hollander AI, Hoyng CB, Cremers FP, Klevering BJ, Keunen JE. The spectrum of retinal dystrophies caused by mutations in the peripherin/RDS gene. Prog Retin Eye Res. 2008;27(2):213–35.
90. Stuck MW, Conley SM, Naash MI. PRPH2/RDS and ROM-1: historical context, current views and future considerations. Prog Retin Eye Res. 2016;52:47–63.
91. Conley SM, Naash MI. Gene therapy for PRPH2-associated ocular disease: challenges and prospects. Cold Spring Harb Perspect Med. 2014;4(11):a017376. https://doi.org/10.1101/cshperspect.a017376.
92. Cheng T, Peachey NS, Li S, Goto Y, Cao Y, Naash MI. The effect of peripherin/rds haploinsufficiency on rod and cone photoreceptors. J Neurosci. 1997;17(21):8118–28.
93. Kedzierski W, Lloyd M, Birch DG, Bok D, Travis GH. Generation and analysis of transgenic mice expressing P216L-substituted rds/peripherin in rod photoreceptors. Invest Ophthalmol Vis Sci. 1997;38(2):498–509.
94. Fahim AT, Daiger SP, Weleber RG. Nonsyndromic retinitis pigmentosa overview. In: GeneReviews®[Internet]. Seattle: University of Washington; 2017.
95. Becirovic E, Böhm S, Nguyen ONP, Riedmayr LM, Koch MA, Schulze E, Kohl S, Borsch O, Santos-Ferreira T, Ader M. In vivo analysis of disease-associated point mutations unveils profound differences in mRNA splicing of peripherin-2 in rod and cone photoreceptors. PLoS Genet. 2016;12(1)
96. Athanasiou D, Aguila M, Bellingham J, Li W, McCulley C, Reeves PJ, Cheetham ME. The molecular and cellular basis of rhodopsin retinitis pigmentosa reveals potential strategies for therapy. Prog Retin Eye Res. 2018;62:1–23. https://doi.org/10.1016/j.preteyeres.2017.10.002.
97. Mendes HF, Van Der Spuy J, Chapple JP, Cheetham ME. Mechanisms of cell death in rhodopsin retinitis pigmentosa: implications for therapy. Trends Mol Med. 2005;11(4):177–85.
98. Warren R, Molday RS. Regulation of the rod photoreceptor cyclic nucleotide-gated channel. Adv Exp Med Biol. 2002;514:205–23. https://doi.org/10.1007/978-1-4615-0121-3_12.
99. Danciger M, Blaney J, Gao YQ, Zhao DY, Heckenlively JR, Jacobson SG, Farber DB. Mutations in the PDE6B gene in autosomal recessive retinitis pigmentosa. Genomics. 1995;30(1):1–7. https://doi.org/10.1006/geno.1995.0001.
100. Dryja TP, Rucinski DE, Chen SH, Berson EL. Frequency of mutations in the gene encoding the alpha subunit of rod cGMP-phosphodiesterase in autosomal recessive retinitis pigmentosa. Invest Ophthalmol Vis Sci. 1999;40(8):1859–65.
101. Ferrari S, Di Iorio E, Barbaro V, Ponzin D, Sorrentino FS, Parmeggiani F. Retinitis pigmentosa: genes and disease mechanisms. Curr Genomics. 2011;12(4):238–49. https://doi.org/10.2174/138920211795860107.
102. Han J, Dinculescu A, Dai X, Du W, Smith WC, Pang J. Review: the history and role of naturally occurring mouse models with Pde6b mutations. Mol Vis. 2013;19:2579–89.
103. McLaughlin ME, Sandberg MA, Berson EL, Dryja TP. Recessive mutations in the gene encoding the beta-subunit of rod phosphodiesterase in patients with retinitis pigmentosa. Nat Genet. 1993;4(2):130–4. https://doi.org/10.1038/ng0693-130.
104. Petersen-Jones SM, Entz DD, Sargan DR. cGMP phosphodiesterase-alpha mutation causes progressive retinal atrophy in the Cardigan Welsh corgi dog. Invest Ophthalmol Vis Sci. 1999;40(8):1637–44.
105. Dvir L, Srour G, Abu-Ras R, Miller B, Shalev SA, Ben-Yosef T. Autosomal-recessive early-onset retinitis pigmentosa caused by a mutation in PDE6G, the gene encoding the gamma subunit of rod cGMP phosphodiesterase. Am J Hum Genet. 2010;87(2):258–64. https://doi.org/10.1016/j.ajhg.2010.06.016.
106. Peng C, Rich ED, Varnum MD. Achromatopsia-associated mutation in the human cone photoreceptor cyclic nucleotide-gated channel CNGB3 subunit alters the ligand sensitivity and pore properties of heteromeric channels. J Biol Chem. 2003;278(36):34533–40. https://doi.org/10.1074/jbc.M305102200.
107. Kaupp UB, Seifert R. Cyclic nucleotide-gated ion channels. Physiol Rev. 2002;82(3):769–824. https://doi.org/10.1152/physrev.00008.2002.
108. Bareil C, Hamel CP, Delague V, Arnaud B, Demaille J, Claustres M. Segregation of a mutation in CNGB1 encoding the beta-subunit of the rod cGMP-gated channel in a family with autosomal recessive retinitis pigmentosa. Hum Genet. 2001;108(4):328–34. https://doi.org/10.1007/s004390100496.
109. Dryja TP, Finn JT, Peng YW, McGee TL, Berson EL, Yau KW. Mutations in the gene encoding the alpha subunit of the rod cGMP-gated channel in autosomal recessive retinitis pigmentosa. Proc Natl Acad Sci U S A. 1995;92(22):10177–81. https://doi.org/10.1073/pnas.92.22.10177.
110. Kohl S, Baumann B, Broghammer M, Jägle H, Sieving P, Kellner U, Spegal R, Anastasi M, Zrenner E, Sharpe LT, Wissinger B. Mutations in the CNGB3

gene encoding the beta-subunit of the cone photoreceptor cGMP-gated channel are responsible for achromatopsia (ACHM3) linked to chromosome 8q21. Hum Mol Genet. 2000;9(14):2107–16. https://doi.org/10.1093/hmg/9.14.2107.
111. Wissinger B, Gamer D, Jägle H, Giorda R, Marx T, Mayer S, Tippmann S, Broghammer M, Jurklies B, Rosenberg T, Jacobson SG, Sener EC, Tatlipinar S, Hoyng CB, Castellan C, Bitoun P, Andreasson S, Rudolph G, Kellner U, Lorenz B, Wolff G, Verellen-Dumoulin C, Schwartz M, Cremers FP, Apfelstedt-Sylla E, Zrenner E, Salati R, Sharpe LT, Kohl S. CNGA3 mutations in hereditary cone photoreceptor disorders. Am J Hum Genet. 2001;69(4):722–37. https://doi.org/10.1086/323613.
112. Haeseleer F, Imanishi Y, Maeda T, Possin DE, Maeda A, Lee A, Rieke F, Palczewski K. Essential role of Ca2+-binding protein 4, a Cav1.4 channel regulator, in photoreceptor synaptic function. Nat Neurosci. 2004;7(10):1079–87. https://doi.org/10.1038/nn1320.
113. Jalkanen R, Bech-Hansen NT, Tobias R, Sankila EM, Mantyjarvi M, Forsius H, de la Chapelle A, Alitalo T. A novel CACNA1F gene mutation causes Aland Island eye disease. Invest Ophthalmol Vis Sci. 2007;48(6):2498–502. https://doi.org/10.1167/iovs.06-1103.
114. Jalkanen R, Mäntyjärvi M, Tobias R, Isosomppi J, Sankila EM, Alitalo T, Bech-Hansen NT. X linked cone-rod dystrophy, CORDX3, is caused by a mutation in the CACNA1F gene. J Med Genet. 2006;43(8):699–704. https://doi.org/10.1136/jmg.2006.040741.
115. Strom TM, Nyakatura G, Apfelstedt-Sylla E, Hellebrand H, Lorenz B, Weber BH, Wutz K, Gutwillinger N, Ruther K, Drescher B, Sauer C, Zrenner E, Meitinger T, Rosenthal A, Meindl A. An L-type calcium-channel gene mutated in incomplete X-linked congenital stationary night blindness. Nat Genet. 1998;19(3):260–3. https://doi.org/10.1038/940.
116. Travis GH, Golczak M, Moise AR, Palczewski K. Diseases caused by defects in the visual cycle: retinoids as potential therapeutic agents. Annu Rev Pharmacol Toxicol. 2007;47:469–512. https://doi.org/10.1146/annurev.pharmtox.47.120505.105225.
117. den Hollander AI, Roepman R, Koenekoop RK, Cremers FP. Leber congenital amaurosis: genes, proteins and disease mechanisms. Prog Retin Eye Res. 2008;27(4):391–419.
118. Morimura H, Fishman GA, Grover SA, Fulton AB, Berson EL, Dryja TP. Mutations in the RPE65 gene in patients with autosomal recessive retinitis pigmentosa or Leber congenital amaurosis. Proc Natl Acad Sci U S A. 1998;95(6):3088–93.
119. Stenson PD, Mort M, Ball EV, Evans K, Hayden M, Heywood S, Hussain M, Phillips AD, Cooper DN. The Human Gene Mutation Database: towards a comprehensive repository of inherited mutation data for medical research, genetic diagnosis and next-generation sequencing studies. Hum Genet. 2017;136(6):665–77. https://doi.org/10.1007/s00439-017-1779-6.
120. Naso MF, Tomkowicz B, Perry WL 3rd, Strohl WR. Adeno-associated virus (AAV) as a vector for gene therapy. BioDrugs. 2017;31(4):317–34. https://doi.org/10.1007/s40259-017-0234-5.
121. Yu-Wai-Man P. Genetic manipulation for inherited neurodegenerative diseases: myth or reality? Br J Ophthalmol. 2016;100(10):1322–31. https://doi.org/10.1136/bjophthalmol-2015-308329.
122. Patel U, Boucher M, de Léséleuc L, Visintini S. Voretigene neparvovec: an emerging gene therapy for the treatment of inherited blindness. In: CADTH issues in emerging health technologies. Canadian Agency for Drugs and Technologies in Health; 2018.
123. Russell S, Bennett J, Wellman JA, Chung DC, Yu Z-F, Tillman A, Wittes J, Pappas J, Elci O, McCague S, Cross D, Marshall KA, Walshire J, Kehoe TL, Reichert H, Davis M, Raffini L, George LA, Hudson FP, Dingfield L, Zhu X, Haller JA, Sohn EH, Mahajan VB, Pfeifer W, Weckmann M, Johnson C, Gewaily D, Drack A, Stone E, Wachtel K, Simonelli F, Leroy BP, Wright JF, High KA, Maguire AM. Efficacy and safety of voretigene neparvovec (AAV2-hRPE65v2) in patients with RPE65-mediated inherited retinal dystrophy: a randomised, controlled, open-label, phase 3 trial. Lancet (London, England). 2017;390(10097):849–60. https://doi.org/10.1016/S0140-6736(17)31868-8.
124. Testa F, Maguire AM, Rossi S, Pierce EA, Melillo P, Marshall K, Banfi S, Surace EM, Sun J, Acerra C, Wright JF, Wellman J, High KA, Auricchio A, Bennett J, Simonelli F. Three-year follow-up after unilateral subretinal delivery of adeno-associated virus in patients with Leber congenital Amaurosis type 2. Ophthalmology. 2013;120(6):1283–91. https://doi.org/10.1016/j.ophtha.2012.11.048.
125. Tang Y, Wu S, Liu Q, Xie J, Zhang J, Han D, Lu Q, Lu Q. Mertk deficiency affects macrophage directional migration via disruption of cytoskeletal organization. PLoS One. 2015;10(1):e0117787. https://doi.org/10.1371/journal.pone.0117787.
126. Feng W, Yasumura D, Matthes MT, LaVail MM, Vollrath D. Mertk triggers uptake of photoreceptor outer segments during phagocytosis by cultured retinal pigment epithelial cells. J Biol Chem. 2002;277(19):17016–22.
127. Gal A, Li Y, Thompson DA, Weir J, Orth U, Jacobson SG, Apfelstedt-Sylla E, Vollrath D. Mutations in MERTK, the human orthologue of the RCS rat retinal dystrophy gene, cause retinitis pigmentosa. Nat Genet. 2000;26(3):270–1. https://doi.org/10.1038/81555.
128. Allikmets R. A photoreceptor cell-specific ATP-binding transporter gene (ABCR) is mutated in recessive Stargardt macular dystrophy. Nat Genet. 1997;17(1):122. https://doi.org/10.1038/ng0997-122a.

129. Weng J, Mata NL, Azarian SM, Tzekov RT, Birch DG, Travis GH. Insights into the function of Rim protein in photoreceptors and etiology of Stargardt's disease from the phenotype in abcr knockout mice. Cell. 1999;98(1):13–23. https://doi.org/10.1016/s0092-8674(00)80602-9.
130. Molday RS. ATP-binding cassette transporter ABCA4: molecular properties and role in vision and macular degeneration. J Bioenerg Biomembr. 2007;39(5-6):507–17. https://doi.org/10.1007/s10863-007-9118-6.
131. Abd El-Aziz MM, Barragan I, O'Driscoll CA, Goodstadt L, Prigmore E, Borrego S, Mena M, Pieras JI, El-Ashry MF, Safieh LA, Shah A, Cheetham ME, Carter NP, Chakarova C, Ponting CP, Bhattacharya SS, Antinolo G. EYS, encoding an ortholog of Drosophila spacemaker, is mutated in autosomal recessive retinitis pigmentosa. Nat Genet. 2008;40(11):1285–7. https://doi.org/10.1038/ng.241.
132. Collin RWJ, Littink KW, Klevering BJ, van den Born LI, Koenekoop RK, Zonneveld MN, Blokland EAW, Strom TM, Hoyng CB, den Hollander AI, Cremers FPM. Identification of a 2 Mb human ortholog of Drosophila eyes shut/spacemaker that is mutated in patients with retinitis pigmentosa. Am J Hum Genet. 2008;83(5):594–603. https://doi.org/10.1016/j.ajhg.2008.10.014.
133. Husain N, Pellikka M, Hong H, Klimentova T, Choe KM, Clandinin TR, Tepass U. The agrin/perlecan-related protein eyes shut is essential for epithelial lumen formation in the Drosophila retina. Dev Cell. 2006;11(4):483–93. https://doi.org/10.1016/j.devcel.2006.08.012.
134. Lu Z, Hu X, Liu F, Soares DC, Liu X, Yu S, Gao M, Han S, Qin Y, Li C, Jiang T, Luo D, Guo A-Y, Tang Z, Liu M. Ablation of EYS in zebrafish causes mislocalisation of outer segment proteins, F-actin disruption and cone-rod dystrophy. Sci Rep. 2017;7:46098. https://doi.org/10.1038/srep46098.
135. Yu M, Liu Y, Li J, Natale BN, Cao S, Wang D, Amack JD, Hu H. Eyes shut homolog is required for maintaining the ciliary pocket and survival of photoreceptors in zebrafish. Biology Open. 2016;5(11):1662–73. https://doi.org/10.1242/bio.021584.
136. Iwanami M, Oshikawa M, Nishida T, Nakadomari S, Kato S. High prevalence of mutations in the EYS gene in Japanese patients with autosomal recessive retinitis pigmentosa. Invest Ophthalmol Vis Sci. 2012;53(2):1033–40. https://doi.org/10.1167/iovs.11-9048.
137. Littink KW, Koenekoop RK, van den Born LI, Collin RW, Moruz L, Veltman JA, Roosing S, Zonneveld MN, Omar A, Darvish M, Lopez I, Kroes HY, van Genderen MM, Hoyng CB, Rohrschneider K, van Schooneveld MJ, Cremers FP, den Hollander AI. Homozygosity mapping in patients with cone-rod dystrophy: novel mutations and clinical characterizations. Invest Ophthalmol Vis Sci. 2010;51(11):5943–51. https://doi.org/10.1167/iovs.10-5797.
138. Katagiri S, Akahori M, Hayashi T, Yoshitake K, Gekka T, Ikeo K, Tsuneoka H, Iwata T. Autosomal recessive cone-rod dystrophy associated with compound heterozygous mutations in the EYS gene. Doc Ophthalmol. 2014;128(3):211–7. https://doi.org/10.1007/s10633-014-9435-0.
139. Imani S, Ijaz I, Shasaltaneh MD, Fu S, Cheng J, Fu J. Molecular genetics characterization and homology modeling of the CHM gene mutation: a study on its association with choroideremia. Mutat Res. 2018;775:39–50. https://doi.org/10.1016/j.mrrev.2018.02.001.
140. Strunnikova NV, Barb J, Sergeev YV, Thiagarajasubramanian A, Silvin C, Munson PJ, Macdonald IM. Loss-of-function mutations in Rab escort protein 1 (REP-1) affect intracellular transport in fibroblasts and monocytes of choroideremia patients. PLoS One. 2009;4(12):e8402. https://doi.org/10.1371/journal.pone.0008402.
141. Marmorstein AD, Marmorstein LY, Rayborn M, Wang X, Hollyfield JG, Petrukhin K. Bestrophin, the product of the Best vitelliform macular dystrophy gene (VMD2), localizes to the basolateral plasma membrane of the retinal pigment epithelium. Proc Natl Acad Sci U S A. 2000;97(23):12758–63. https://doi.org/10.1073/pnas.220402097.
142. Marmorstein AD, Kinnick TR, Stanton JB, Johnson AA, Lynch RM, Marmorstein LY. Bestrophin-1 influences transepithelial electrical properties and Ca2+ signaling in human retinal pigment epithelium. Mol Vis. 2015;21:347–59.
143. Milenkovic A, Brandl C, Milenkovic VM, Jendryke T, Sirianant L, Wanitchakool P, Zimmermann S, Reiff CM, Horling F, Schrewe H, Schreiber R, Kunzelmann K, Wetzel CH, Weber BH. Bestrophin 1 is indispensable for volume regulation in human retinal pigment epithelium cells. Proc Natl Acad Sci U S A. 2015;112(20):E2630–9. https://doi.org/10.1073/pnas.1418840112.
144. Guziewicz KE, Sinha D, Gómez NM, Zorych K, Dutrow EV, Dhingra A, Mullins RF, Stone EM, Gamm DM, Boesze-Battaglia K, Aguirre GD. Bestrophinopathy: an RPE-photoreceptor interface disease. Prog Retin Eye Res. 2017;58:70–88. https://doi.org/10.1016/j.preteyeres.2017.01.005.
145. Johnson AA, Guziewicz KE, Lee CJ, Kalathur RC, Pulido JS, Marmorstein LY, Marmorstein AD. Bestrophin 1 and retinal disease. Prog Retin Eye Res. 2017;58:45–69. https://doi.org/10.1016/j.preteyeres.2017.01.006.

Approach to Inherited Retinal Diseases

2

Eun Kyoung Lee

Abstract

Inherited retinal diseases (IRDs) are a genetically and phenotypically heterogeneous group of neurodegenerative disorders. An accurate assessment and diagnosis of IRDs are important, as it allows the patient to be aware of their visual limitations and helps to determine their visual prognosis. Furthermore, through appropriate examination, physicians will be able to detect and manage treatable complications, such as cataract and cystoid macular edema, monitor for other systemic involvement, provide information on the genetic nature of the disease, and provide aids and services for low vision. This chapter introduces various testing procedures and how to approach and evaluate patients with IRDs.

Keywords

Electroretinography · Fundus autofluorescence · Inherited retinal disease · Optical coherence tomography · Visual field testing

E. K. Lee (✉)
Department of Ophthalmology, Seoul National University Hospital, Seoul, Korea

H.-G. Yu (ed.), *Inherited Retinal Disease*, https://doi.org/10.1007/978-981-16-7337-5_2

2.1 Introduction

Inherited retinal diseases (IRDs) are a rare group of neurodegenerative disorders that are genetically and phenotypically heterogeneous and result in progressive visual impairment. IRDs are estimated to affect around 1 in 2000 individuals and thereby are the leading cause of vision loss in persons between 15 and 45 years of age [1, 2]. They affect approximately 200,000 people in the USA and 4.5 million worldwide. Over 270 causative genes have been identified, the mutations of which can cause one or more of the clinical subtypes of IRD (RetNet: https://sph.uth.edu/retnet/, last updated February 14, 2020). IRDs can be clinically classified based on disease progression and the retinal cell types that are primarily involved in disease pathogenesis. IRDs can be sporadic or familial. They can be stationary, such as in congenital stationary night blindness (CSNB) and achromatopsia (ACHM), or progressive, such as in retinitis pigmentosa (RP) and Stargardt disease (STGD). IRDs can be nonsyndromic (isolated), such as in RP and STGD, or syndromic, such as in Usher syndrome, which affects hearing and vision, and Bardet–Biedl syndrome, which affects vision as well as many other metabolic and physical characteristics. Most forms of IRD primarily affect photoreceptors, while other forms mainly affect the retinal pigment epithelium (RPE) or the inner retina. IRDs can be inherited through all modes of inheritance; autosomal dominant (AD), autosomal recessive (AR), X-linked (XL) or mitochondrial.

2.2 Examination of Patients with IRDs

A complete record of ocular and medical history, as well as the family history of eye disease, is to be obtained at the first visit. Important components of patient history include specific symptoms such as central scotoma or night blindness (nyctalopia); the age of onset, which determines the severity of the disease; and family history to establish the pattern of inheritance. Examining other family members is often useful. A complete knowledge of past medical history and intensive physical examination are important to establish systemic associations. It is also important to exclude patients with suspected IRDs from other toxic, infectious, and autoimmune disorders that can mimic IRDs (Fig. 2.1). The clinical assessment includes measurement of best-corrected visual acuity and intraocular pressure, biomicroscopy, and dilated ophthalmoscopy. The American Academy of Ophthalmology's (AAO) clinical statement provides recommendations for the evaluation and clinical assessment of patients with IRDs [3]. Various testing procedures are recommended in Table 2.1.

2.2.1 Color Fundus Photography and Fundus Autofluorescence Imaging

Standard color or wide-field fundus photography should be performed at the initial visit to procure documentation of the disease state as well as the context to align and compare data from other fundus modalities such as fundus autofluorescence (FAF) images. Serial fundus photography is useful for recording the progress of a disease over time (Fig. 2.2). For patients with nyctalopia or peripheral visual field loss, wide-field imaging is advantageous because the primary site of disease is not in the macula in the initial stages of the disease.

In macular and diffuse retinal dystrophies, various associated abnormalities in FAF have been described [4]. Pale yellowish deposits, visible on the fundus photographs, at the level of RPE/Bruch's membrane in Best disease (Fig. 2.3), adult vitelliform macular dystrophy, and other pattern dystrophies, as well as STGD (Fig. 2.4), are associated with an intense focally increased FAF signal [5, 6].

Discrete, well-defined lines of increased FAF may occur in various forms of retinal dystrophies [6–8]. These lines appear as a ring-like structure in RP or macular dystrophies or along the retinal veins in pigmented paravenous chorioretinal atrophy (PPCRA) (Fig. 2.5). Although the orientation of these lines in different entities varies,

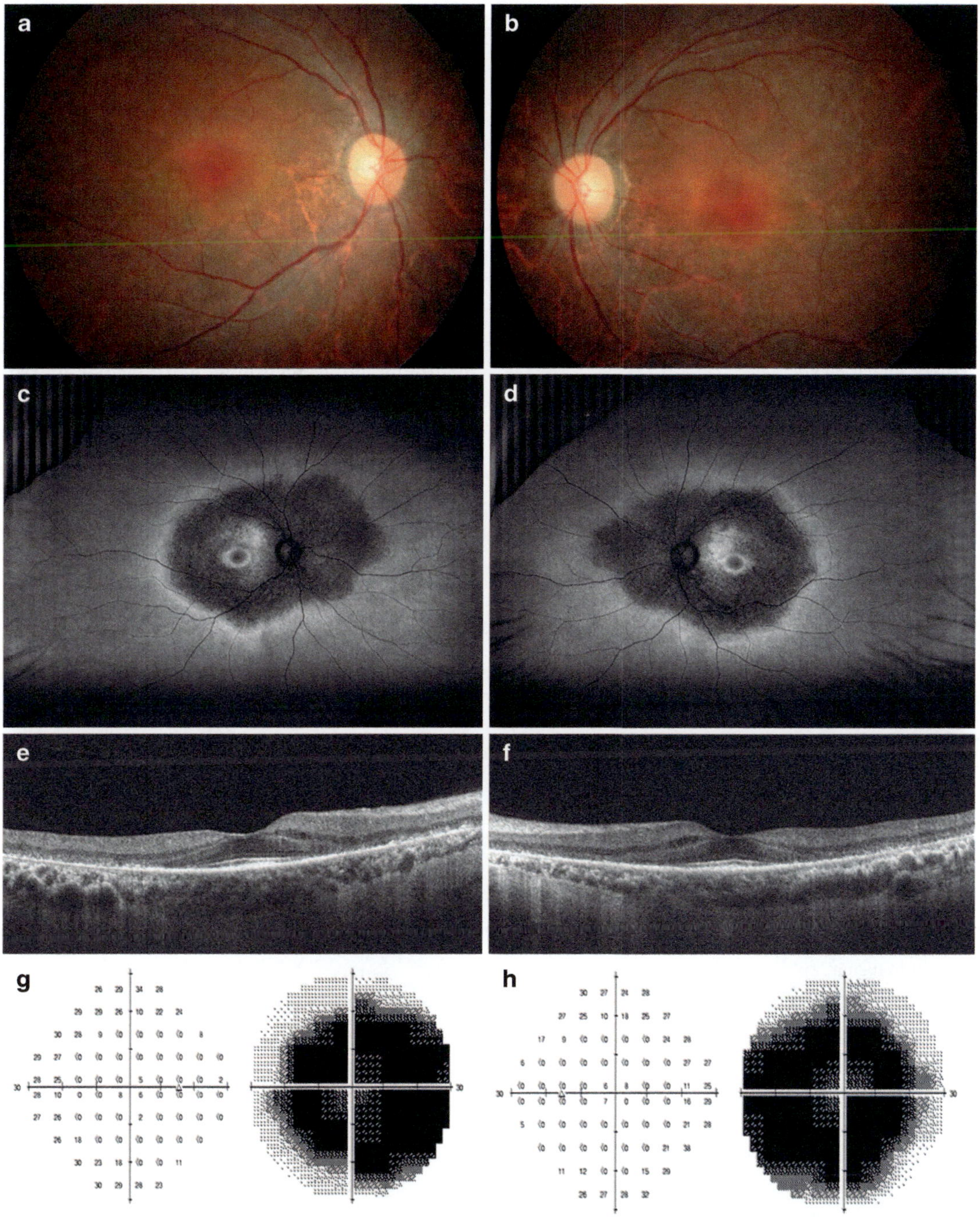

Fig. 2.1 (**a**, **b**) Fundus photographs of the eyes of a 37-year-old female with hydroxychloroquine retinopathy, mimicking sectoral retinitis pigmentosa. The patient had been taking 400 mg of hydroxychloroquine daily for 20 years for the management of systemic lupus erythematosus. (**c**, **d**) Wide-field fundus autofluorescence demonstrates diffuse pericentral and nasal hypoautofluorescence. (**e**, **f**) Spectral domain-optical coherence tomography reveals disruption and irregularity of the retinal pigment epithelium and perifoveal loss of the retinal ellipsoid zone. (**g**, **h**) Humphrey 30-2 visual field tests show dense visual field defects in both eyes

Table 2.1 Clinical evaluation of patients with inherited retinal diseases [3]

Assessment
History • Ocular (including current needs) • Medical (including current medications and history of retinotoxic medication use)
Pedigree (family history)
Clinical ophthalmologic examination • Best-corrected visual acuity • Slit-lamp biomicroscopy • Intraocular pressure • Indirect ophthalmoscopy
Imaging • Color fundus photos • Spectral domain-optical coherence tomography • Fundus autofluorescence: Short-wavelength with reduced illumination when possible • Infrared autofluorescence (when available)
Visual fields • Kinetic • Static • Microperimetry (when available)
Electroretinography • Full-filed ERG (when appropriate) • Multifocal ERG (when appropriate)
Genetic diagnostic testing

the agreement between similar appearance and functional findings in FAF images indicates that these lines in heterogeneous diseases share a common underlying pathophysiological mechanism [7]. Previous studies have reported abnormal FAF in the form of a parafoveal ring of increased signal in RP patients [9, 10] (Fig. 2.6). The ring demarcates the areas of preserved central photopic function and also seems to be of prognostic value as it is useful in assessing the degree of macular dysfunction in patients with RP [8, 9, 11]. Functional assessment in cone-rod dystrophy, cone dystrophy, and macular dystrophies exhibiting a parafoveal ring of increased FAF revealed opposing results compared to RP (Fig. 2.7). In patients with macular dystrophy, there was severe retinal dysfunction within the ring, and the FAF signal and retinal sensitivity were almost normal outside the ring. Although the pathophysiological mechanism for this effect is unknown, the increase in FAF signals observed in various retinal dystrophies is associated with an accumulation of lipofuscin in the transition zone [7, 11].

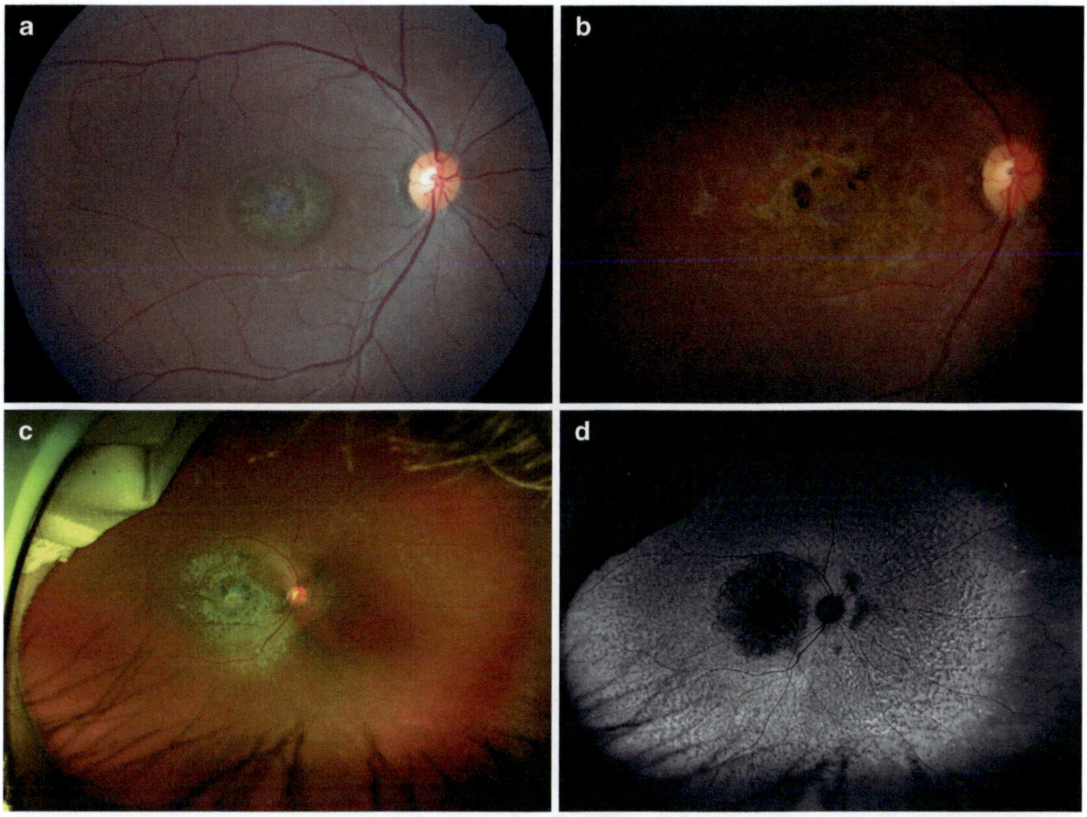

Fig. 2.2 (**a**) Fundus photograph of the right eye of a 12-year-old female with compound heterozygous mutations in *ABCA4* (Leu2241Arg/His1865Tyr) causing Stargardt disease. Her visual acuity was 8/200. The small patch of geographic atrophy has a shiny base that glistens in this photograph. Multiple small flecks can also be seen. (**b**) At age 21, there has been a modest enlargement of the central atrophy, and some clumps of dark pigment have developed, but visual acuity remains 8/200. (**c**) At age 28, the area of central atrophy has continued to enlarge, but visual acuity remains 8/200. (**d**) Wide-field fundus autofluorescence imaging reveals a loss of autofluorescence in the area of central atrophy and numerous flecks in the mid periphery retina

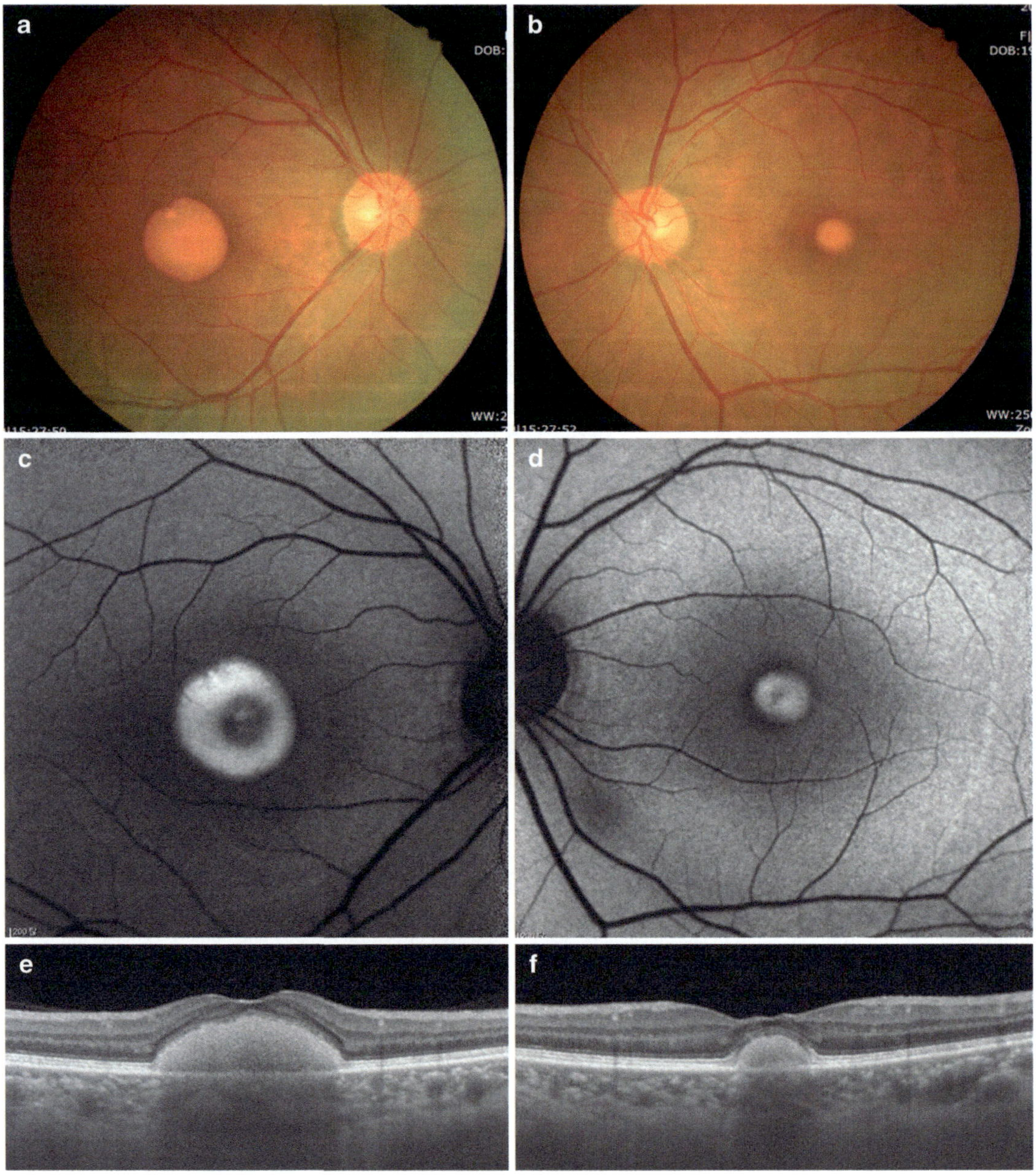

Fig. 2.3 (**a**, **b**) Fundus photographs of the eyes of a 53-year-old male with Best macular dystrophy. There are classic vitelliform lesions in both eyes. (**c**, **d**) A sharply demarcated area of increased fundus autofluorescence (FAF) is visible in the macular area. In the center of the lesion there is reduced FAF. (**e**, **f**) Spectral domain-optical coherence tomography demonstrates hyper-reflectivity of the vitelliform material in the subretinal space in both eyes

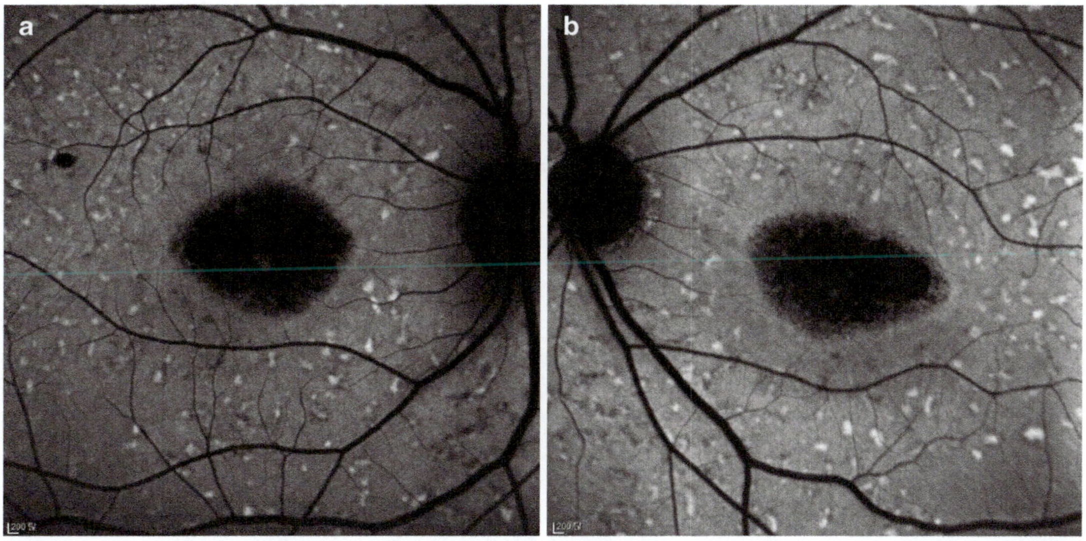

Fig. 2.4 (**a**, **b**) Fundus autofluorescence (FAF) images of the eyes of a 44-year-old female with Stargardt disease. Focal flecks visible on the fundoscope show a bright and increased FAF signal. Focal areas of decreased FAF correspond with retinal pigment epithelial atrophy

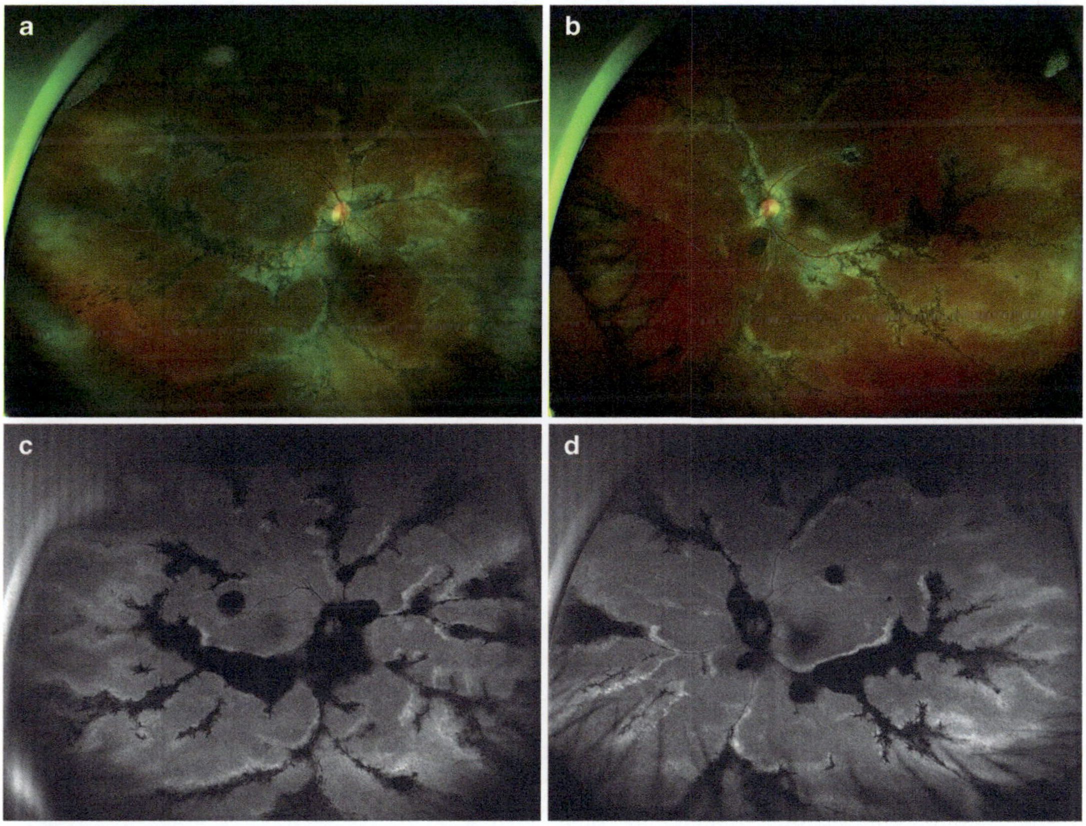

Fig. 2.5 (**a**, **b**) Wide-field fundus photographs of the eyes of a 48-year-old female with pigmented paravenous chorioretinal atrophy. (**c**, **d**) Wide-field fundus autofluorescence images show well-demarcated contiguous areas of hypoautofluorescence corresponding to the areas of chorioretinal atrophy. Hyperautofluorescent lines appear at the edge of affected areas with hypoautofluorescent signal

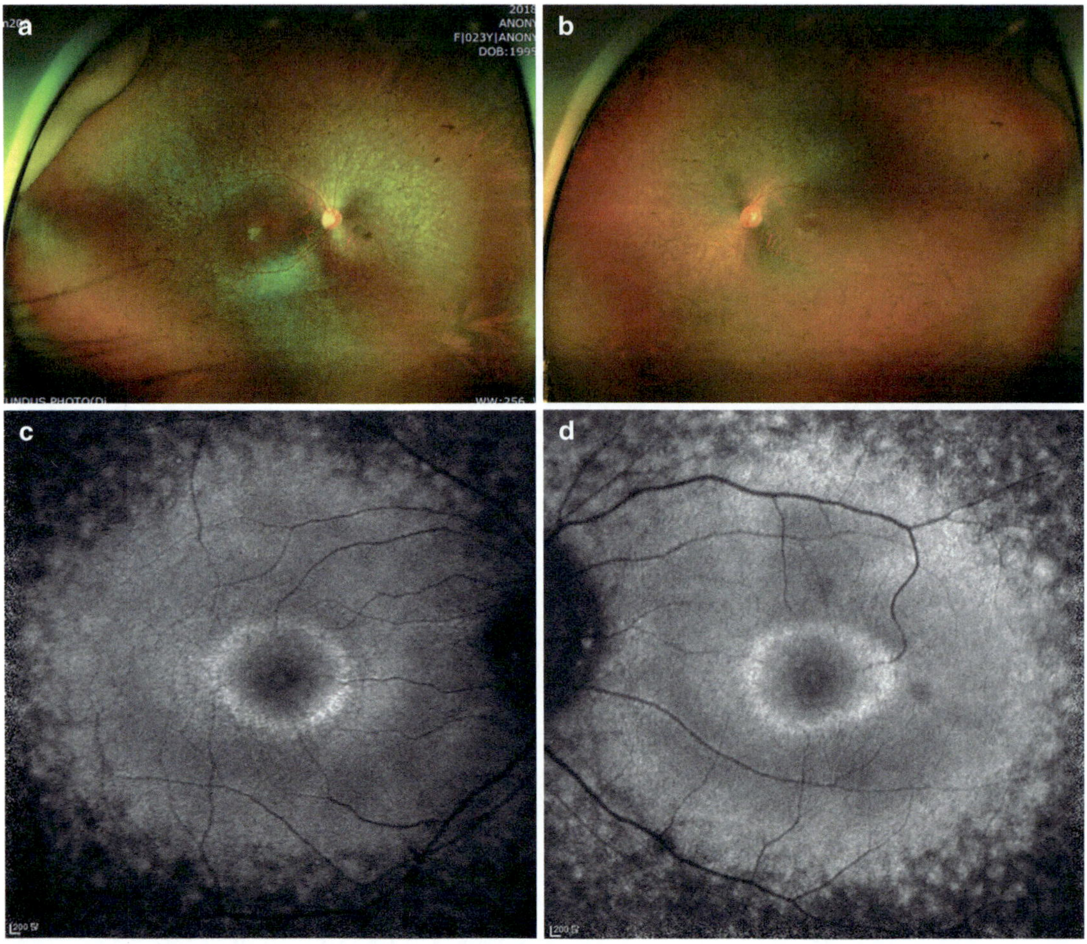

Fig. 2.6 (**a**, **b**) Wide-field fundus photographs of the eyes of a 25-year-old female with retinitis pigmentosa. (**c**, **d**) Fundus autofluorescence images demonstrate a diffuse peripheral hypoautofluorescence and a hyperautofluorescent ring

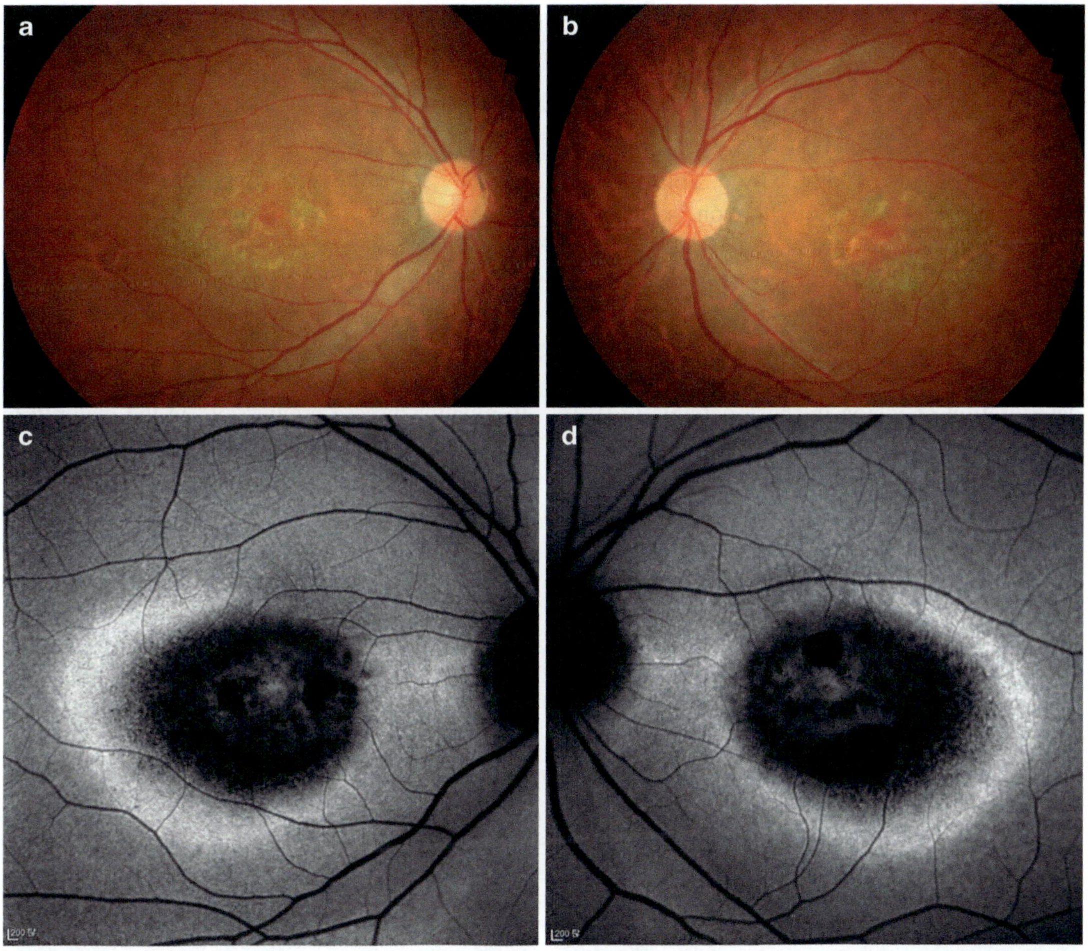

Fig. 2.7 (**a**, **b**) Fundus photographs of the eyes of a 50-year-old female with macular dystrophy. (**c**, **d**) Fundus autofluorescence (FAF) images show areas of hypoautofluorescence corresponding to the areas of retinal pigment epithelial atrophy and the arc of increased FAF

2.2.2 Optical Coherence Tomography

Optical coherence tomography (OCT) provides detailed in vivo images and quantitative morphometric information of the retinal structure [12]. It offers cross-sectional imaging of the photoreceptors, RPE, and inner retinal layers, including the retinal nerve fiber layer. The introduction of spectral domain-OCT (SD-OCT) makes the assessment of accompanying retinal pathology, such as epiretinal membranes [13, 14], cystoid macular edema [15, 16], or retinal layer schisis [17, 18] possible in great detail.

In STGD, OCT can reveal the extent of outer retinal loss and atrophy of the RPE and can also accurately distinguish the anatomic level of flecks [19, 20]. Retinal flecks have an appearance of hyper-reflective deposits opposed to the RPE, or rarely, further away in the outer nuclear layer. They are encountered in advanced or severe stages, with the loss of the photoreceptor layer within the foveal zone, ultimately leading to foveal atrophy (Fig. 2.8). In the case of Best disease, the yellow material of the classic egg-yolk lesion is in the subretinal space and appears fairly homogeneous on OCT [21–23] (Fig. 2.3e, f). In some patients, some of the yellow pigment disappears over time and is replaced by clear fluid. The yellow pigment is denser than the clear fluid, and gravity causes it to settle at the bottom of the egg-yolk lesion, creating a fairly sharp horizontal line that marks the boundary between the pigment and the fluid. This configuration, known as "pseudohypopyon," causes the yellow pigment to appear hyper-reflective on OCT while the clear subretinal fluid appears hypo-reflective (Fig. 2.9).

OCT can identify vitreoretinal abnormalities associated with RP that often contribute to the deterioration of vision in these patients [24]. In RP, SD-OCT demonstrates loss of the ellipsoid zone at peripheral locations from early stages [24, 25]. Cystoid macular edema (CME), which is commonly associated with RP, can also be easily seen in SD-OCT, and it is especially useful for detecting and monitoring CME following treatment (Fig. 2.10). In X-linked retinoschisis (XLRS), OCT helps to enhance the visualization of macular pathologic features [26] (Fig. 2.11). The schisis can occur in different layers of the neural retina. OCT findings may vary depending on the disease stage [27].

2.2.3 Visual Field Testing

Visual field assessment is an important aspect in the management of RP patients. Visual field testing is crucial for documenting the functional extent of the visual field from central to the far periphery for determination of legal blindness and disability, and to monitor disease progression. In the majority of RP patients, the earliest visual field defect in kinetic perimetry is the relative scotoma in the mid periphery, between 30 and 50° from fixation. Scotomas enlarge, deepen, and coalesce to form a ring of visual field loss (Fig. 2.12). As ring scotomas expand toward the far periphery, islands of the relatively normal visual field remain, usually temporal but occasionally inferior or nasal. The outer edge of the ring scotoma expands relatively quickly to the

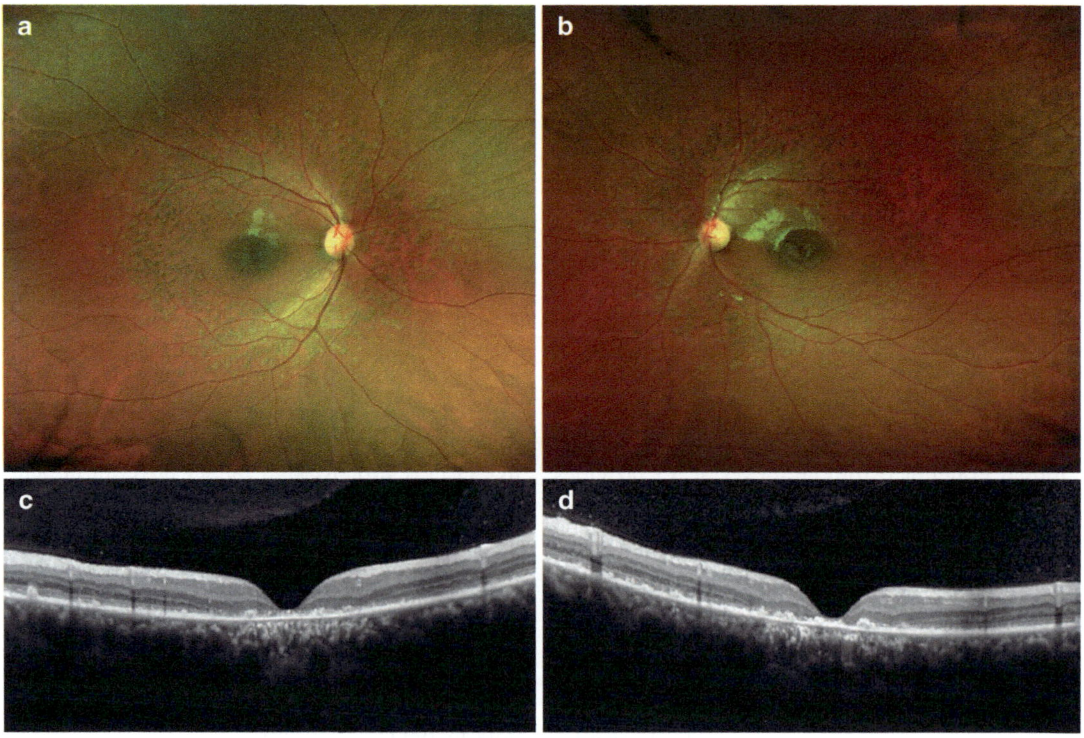

Fig. 2.8 (**a**, **b**) Fundus photographs of the eyes of a 12-year-old female with Stargardt disease. The small patch of geographic atrophy with a uniform light brown color is seen. There are numerous flecks throughout the posterior pole. (**c**, **d**) Spectral domain-optical coherence tomography reveals the loss of foveal photoreceptors and hyper-reflective deposits corresponding with retinal flecks

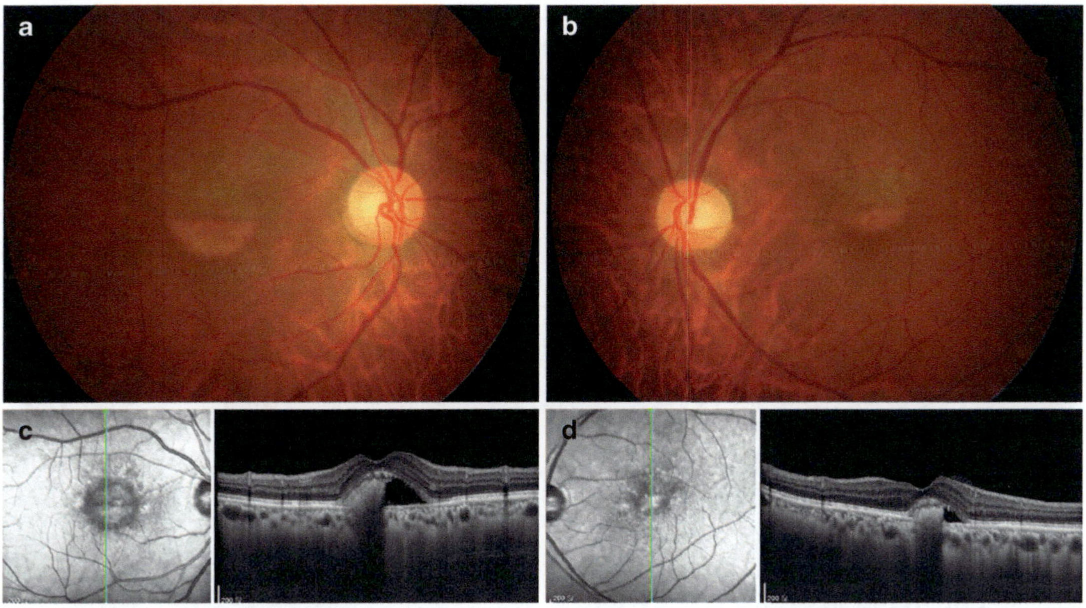

Fig. 2.9 (**a**, **b**) Fundus photographs of the eyes of a 65-year-old male with Best disease. There are vitelliform lesions with a pseudohypopyon appearance in both eyes. (**c**, **d**) Spectral domain-optical coherence tomography demonstrates hyper-reflective deposit corresponding with yellow pigment and hypo-reflective material corresponding with clear subretinal fluid

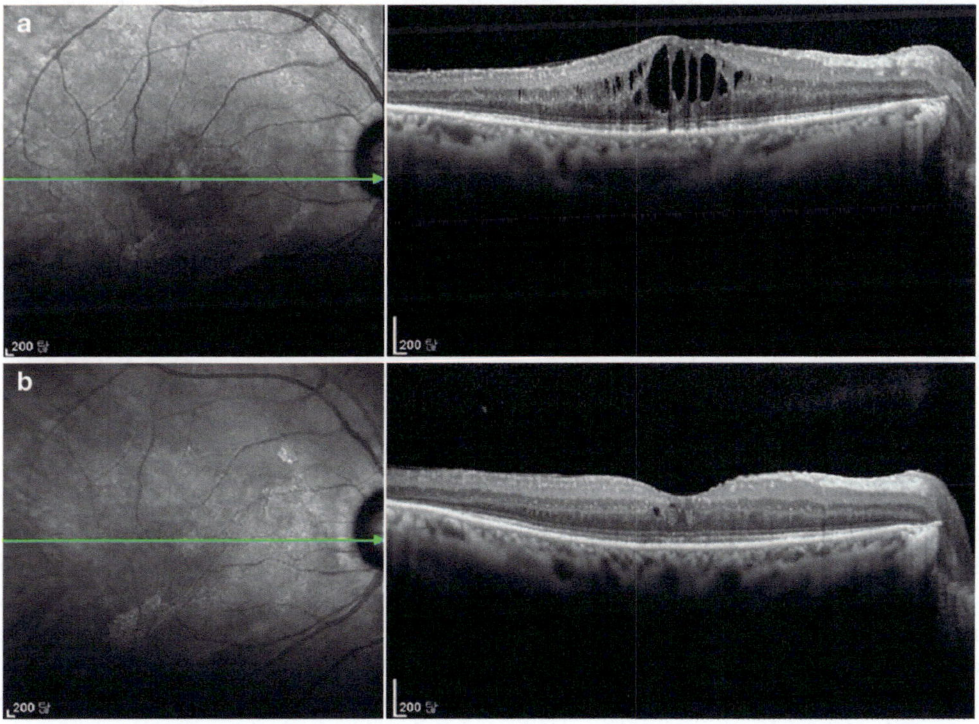

Fig. 2.10 (**a**) The spectral domain-optical coherence tomography images of the eyes of a 61-year-old male retinitis pigmentosa (RP) patient with cystoid macular edema in his right eye. Intravitreal dexamethasone (Ozurdex®) implant injection was performed. (**b**) One month after Ozurdex® injection, cystoid macular edema substantially decreased

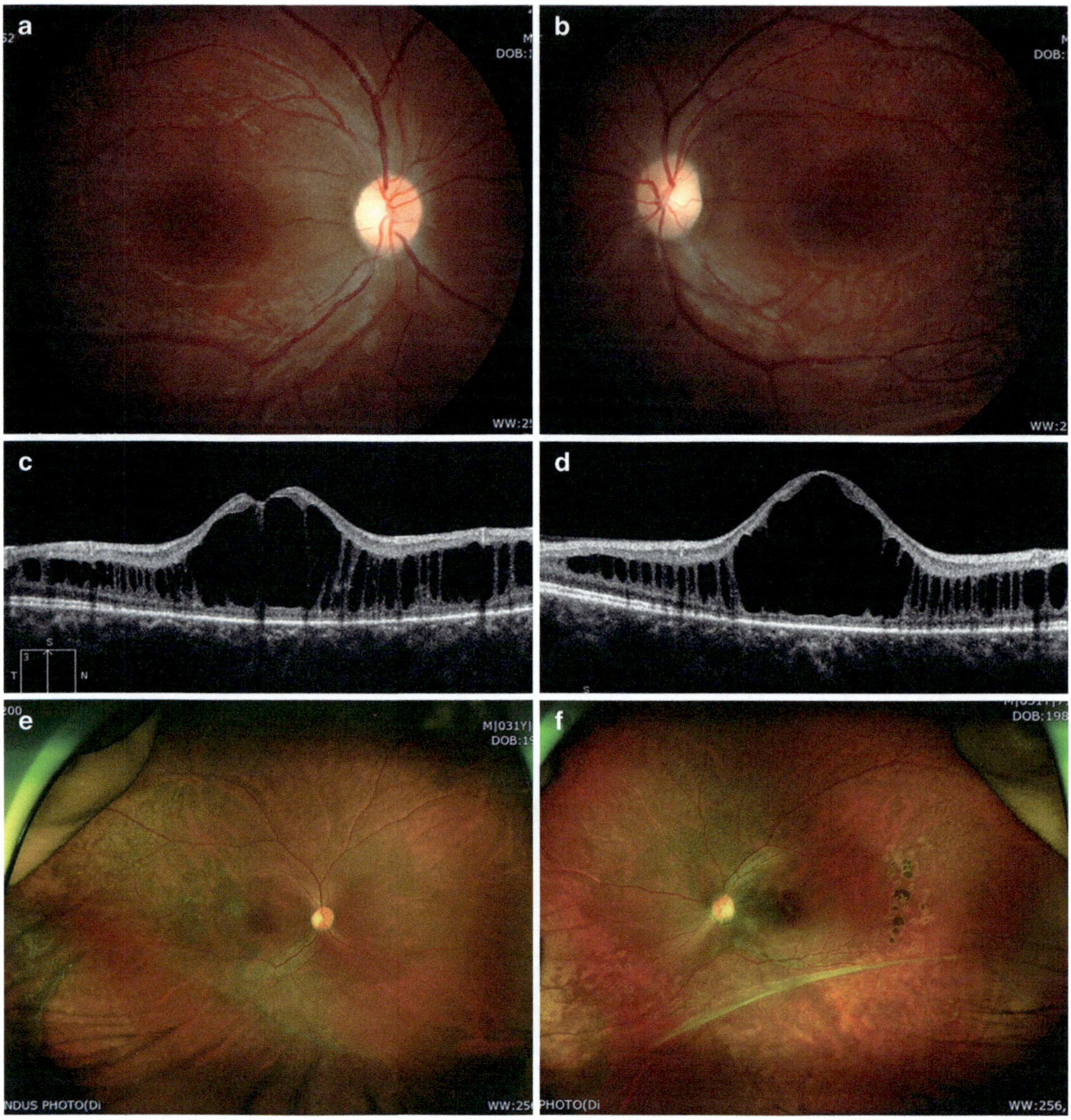

Fig. 2.11 (**a**, **b**) Fundus photographs of the eyes of an 18-year-old male with X-linked retinoschisis reveal foveal cysts in a spoke wheel pattern (**c**, **d**) Spectral domain-optical coherence tomography demonstrates splitting of the inner and outer retinal layers. (**e**, **f**) Wide-field fundus photographs reveal peripheral retinoschisis in the inferotemporal region in both eyes

far periphery, while the inner edge constricts slowly toward fixation [28]. Patients often have a good central vision from a small central island, called "tunnel vision," until they reach their 50s or 60s [29].

For RP patients who drive vehicles, regular visual field evaluation is mandatory, and should be performed at least every 2 years. Although the static perimetry using the Humphrey 30-2 protocol is acceptable for the determination of legal blindness and vision-related disability, kinetic perimetry using Goldmann perimetry is the most common method used for the assessment of peripheral vision and for licensing requirements for driving and disability. Almost all RP patients have to restrict their night driving and eventually stop driving altogether. Regular evaluation of full-field kinetic perimetry helps provide patients with knowledge of their visual limitations. Regular evaluation also prepares patients on when to restrict as well as when to stop driving.

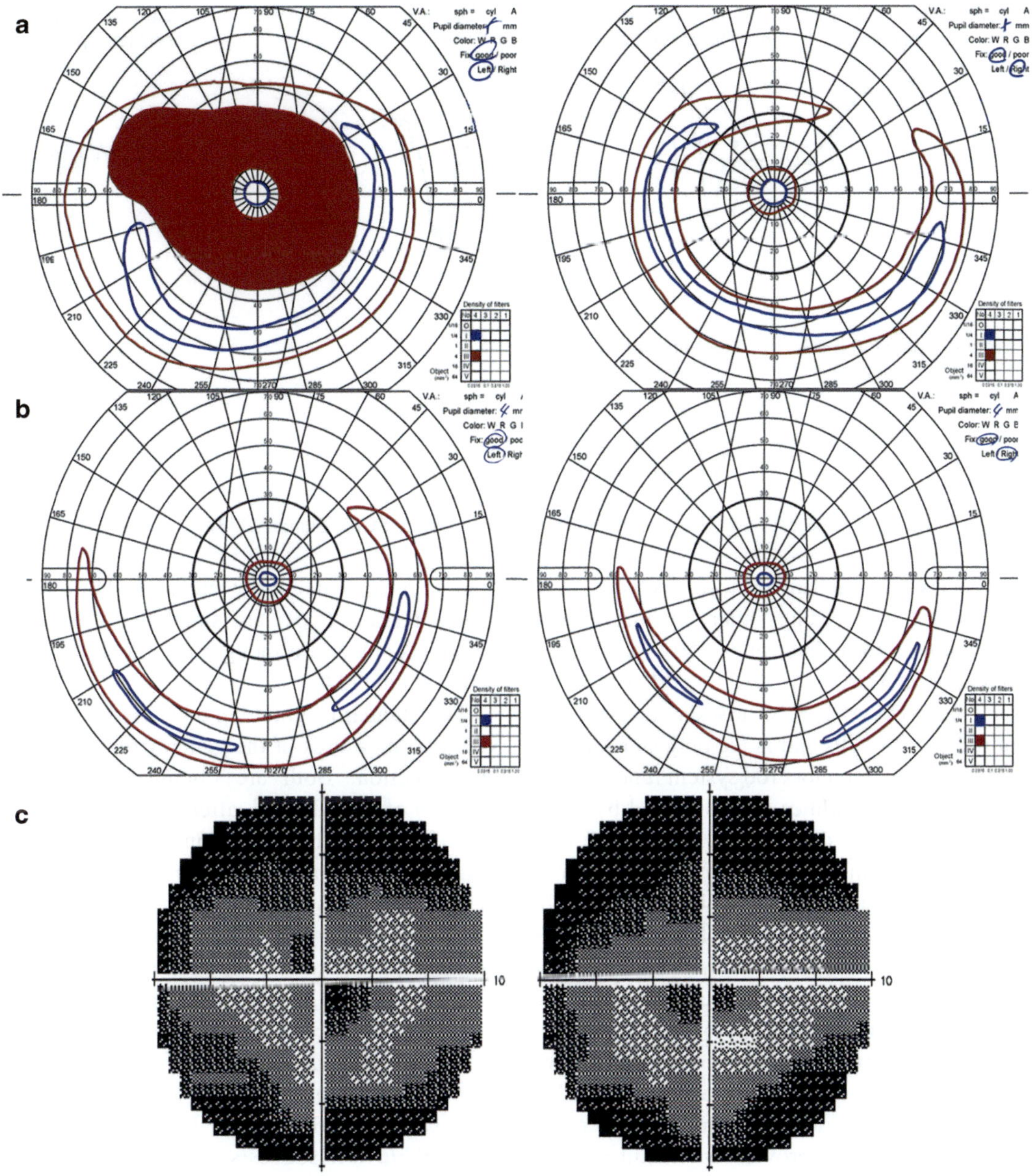

Fig. 2.12 Goldmann kinetic perimetry for a patient with retinitis pigmentosa at age 53 (**a**) and 55 years (**b**). There are scotomas in the midperiphery. As scotomas enlarge toward the periphery, central 10° visual field with inferior peripheral visual field remains. (**c**) Humphrey 10-2 perimetry at age 60 reveals constriction of the central island and deepening of scotomas

2.2.4 Electroretinography

Full-field electroretinography (ERG) is important for the diagnosis and staging of IRDs and is helpful for many patients with diffuse photoreceptor disease to evaluate the function of rods and cones. Standardized conditions and evaluation protocols have been established for electrodiagnostic investigations [30, 31]. ISCEV (International Society for Clinical Electrophysiology of Vision) has published and updated standards that enable electroretinography recordings to be compared between institutions and examiners [32, 33] (Fig. 2.13).

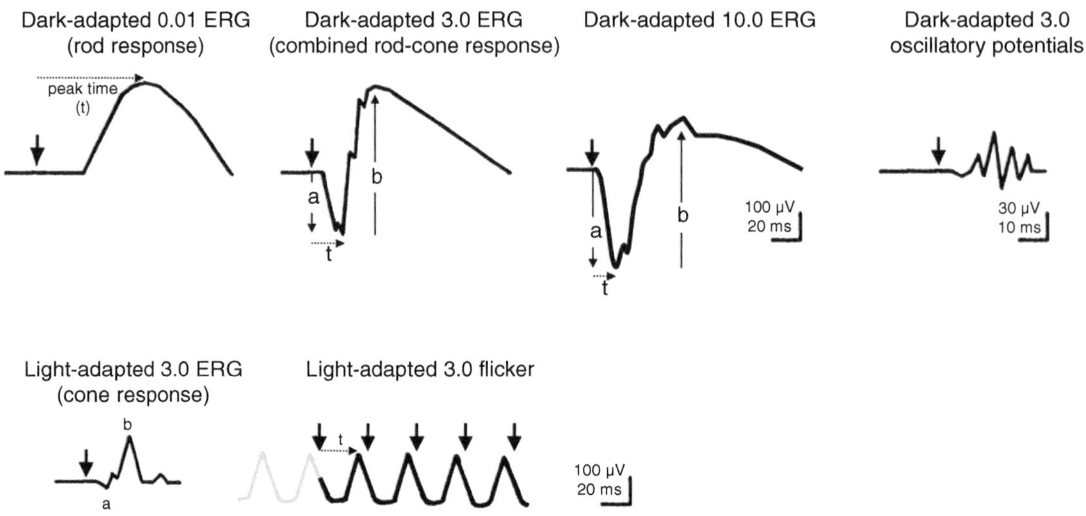

Fig. 2.13 Diagram of the six basic electroretinographies defined by the ISCEV Standard [33]

The ISCEV standard protocol includes dark-adapted (DA) recordings after 20 min of dark adaptation to flash intensities of 0.01, 3.0, and 10.0 cd s m^{-2} (DA 0.01; DA 3.0; DA 10.0). The weak flash (DA 0.01) ERG arises in the inner retinal rod bipolar cells and is the only standard test that selectively monitors rod system function. DA 0.01 ERG abnormalities can be caused by either rod photoreceptor dysfunction or selective dysfunction occurring post-phototransduction or at the level of the inner retinal rod bipolar cells. The DA 3.0 (standard flash) and DA 10.0 (strong flash) ERGs have inputs from both rod and cone systems, but the DA rod system contribution dominates in a normal retina. Approximately the first 8 ms of the cornea-negative a-wave reflects rod hyperpolarizations, and as the a-wave in the DA 10.0 ERG is of shorter peak time and larger than in the DA 3.0 ERG, it provides a better measure of rod photoreceptor function. The subsequent cornea-positive b-wave arises mainly in the rod ON-bipolar cells and reflects a function that is post-phototransduction. Therefore, DA strong flash ERG enables localization of dysfunction to the rod photoreceptors or to a level that is post-phototransduction or inner retina. The DA oscillatory potentials (Ops) are small high-frequency components that are thought to reflect amacrine cell signaling [34].

The standard light-adapted (LA) ERGs provide two measures of the generalized cone system function. Both are obtained to a flash strength of 3.0 cd s m^{-2}, after a standard period of 10 min of light adaptation in the Ganzfeld, with a constant background luminance of 30 cd m^{-2}. A 30 Hz flash stimulus is used to elicit the LA 30 Hz flicker ERG, generated primarily by post-receptoral retinal structures. The single flash cone (LA 3.0) ERG consists mainly of a- and b-waves. The LA 3.0 ERG a-wave arises in the cone photoreceptors and OFF-bipolar cells; the b-wave is dominated by a combination of cone ON- and OFF-bipolar cell activity, and a reduced b/a ratio suggests cone system dysfunction [34].

The full-field ERG is usually the first ancillary test for classifying IRDs (Fig. 2.14). A multifocal ERG can be useful for detecting and monitoring disease progression of diseases that primarily affect the macula [32].

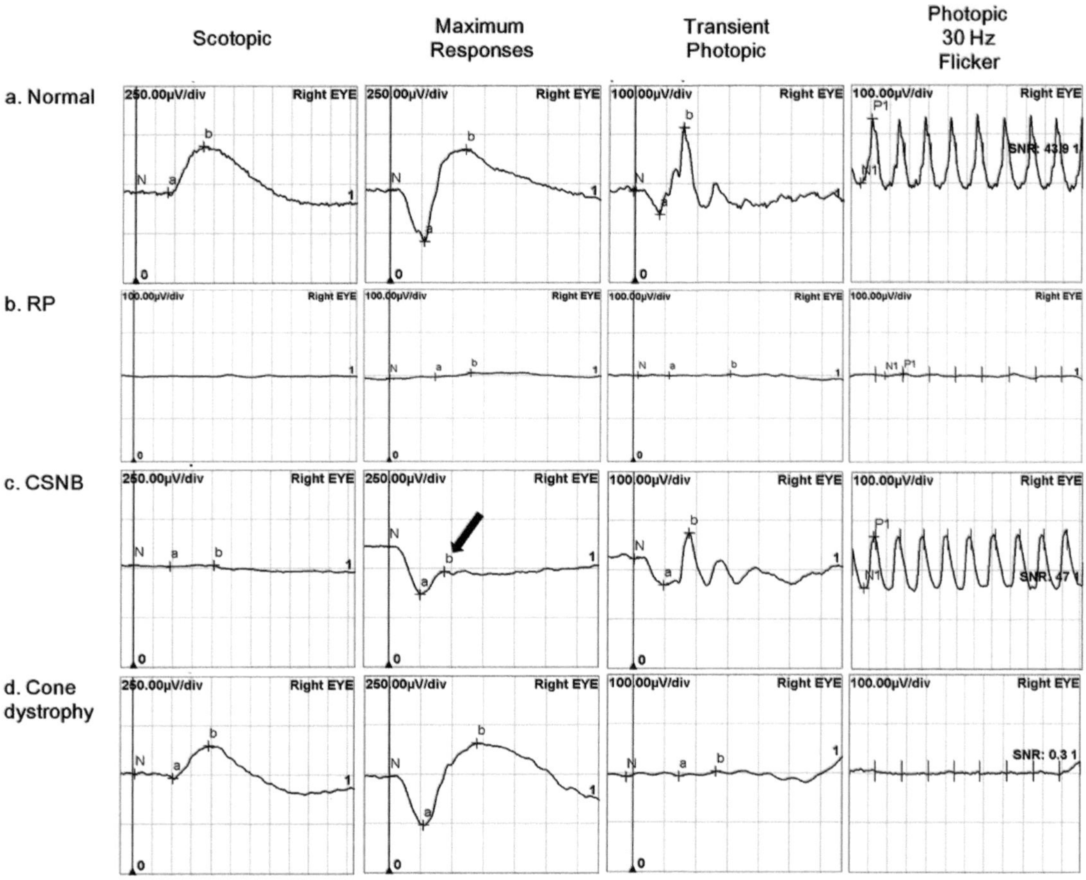

Fig. 2.14 Representative full-field electroretinography (ERG) in a normal subject (**a**), in a subject with retinitis pigmentosa (RP) (**b**), congenital stationary night blindness (CSNB) (**c**), and cone dystrophy (**d**). (**a**) Normal cone and rod responses. (**b**) The ERG response was nearly totally extinguished and nonrecordable. (**c**) Note the undetectable rod response and electronegative b-wave (black arrow). (**d**) Note the undetectable transient photopic responses and 30 Hz flicker

2.3 Inherited Retinal Disease Categories

IRDs can be classified based on the retinal cell types (rods or cones) that are primarily involved in disease pathogenesis and thus predominantly affect the macular or the peripheral retina, respectively. Other ways to classify IRDs are based on the onset time and progression of vision loss. Table 2.2 presents one of the ways to classify IRDs [35]. There has been tremendous progress in the past few years in understanding the molecular basis of IRDs, and it is now evident that the disease is characterized by both clinical and genetic heterogeneity. IRDs show substantial clinical and genetic overlap [36]. The distinction between some IRDs can be very subtle or even arbitrary, and mutations in a single gene can result in varied clinical diagnoses [36]. The identification of pathogenic genes and mutations in humans has allowed knockout, overexpression, and, more recently, gene editing techniques to be used to develop models in rodents and larger animals. Further progress in the molecular genetics of IRDs will enable a comprehensive understanding of the disease pathogenesis and better disease classification, ultimately moving closer to the successful treatment of IRDs.

Table 2.2 Classification of inherited retinal diseases [35]

1. Photoreceptor disease
   - (a) Isolated
     - (I) Acquired/progressive
       - (A) Retinitis pigmentosa
         - (i) X-linked
         - (ii) Autosomal dominant
         - (iii) Autosomal recessive
         - (iv) Other multiplex
       - (B) Cone and cone-rod dystrophy
         - (i) X-linked
         - (ii) Autosomal dominant
         - (iii) Autosomal recessive
         - (iv) Other multiplex
     - (II) Congenital/stationary
       - (A) Leber congenital amaurosis
       - (B) Severe early childhood-onset retinal dystrophy
       - (C) Early childhood-onset retinal dystrophy
       - (D) Achromatopsia (congenital stationary cone dysfunction)
       - (E) Blue cone monochromacy
       - (F) Congenital stationary night blindness
         - (i) X-linked
         - (ii) Autosomal dominant
         - (iii) Autosomal recessive with normal fundus
         - (iv) Enhanced S-cone syndrome
         - (v) Fundus albipunctatus
         - (vi) Oguchi disease
       - (G) Congenital stationary synaptic dysfunction
       - (H) Delayed retinal maturation
   - (b) Syndromic
     - (I) Usher syndrome
       - (A) Type I
       - (B) Type II
       - (C) Type III
     - (II) Bardet-Biedl syndrome
     - (III) Neuronal ceroid lipofuscinosis
     - (IV) Senior-Loken syndrome
     - (V) Joubert syndrome
     - (VI) Microcephaly with or without chorioretinopathy lymphedema and mental retardation
     - (VII) Retinitis pigmentosa with ataxia
     - (VIII) Peroxisomal biogenesis disorders
     - (IX) Cohen syndrome
2. Macular dystrophies
   - (a) Autosomal recessive Stargardt disease
   - (b) Best disease
   - (c) Pattern dystrophy
   - (d) Autosomal dominant Stargardt disease
   - (e) Sorsby fundus dystrophy
   - (f) Malattia leventinese
   - (g) North Carolina macular dystrophy
   - (h) Syndromic macular diseases
     - (I) Maternally inherited diabetes and deafness
     - (II) Pseudoxanthoma elasticum
     - (III) Homocystinuria with macular atrophy
     - (IV) Spinocerebellar atrophy
   - (i) Benign fleck retina

Table 2.2 (continued)

3. Third branch disorders
   - (a) Choroidopathies
     - (I) Choroideremia
     - (II) Gyrate atrophy
     - (III) Late-onset retinal dystrophy
     - (IV) Nummular choroidal atrophy
     - (V) Helicoid peripapillary chorioretinal degeneration
   - (b) Retinoschisis
     - (I) X-linked
     - (II) Recessive
   - (c) Optic neuropathies
     - (I) Nonsyndromic
       - (A) Autosomal dominant
       - (B) Autosomal recessive
       - (C) Leber hereditary optic neuropathy
     - (II) Syndromic
       - (A) Wolfram syndrome
       - (B) Hearing loss
   - (d) Tumors
     - (I) von Hippel-Lindau
     - (II) Retinoblastoma
     - (III) Tuberous sclerosis
     - (IV) Gardner syndrome
   - (e) Vitreoretinopathies
     - (I) Stickler syndrome
     - (II) Familial exudative vitreoretinopathy
       - (A) Norrie disease
       - (B) Autosomal dominant
     - (III) Autosomal dominant neovascular inflammatory vitreoretinopathy
     - (IV) Wagner disease (erosive vitreoretinopathy)
     - (V) Knobloch syndrome
     - (VI) Heritable vascular tortuosity
       - (A) Autosomal dominant retinal vascular tortuosity
       - (B) Cerebroretinal vasculopathy
       - (C) Facioscapulohumeral dystrophy
   - (f) Albinism
     - (I) X-linked ocular albinism
     - (II) Oculocutaneous albinism
       - (A) Nonsyndromic
       - (B) Hermansky-Pudlak
       - (C) Chediak-Higashi
   - (g) Isolated foveal hypoplasia

References

1. Rattner A, Sun H, Nathans J. Molecular genetics of human retinal disease. Annu Rev Genet. 1999;33:89–131.
2. Sohocki MM, Daiger SP, Bowne SJ, et al. Prevalence of mutations causing retinitis pigmentosa and other inherited retinopathies. Hum Mutat. 2001;17(1):42–51.
3. AAO Clinical Statement. Recommendations on clinical assessment of patients with inherited retinal

degenerations. 2016. https://www.aao.org/clinical-statement/recommendations-on-clinical-assessment-of-patients. Accessed 25 May 2020.
4. von Rückmann A, Fitzke F, Schmitz-Valckenberg S, et al. Macular and retinal dystrophies. In: Holz FG, Schmitz-Valckenberg S, Spaide R, et al., editors. Atlas of fundus autofluorescence imaging. Berlin: Springer; 2007.
5. Delori FC, Dorey CK, Staurenghi G, Arend O, Goger DG, Weiter JJ. In vivo fluorescence of the ocular fundus exhibits retinal pigment epithelium lipofuscin characteristics. Invest Ophthalmol Vis Sci. 1995;36(3):718–29.
6. von Rückmann A, Fitzke FW, Bird AC. In vivo fundus autofluorescence in macular dystrophies. Arch Ophthalmol. 1997;115(5):609–15.
7. Fleckenstein M, Charbel Issa P, Fuchs HA, et al. Discrete arcs of increased fundus autofluorescence in retinal dystrophies and functional correlate on microperimetry. Eye (Lond). 2009;23(3):567–75.
8. Robson AG, Michaelides M, Saihan Z, et al. Functional characteristics of patients with retinal dystrophy that manifest abnormal parafoveal annuli of high density fundus autofluorescence; a review and update. Doc Ophthalmol. 2008;116(2): 79–89.
9. Robson AG, Egan C, Holder GE, Bird AC, Fitzke FW. Comparing rod and cone function with fundus autofluorescence images in retinitis pigmentosa. Adv Exp Med Biol. 2003;533:41–7.
10. Robson AG, El-Amir A, Bailey C, et al. Pattern ERG correlates of abnormal fundus autofluorescence in patients with retinitis pigmentosa and normal visual acuity. Invest Ophthalmol Vis Sci. 2003;44(8):3544–50.
11. Lenassi E, Troeger E, Wilke R, Hawlina M. Correlation between macular morphology and sensitivity in patients with retinitis pigmentosa and hyperautofluorescent ring. Invest Ophthalmol Vis Sci. 2012;53(1):47–52.
12. Ko TH, Fujimoto JG, Schuman JS, et al. Comparison of ultrahigh- and standard-resolution optical coherence tomography for imaging macular pathology. Ophthalmology. 2005;112(11):1922.e1–15.
13. Fragiotta S, Rossi T, Carnevale C, et al. Vitreomacular interface disorders in retinitis pigmentosa. Graefes Arch Clin Exp Ophthalmol. 2019;257(10): 2137–46.
14. Liu J, Lyu J, Zhang X, Zhao P. Lamellar hole-associated epiretinal membrane is a common feature of macular holes in retinitis pigmentosa [published correction appears in Eye (Lond). 2020 Jan 15]. Eye (Lond). 2020;34(4):643–9.
15. Huckfeldt RM, Comander J. Management of cystoid macular edema in retinitis pigmentosa. Semin Ophthalmol. 2017;32(1):43–51.
16. Strong S, Liew G, Michaelides M. Retinitis pigmentosa-associated cystoid macular oedema: pathogenesis and avenues of intervention. Br J Ophthalmol. 2017;101(1):31–7.
17. Eriksson U, Larsson E, Holmström G. Optical coherence tomography in the diagnosis of juvenile X-linked retinoschisis. Acta Ophthalmol Scand. 2004;82(2):218–23.
18. Hu QR, Huang LZ, Chen XL, Xia HK, Li TQ, Li XX. X-linked retinoschisis in juveniles: follow-up by optical coherence tomography. Biomed Res Int. 2017;2017:1704623.
19. Ergun E, Hermann B, Wirtitsch M, et al. Assessment of central visual function in Stargardt's disease/fundus flavimaculatus with ultrahigh-resolution optical coherence tomography. Invest Ophthalmol Vis Sci. 2005;46(1):310–6.
20. Lenassi E, Jarc-Vidmar M, Glavac D, Hawlina M. Pattern electroretinography of larger stimulus field size and spectral-domain optical coherence tomography in patients with Stargardt disease. Br J Ophthalmol. 2009;93(12):1600–5.
21. Ferrara DC, Costa RA, Tsang S, Calucci D, Jorge R, Freund KB. Multimodal fundus imaging in Best vitelliform macular dystrophy. Graefes Arch Clin Exp Ophthalmol. 2010;248(10):1377–86.
22. Pianta MJ, Aleman TS, Cideciyan AV, et al. In vivo micropathology of Best macular dystrophy with optical coherence tomography. Exp Eye Res. 2003;76(2):203–11.
23. Querques G, Regenbogen M, Quijano C, Delphin N, Soubrane G, Souied EH. High-definition optical coherence tomography features in vitelliform macular dystrophy. Am J Ophthalmol. 2008;146(4):501–7.
24. Triolo G, Pierro L, Parodi MB, et al. Spectral domain optical coherence tomography findings in patients with retinitis pigmentosa. Ophthalmic Res. 2013;50(3):160–4.
25. Aizawa S, Mitamura Y, Baba T, et al. Correlation between visual function and photoreceptor inner/outer segment junction in patients with retinitis pigmentosa. Eye. 2009;23:304–8.
26. Muscat S, Fahad B, Parks S, Keating D. Optical coherence tomography and multifocal electroretinography of X-linked juvenile retinoschisis. Eye (Lond). 2001;15(Pt 6):796–9.
27. Yu J, Ni Y, Keane PA, Jiang C, Wang W, Xu G. Foveomacular schisis in juvenile X-linked retinoschisis: an optical coherence tomography study. Am J Ophthalmol. 2010;149(6):973–8.e2.
28. Sujirakul T, Lin MK, Duong J, Wei Y, Lopez-Pintado S, Tsang SH. Multimodal imaging of central retinal disease progression in a 2-year mean follow-up of retinitis pigmentosa. Am J Ophthalmol. 2015;160(4):786–98.e4.
29. Grover S, Fishman GA, Brown J Jr. Patterns of visual field progression in patients with retinitis pigmentosa. Ophthalmology. 1998;105(6):1069–75.
30. Marmor MF. An updated standard for clinical electroretinography. Arch Ophthalmol. 1995;113(11):1375–6.
31. Marmor MF, Fulton AB, Holder GE, et al. ISCEV Standard for full-field clinical electroretinography (2008 update). Doc Ophthalmol. 2009;118(1):69–77.

32. Hood DC, Bach M, Brigell M, et al. ISCEV standard for clinical multifocal electroretinography (mfERG) (2011 edition). Doc Ophthalmol. 2012;124(1):1–13.
33. McCulloch DL, Marmor MF, Brigell MG, et al. ISCEV Standard for full-field clinical electroretinography (2015 update) [published correction appears in Doc Ophthalmol. 2015 Aug;131(1):81-3]. Doc Ophthalmol. 2015;130(1):1–12.
34. Robson AG, Nilsson J, Li S, et al. ISCEV guide to visual electrodiagnostic procedures. Doc Ophthalmol. 2018;136(1):1–26.
35. Stone EM, Andorf JL, Whitmore SS, et al. Clinically focused molecular investigation of 1000 consecutive families with inherited retinal disease. Ophthalmology. 2017;124(9):1314–31.
36. den Hollander AI, Black A, Bennett J, Cremers FP. Lighting a candle in the dark: advances in genetics and gene therapy of recessive retinal dystrophies [published correction appears in J Clin Invest. 2011 Jan 4;121(1):456–7]. J Clin Invest. 2010;120(9):3042–53.

Stem Cell and Gene Therapy for Inherited Retinal Diseases

3

Philip DeSouza, Un Chul Park, and Susanna S. Park

3.1 Introduction

The neurosensory retina has a complex architecture of different cell types and proteins that function in the biochemical processes of the visual cycle. The retinal pigment epithelium (RPE), adjacent to the outer neurosensory retina, is essential to the phototransduction process by supporting the metabolism of the highly active retinal cells. Mutations to any of these interdependent cells can lead to inherited retinal diseases (IRDs). These IRDs result in progressive and irreversible vision loss.

Stem cell therapy and gene therapy are promising therapeutic approaches for the treatment of retinal degenerative conditions including IRDs. There are several features of the eye that provide unique advantages for studying the effect of stem cell or gene therapy on retinal degeneration. First, the transplantation site, whether intravitreal, subretinal, suprachoroidal or periocular, can be easily accessed. Second, given that the eye is a small enclosed organ, only a small amount of stem cells or gene therapy products may be required to achieve a therapeutic response when compared to other larger organs. Third, the immune privilege status of the eye may minimize the risk of immune rejection of grafted stem cells or gene therapy products. Last, but not least, the effects of stem cell and gene therapy can be monitored easily noninvasively via eye examination and in vivo imaging modalities given the optical clarity of the ocular media. Various established visual functional tests, such as visual acuity, electroretinography (ERG), or visual field testing, have been used to access efficacy and safety of these novel therapies. Since IRD usually involves both eyes, the untreated contralateral eye often serves as an internal control in clinical trials.

This chapter is an up-to-date overview of advances in stem cell therapy and gene therapy for treatment of IRD. An updated list of completed and ongoing clinical trials and relevant preclinical observations are provided as rationale for exploring specific therapies.

3.2 Stem Cell Therapy

In general, two strategies were adopted for stem cell therapy to treat IRD. One is to replace the diseased or lost cell populations by transplanting differentiated photoreceptors or retinal pigment epithelial (RPE) cells. The other is to indirectly promote the survival of host retinal cells and to delay disease progression via paracrine trophic effects of the transplanted cells. For stem cell treatment of IRD, both approaches can be imple-

P. DeSouza · S. S. Park (✉)
Department of Ophthalmology & Vision Science, University of California Davis, Sacramento, CA, USA
e-mail: sscpark@ucdavis.edu

U. C. Park
Department of Ophthalmology, Seoul National University, Seoul, South Korea

H.-G. Yu (ed.), *Inherited Retinal Disease*, https://doi.org/10.1007/978-981-16-7337-5_3

mented irrespective of the underlying genetic defects. This is the main advantage of stem cell therapy when compared to gene therapy, which aims to correct the specific genetic defect. A majority of intraocular stem cell therapy clinical trials to date have been focused on age-related macular degeneration (AMD), but those targeting IRD are increasing as summarized in Table 3.1. In this section of the chapter, results of cornerstone preclinical and clinical studies and recent progress in stem cell therapy for IRDs are summarized.

3.2.1 Strategies for Stem Cell Therapy for Eyes with Retinal Degeneration

In order to rescue degenerating retina using stem cells, various strategies have been explored. As shown in Table 3.1, different sources of stem cells have been explored including embryonic stem cells (ESCs), induced pluripotent stem cells (iPSCs), fetal retinal progenitor cells, bone marrow-derived mononuclear and CD34+ cells, and mesenchymal stem cells from various sources. In addition, different routes of stem cell administration are being explored including subretinal, intravitreal, and periocular administration. Furthermore, various preparations of cells have been explored including single-cell suspension, cellular sheets, and retinal tissue.

The cells in the RPE play a critical role in maintaining the health of the overlying photoreceptor cells. As such, replacing the diseased RPE cells with healthy RPE cells may slow down the progression of retinal degeneration in eyes with IRD or AMD [1]. In an animal model of retinal degeneration, intravitreally injected human ESC-derived RPE cells failed to show regenerative effects while subretinal injection resulted in rescue effects [12, 13]. For subretinal transplantation of RPE cells, various groups have developed cellular sheets of RPE cells which may be a preferable form of RPE transplantation than cellular suspension since delivery of RPE cells as a monolayer sheet may allow more physiologic orientation of the cells relative to Bruch membrane and overlying photoreceptors [13, 14]. This may be important for RPE cell adhesion, differentiation, and migration and more effective support of the overlying photoreceptor cells [13, 14]. Various materials have been tested as a supportive scaffold to mimic Bruch membrane, usually in the form of electrospun nanofibrous membranes [15–17]. The scaffold must be non-immunogenic, ultrathin, and not compromise RPE cellular function. An RPE monolayer sheet has been developed and explored in early phase clinical trials for eyes with nonexudative and exudative AMD suggesting feasibility and safety [18–20]. To date there are no published clinical trial reports using transplantation of RPE sheet or patch in human eyes with IRDs. However, an early phase clinical trial in France has started enrolling patients with Retinitis Pigmentosa (RP) for subretinal transplantation of RPE monolayer derived from human ESCs (Table 3.1; NCT03963154).

Another cell therapy approach to treat IRD is via transplantation of photoreceptor progenitor cells. This may be the preferred approach for retinal degenerative conditions with primarily photoreceptor loss. Rod precursors isolated from the developing retina of mouse could differentiate into rod photoreceptors, and integrate into the donor retina forming apparent synaptic connections in a murine model of retinal degeneration [21, 22]. Photoreceptor progenitor cells derived from human ESC also showed apparent integration and differentiation into functional photoreceptors after transplantation into the subretinal space of *Crx-/-*mice [23]. Retinal progenitor cells have been cultured and harvested from human fetal neural tissue also showing regenerative potential in RCS rats and tolerability in early phase clinical trial [24]. Due to a limited supply and genetic heterogeneity of human fetal tissue, photoreceptor cells derived from induced pluripotent stem cells (iPSCs) are being explored also as potential source for photoreceptor replacement for eyes with retinal degenerative disease [25, 26].

Although photoreceptor progenitor cells transplanted into the subretinal space were thought initially to integrate into the recipient retina, recent data suggest that the mechanism for

Table 3.1 Current and completed stem cell clinical trials for inherited retinal disease

Clinicaltrials.gov identifier	Retinal dystrophy	Stem cell	Route and cell number	Sample size (enrollment status)	Study design	Treatment center
NCT01345006 [1]	Stargardt	ESC-derived RPE cells (MA09-hRPE)	Subretinal (50K–200K cells)	13 (completed)	Phase 1/2a open-labeled multicenter	Jules Stein/University of California Los Angeles Astellas Institute for Regenerative Medicine
NCT02445612 [2]	Stargardt	ESC-derived RPE cells (MA09-hRPE)	Subretinal (50K to 200K cells)	13 (completed)	5-year follow-up of phase 1/2a study	Jules Stein/University of California Los Angeles Astellas Institute for Regenerative Medicine
NCT01469832 [3]	Stargardt	ESC-derived RPE cells (MA09-hRPE)	Subretinal (50K–200K cells)	12 (completed)	Phase 1/2a open labeled, muticenter	Moorefields Eye Hospital, UK Astellas Institute for Regenerative Medicine
NCT02941991	Stargardt	ESC-derived RPE cells (MA09-hRPE)	Subretinal (50K–200K cells)	12 (completed)	5-year Follow-up study of Phase 1/2a study	Moorefields Eye Hosptial, UK Astellas Institute for Regenerative Medicine
NCT03963154	Retinitis pigmentosa	ESC-derived RPE cell monolayer	Subretinal	12 (enrolling)	Phase I/2	Centre Hospitalier National d'Ophtalmologie (CHNO) des Quinze-Vingts, Paris, France
NCT03944239	Retinitis pigmentosa	ESC-derived RPE cells	Subretinal	10 (enrolling)	Phase 1, open labeled, single arm	Capital Medical University, Beijing, China
NCT04284293	Retintis Pigmentosa	Fetal cortical Neural progenitor cells (CNS10-NPC)	Subretinal	16 (enrolling)	Phase 1/2a dose escalating open labeled	Cedar-Sinai Medical Center
NCT02464436	Retinitis pigmentosa	Fetal retinal progenitor cells (ReNeuron)	Subretinal	12 (enrolling)	Phase 1/2a	Retina Research Institute, AZ Massachusetts Eye & Ear Infirmary, MA ReNeuron LTD
NCT02320812	Retinitis pigmentosa	Allogeneic fetal retinal progenitor cells (jCells)	Intravitreal (0.5 to 3 million cells)	28 (enrollment completed)	Phase 1/2 open labeled, multicenter study	University of California Irvine
NCT0106856153	Retinitis pigmentosa	Autologous bone marrow mononuclear cells	intravitreal	5 (study completed)	Phase I	San Paulo University, Brazil

(continued)

Table 3.1 (continued)

Clinicaltrials.gov identifier	Retinal dystrophy	Stem cell	Route and cell number	Sample size (enrollment status)	Study design	Treatment center
NCT01736059 [4]	Retinitis pigmentosa, Stargardt	Autologous bone marrow CD34+ cells	Intravitreal	15 (enrollment by invitation)	Phase 1, open labeled, single arm	University of California Davis
NCT03772938	Retinitis Pigmentosa; Stargardt	Autologous bone marrow derived progenitor cells	Intravitreal	30 (enrollment by invitation)	Phase 1 nonrandomized study	Pometanian Medical University, Szczecin, Poland
NCT01531348	Retinitis pigmentosa	Bone marrow-derived MSCs	Intravitreal (1 million cells)	10 (enrollment by invitation)	Phase 1, open labeled, single arm	Mahidol University, Thailand
NCT02280135	Retinitis pigmentosa	Autologous bone marrow-derived mononuclear cells	Intravitreal (5–60 million cells)	8 (enrollment completed)	Phase 1, open labeled	Hospital Universitario Virgen de la Arrixaca, Spain

www.clinicaltrials.gov listing of actively enrolling or completed clinical trials for using stem cells for retina dystrophy as of May, 2020
ESC, embryonic stem cell; RPE, retinal pigment epithelial cell

photoreceptor integration may likely involve bidirectional material exchange between the transplanted and recipient cells rather than somatic integration [27–30]. Other possible mechanisms involving material exchange between transplanted and recipient cells are direct cell membrane fusion, free uptake of protein or nucleic acid, and intercellular trafficking such as exosomes [13, 31]. Based on these novel findings, our understanding of the mechanism underlying the photoreceptor rescue associated with cell therapy is being re-evaluated [27, 28].

In eyes with mainly retinal damage from IRD or other types of retinal degeneration, transplantation of just photoreceptor progenitor cells may not be enough to restore retinal function and morphology since there is secondary remodeling of the retina beyond the photoreceptor layer [32]. Researchers are exploring retinal regeneration using tissue with multiple different types of retinal cells arranged in their proper layers to treat such eyes with advanced retinal degeneration. Recent development of 3-dimensional (3D) retinal organoids derived from ESC and iPSC enabled preparation of such retinal tissue for implantation [33, 34]. Transplantation of ESC or iPSC-induced 3D retinal sheet in *rd1* mouse or human ESC-derived retinal tissue in primate retinal degeneration model resulted in structured outer nuclear layers and apparent host-graft synaptic connections [35, 36]. Such studies provide proof-of-concept evidence in support of transplantation of "retinal tissue" for eyes with advanced retinal degeneration.

Table 3.1 summarizes the completed and ongoing clinical trials using stem cells for treatment of IRD. The major sources of stem cells that are being explored for IRD are as follows: embryonic stem cells, induced pluripotent stem cells, bone marrow stem cells, and fetal stem cells. The observations made using these major groups of stem cells in treating IRD are described.

3.2.2 Human Embryonic Stem Cells

Human ESCs are derived from the inner cell mass of a blastocyst of 5-day-old preimplantation embryos. Although there are ethical issues and debates regarding the therapeutic use of human ESCs, these cells are an unlimited source of pluripotent stem cells for cell therapy. Since transplantation of pluripotent stem cells, including ESCs, can result in abnormal cellular proliferation and development of teratomas, many groups have developed partially differentiated RPE cells from human ESCs to use for retinal regeneration [12, 37–39]. These RPE cells derived from human ESC are very similar to primary human RPE cells [40]. In preclinical studies, transplantation of human ESC-derived RPE cells in the subretinal space showed improved visual function in Royal College of Surgeon (RCS) rats [12, 41, 42], and showed long-term survival (>200 days) of transplanted cells without teratoma formation [39]. Recent preclinical studies showed rescue effects of GMP (Good Manufacturing Practice) grade RPE cells derived from human ESC under xeno-free condition up to 150 days after subretinal transplantation in RCS rats [43].

The first human clinical trial explored the safety and tolerability of subretinal transplantation of human ESC-derived RPE cells in eyes with vision loss from Stargardt disease (NCT01345006) and atrophic AMD (NCT01344993). This allogeneic cell transplantation was well tolerated in most eyes although epiretinal membrane formation was noted in a few eyes and several participants had adverse effects from systemic immunosuppression administered to minimize rejection of the cells [1, 2]. In 13 of 18 eyes treated with subretinal human ESC-derived RPE cells, patches of increasing subretinal pigmentation in an area previously without RPE were observed. This observation may suggest replacement of damaged RPE after cell transplantation, but it could also reflect the released pigment after death of injected human ESC-derived RPE cells [3]. In this open-labeled phase I/II study, seven of eight eyes with Stargardt disease had stable or improved visual acuity at 6 months follow-up. In contrast, a phase I/II study conducted in the UK using the same cells showed no significant visual benefit in eyes with Stargardt disease even after 12 months follow-up [3]. The study findings highlight the importance of conducting a prospective randomized sham-controlled study to evaluate efficacy of any novel therapy.

Human ESCs can also differentiate into retinal progenitor cells or photoreceptor cells under appropriate culture conditions [44]. Human ESC-derived retinal progenitor cells transplanted in the subretinal space of nonhuman primates survived at least 3 months without immunosuppression and showed extended axonal projections into the host retina [45]. Based on these promising preclinical findings, clinical trials using human ESC-derived retinal cells may be started exploring this cell therapy for IRD.

3.2.3 Induced Pluripotent Stem Cells

In a seminal work in 2006, Takahashi and Yamanaka reprogrammed differentiated somatic cells to iPSCs, which acquired the ability to self-renew and differentiate to any type of cells in the body [46]. Generating pluripotent stem cells without harvesting them from an embryo or fetus enables patient-specific autologous stem cell therapy and avoids the issue of immunogenic rejection of transplanted cells. Several groups reported successful differentiation of iPSCs to RPE cells [47–49]. The RPE cells derived from iPSCs can form a monolayer of pigmented cells with tight junctions and show phagocytotic ability, growth factor secretion, and gene-expression pattern similar to genuine RPE cells [47, 48, 50].

The first clinical application of autologous RPE cells derived from iPSCs was performed in a patient with vision loss from neovascular AMD. The RPE cell sheet generated from iPSCs derived from the patient's skin fibroblasts was surgically transplanted in the submacular space after removal of the submacular neovascular membrane [20, 51]. After 1 year, no ocular or systemic adverse event was noted. Visual acuity remained stable and optical coherence tomography (OCT) showed good retinal integrity over the graft. This single case provides proof of concept that subretinal delivery of autologous RPE cells generated from iPSCs is possible. Unfortunately, the clinical trial was placed on hold since some genetic instability was noted in subsequently generated iPSC lines [52].

Retinal cell lines derived from iPSCs also may be explored for IRD. A preclinical study by the same group showed direct contact between the host and grafted retinal cells and light-induced behavioral change after transplantation of iPSC-derived retinal tissue in a *rd1* mouse model [53]. In patients with IRD, autologous iPSC-derived retinal cells can supply an unlimited cell source for transplantation [54], but the derived cells still have innate genetic defects responsible for the retinal degeneration. Thus, allogenic transplantation of iPSC-derived retinal and RPE cells is also being explored. Allogenic RPE cells can be immunogenic, but in HLA-A, -B, and DRB1-matched iPSC-derived RPE cells from HLA homozygous donors, a lack of T cell response was observed in vitro [55]. In a primate model, no signs of rejection were observed in MHC-matched iPSC-derived RPE allograft although immune response was detected around the MHC-mismatched grafts [56]. Based on these findings, investigators in Japan are establishing banks of iPSC cell lines bearing common HLA combination in the Japanese population for future allogeneic cell therapy clinical trials [31].

3.2.4 Human Retinal Progenitor Cells

Retinal progenitor cells (RPCs) can be isolated from developing fetal neural retina. They are mitotically active and have the potential for expansion in culture. In particular, they have potential to differentiate to photoreceptor cells [57]. These fetal cells are being explored in early phase clinical trials for IRD (Table 3.1). Initially, RPCs were used as a fetal retinal sheet transplanted in the subretinal space of patients with RP (NCT00345917) and AMD [58]. Recent observations showed that multipotency and self-renewal properties of RPCs are maintained under low oxygen culture conditions [59]. This makes cultured fetal RPCs feasible cell products to explore for allogenic cell transplantation.

One clinical trial underway is a phase I/IIa trial for the safety and tolerability of subretinally transplanted human fetal RPCs in patients with RP (NCT02464436). In this dose-escalating study sponsored by ReNeuron, participants received a single subretinal injection of one of three doses of fetal RPCs. Follow-up is for a year. This clinical trial is based on promising preclinical observations made in RCS rats, showing that subretinal transplantation of RPCs was well-tolerated and resulted in preservation of vision and retinal morphology after 12 weeks [60].

Another approach is intravitreal administration of RPCs. A phase I/IIa clinical trial is evaluating the safety of intravitreal injection of human RPCs (jCell) developed by the stem cell company, jCyte, in human patients with RP (NCT02320812). This trial is based on rationale that injected fetal RPCs secrete factors that would slow RP progression, rather than integrate into the host retina and differentiate to replace the diseased retinal cells. The result of this trial, which is being prepared for publication, showed that the cell injection is well tolerated in all tested doses [31]. Visual acuities of treated eyes were superior to that of untreated eyes, and vision gain was dose dependent. Based on these results, a phase IIb trial (NCT03073733) with a control arm and masking of study groups has been initiated to evaluate for the efficacy of this cell therapy.

3.2.5 Bone Marrow Stem Cells

Bone marrow (BM) consists of a heterogenous cell population consisting mostly of different blood cells, but it is an excellent source of adult stem cells. Since less than 0.1% of total cells harvested from BM have regenerative potential, identifying and harvesting the ideal stem cells from BM can be a challenge. The mononuclear cell fraction of BM is obtained after removal of erythrocytes and polymorphonuclear cells from BM aspirate. It consists mostly of lymphocytes and monocytes. Hematopoietic stem cells (i.e., CD34+ cells in humans) and mesenchymal stem cells (MSCs) are present in the mononuclear cell fraction but constitute <0.2% and 0.01% of this cell fraction respectively [32, 61]. Early phase clinical trials conducted in Brazil demonstrated that intravitreal injection of autologous mononuclear cells obtained from bone marrow appears to be well-tolerated in eyes with RP (NCT01560715) and atrophic AMD (NCT01518127) [61–63]. Some improved visual function in AMD eyes was noted and attributed to possible paracrine effect of CD34+ cells present in the mononuclear cell fraction [64]. However, the concentration of CD34+ cells in the monocular cell fraction is very low.

CD34 is a commonly used cell surface marker to identify human hematopoietic stem cells and endothelial progenitor cells [65]. Using a magnetic cell sorter, CD34+ cells can be harvested from the mononuclear cell fraction, resulting in a purified enriched fraction of CD34+ cell of > 70% concentration. Since human CD34+ cells are mobilized from BM to the sites of tissue ischemia for regeneration and angiogenesis [66], intravitreal injection of harvested CD34+ cells has been investigated as potential therapy for ischemic retinal diseases in preclinical studies. In a model of diabetic retinopathy, homing and integration of these human cells into the inner retina and retinal vasculature with preservation of the retinal vasculature has been demonstrated following intravitreal injection of CD34+ cells [67]. In NOD-SCID murine model of acute ischemia-reperfusion injury, normalization of retinal vessels was noted with no long-term ocular or systemic safety effects following intravitreal injection of human CD34+ cells from bone marrow [68].

The regenerative potential of human CD34+ cells does not appear to be limited to ischemic tissue and has been explored as a potential therapy for IRD. In a murine IRD model, Otani et al. showed that intravitreal injection of autologous BM-derived hematopoietic stem cells had neuroprotective effects [69]. Since injected cells were only observed within retinal vasculature and not in the degenerating photoreceptor layer, a paracrine trophic effect was theorized. Recently, OCT in vivo retinal imaging showed that human BM-derived CD34+ cells rapidly migrate to the degenerating retinal surface after intravitreal injection in a murine model of IRD and systemic immunosuppression [70]. Although functional benefit was not observed with the CD34+ cell injection in this murine model of rapidly progressive retinal degeneration, altered expression of genes that regulate photoreceptor function, maintenance, and apoptosis was observed.

Based on these preclinical studies, a phase I clinical trial was conducted to evaluate the safety and feasibility of intravitreal injection of autologous BM-derived CD34+ cells in eyes with ischemic or degenerative retinal diseases (NCT01736059) [4]. Some of the treated eyes had IRD, including Stargardt disease and RP. A high yield of good quality CD34+ cells was harvested from BM of all participants and injected into the affected eye. No adverse effect was observed during extended follow-up. Although the study was not designed to assess efficacy, various degrees of vision improvement were observed in most treated eyes, and some cellular level changes within the retina were observed using adaptive optics-OCT imaging suggestive of intraretinal incorporation of the injected cells (Fig. 3.1).

Another type of stem cell harvested from BM and explored for retinal regeneration is MSC. MSCs constitute < 0.1% of cells in the mononu-

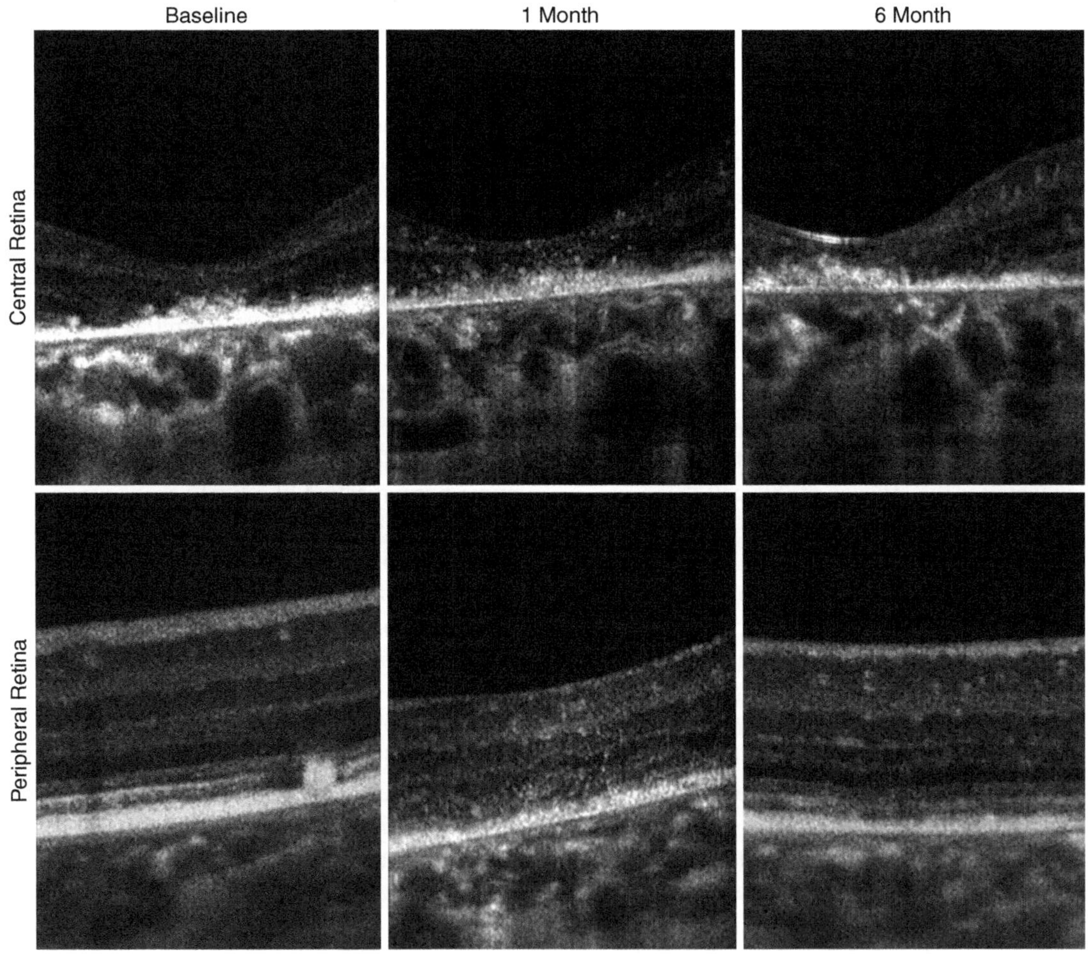

Fig. 3.1 Adaptive optics-optical coherence tomography images of the central and peripheral macula of an eye with Stargardt disease following intravitreal injection of autologous CD34+ bone marrow stem cells. Hyperreflective new foci are seen within the retinal layers suggestive of intraretinal incorporation of injected stem cells at 1 and 6 months following CD34+ stem cell injection [4] (courtesy of Athanasios Parorgias, PhD and John S. Werner, PhD of the Advanced Retinal Imaging Laboratory at University of California Davis)

clear cell fraction of BM but can be harvested and expanded easily in culture [32]. These cells have plasticity to differentiate into cells of mesenchymal origin, but appear to have regenerative effects via paracrine mechanisms [71–73]. Intravitreal and subretinal injection of MSCs showed protective effects in RCS rats [74]. However, clinical application of MSCs for IRD is limited thus far by potential proinflammatory effect and heterogeneity in cell populations [75, 76]. After intravitreal and subretinal injection of MSCs, safety concerns such as reactive gliosis, progressive vitreous haze, and fibrous proliferation leading to retinal detachment, have been reported in preclinical and early phase clinical studies [32, 74–78]. Currently a clinical trial is exploring periocular administration of MSCs as treatment for RP (NCT04224207; Table 3.1).

3.2.6 Three-Dimensional Retinal Organoid

Three-dimensional retinal organoids resemble retinal tissue more closely than cultured retinal cells since they are grown under more physiologic conditions and can partially maintain complex architecture and cell-to-cell interaction within the retina. As such, retinal organoids are being explored as a possible tissue and cell source for retinal replacement therapy in eyes with retinal degeneration, including IRD.

After the spontaneous formation of the optic-cup-like structures from a 3D culture of mouse ESC aggregates in 2011 [79], recent advances in the micro-physiological system enabled 3D organoids to be derived from both iPSCs and ESCs. The use of these organoids is a promising approach to approximating the complex architecture of retinal tissue [80–82]. Retinal organoid resembles rudimentary optic cup- or vesicle-like structures with a stratified retinal tissue that resembles physiologic retina. The retinal tissue contains most of the relevant retinal cell types including photoreceptors [33, 34]. More mature photoreceptors with connecting cilium and photoreceptor outer segments can be generated using retinal organoids [83]. With these strengths, retinal organoids would be a good source of retinal cells and tissue for transplantation in future research [34, 35].

Current retinal organoid technologies still have some limitations that need to be addressed before they can be used effectively for retinal replacement. They include high heterogeneity between cell lines, limited generation of inner nuclear neurons, lack of tissue vascularization, lack of physiological interaction between photoreceptors and RPE, and lack of some essential cells such as microglia. In addition, retinal organoids can develop tissue degeneration in the center due to limited perfusion and can take up to 300 days to culture [84–86]. Advances are being made to overcome some of these limitations. A recent novel micro-physiological model of "retina-on-a-chip" under microfluidic condition enables vasculature-like perfusion of the retinal organoid and interaction between the mature photoreceptors and RPE [87].

Currently, retinal organoids are the most physiological in vitro system that can be used to provide sufficient amounts of clinically relevant retinal cell populations for cell therapies [84, 85]. With further technical advances, retinal organoid platform has potential to be used as a research tool for investigating early retinogenesis, drug toxicity testing and screening, disease modeling, and repair [88–90]. Finally, as defined manufacturing protocols develop for storable retinal organoids and RPE, large-scale production and banking of differentiated retinal tissues can be possible using organoids [91].

3.2.7 Safety and Adverse Events with Stem Cell Therapy

Risk of abnormal cellular proliferation leading to tumor formation is the main safety concern associated with stem cell treatment. This risk is minimized by using partially differentiated cells rather than pluripotent or undifferentiated cells. Nonetheless, injected cells can undergo further differentiation and maturation after subretinal administration induced by the subretinal niche environment [35, 36]. In the case of iPSC-derived RPE cells, the risk of tumor formation or cellular hyperproliferation in athymic nude rats was minimized by removing undifferentiated cells before transplantation [92, 93]. Although no tumor formation has been reported in stem cell clinical trials to date for IRD, epiretinal membrane formation has been described near the subretinal cell injection site [1].

Gene mutation may occur before or after cell transplantation since mutation of established cell lines can occur at each stage of cell division. Thus, the genetic stability of established cell lines is an important safety feature to consider in developing stem cell therapy for IRD. This safety concern was recognized by researchers conducting the landmark clinical trial using autologous iPSC-RPE sheets for eyes with AMD. The trial is currently on hold after identification of a potentially oncogenic mutation in the iPSC line [20].

Immune rejection is also an important issue for allogeneic cell transplantation. The resulting inflammation can damage remnant host retinal tissue as well as the transplanted cells. Although human ESCs express low level of HLA class I molecules in the resting state [94], allogenic transplantation of human ESC-derived retinal cells can cause an immune response, necessitating the use of systemic immunosuppression before and after cell injection. Unfortunately, adverse events were noted using systemic immunosuppression in study participants [3]. Currently, clinical trials are administering varying degrees of immunosuppression since there is some controversy among researchers regarding what constitutes adequate immunosuppression to avoid rejection of transplanted cells and minimize intraocular inflammation. Based on the relative immune-privileged status of the eye, some studies are being conducted using no systemic immunosuppression.

In this regard, autologous cell therapy would be preferred. Autologous intravitreal injection of bone marrow mononuclear cells and CD34+ cells have been conducted in early phase clinical trials without any associated intraocular inflammation reported to date [4, 61]. Retinal cells derived from autologous iPSCs would be another source of autologous cells for treatment of IRD [20], but these cells can be immunogenic. Activation of innate immune system can occur induced by microbial products in the transplants, endogenous proinflammatory factors released during surgical procedure [13, 95] or by increased genomic instability and epigenetic abnormalities that can be developed in the cells during prolonged in vitro culture [52, 96]. In the case of using autologous stem cell for treating IRD, there also are concerns about the putative genetic defect being present within the transplanted cells. A potential solution being explored is the use of established stable allogeneic iPSC lines with the best immunological match to the recipient, selected from a stem cell bank established from healthy donors [97, 98].

Reported ocular adverse events after subretinal injection of RPE cells derived from EPCs include cataract progression, focal RPE loss at the injection site, epiretinal membrane, vitreous inflammation, and endophthalmitis [1]. However, other more serious ocular adverse events have been reported in individuals receiving fee-for-service unregulated autologous "stem cell" treatments. These unregulated treatment centers are injecting uncharacterized cells from adipose tissue in both eyes, and permanent catastrophic bilateral vision loss, as a result, has been reported in some individuals who received these treatments [99]. Since the final cellular product being injected in the eye is not characterized and is prepared using unknown methods, it is unclear what is actually being administered in these fee-for-service "stem cell" treatments. The cellular product may contain unknown and undesired cell populations, such as fibroblasts and adipose cells, and may contain reagents that are toxic to the eye. In the literature, causes of vision loss after injection of "stem cells" as part of a fee-for-service unregulated treatment include retinal detachment secondary to proliferative vitreoretinopathy, epiretinal membrane formation, and retinal vascular occlusion [32, 99–102].

In contrast, in stem cell clinical trials that are regulated by public agencies such as the FDA, the purity, sterility, and health of the cells in the final product is confirmed by vigorous testing before the final cell product is released for clinical use. In order to ensure sterility of the final product, the cells are harvested and manufactured in a GMP laboratory (Fig. 3.2).

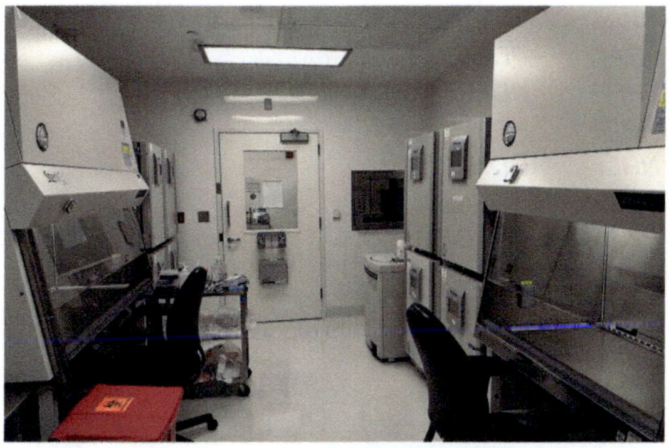

Fig. 3.2 Image of one of six Good Manufacturing Practice (GMP) laboratories inside the GMP facility at the University of California Davis, Institute for Regenerative Cures. This is where CD34+ stem cells and progenitor cells are isolated for clinical trials. It is an ISO7 (Class 10,000) cleanroom laboratory with temperature, air pressure, and humidity control. This assures a tightly controlled and highly reproducible environment avoiding contamination by air particulates. Any person entering this area must undergo a special gowning procedure and have special training pertaining to procedures applied in GMP laboratories (courtesy of Professor Gerhard Bauer, Director of GMP laboratory)

When assessing the appropriateness of stem cell clinical trials for retinal diseases, including IRD, the relative risks and benefits of the treatment should be carefully reviewed with the study participant by the investigators. Registration of a clinical trial on public websites such as www.clinicaltrials.gov does not confirm that the trial is regulated. Since all stem cell treatment for retinal disease is investigational at the current time, individuals should avoid "trials" with the following features: [103] fee-for-service, bilateral simultaneous treatment, multiplicity of target disorders, scientifically inappropriate delivery route, and absence of published preclinical data.

3.3 Gene Therapy

A growing database of over 300 different gene mutations that cause IRD is maintained online (Fig. 3.3) [104]. Recent advances in genomic sequencing techniques (including next-

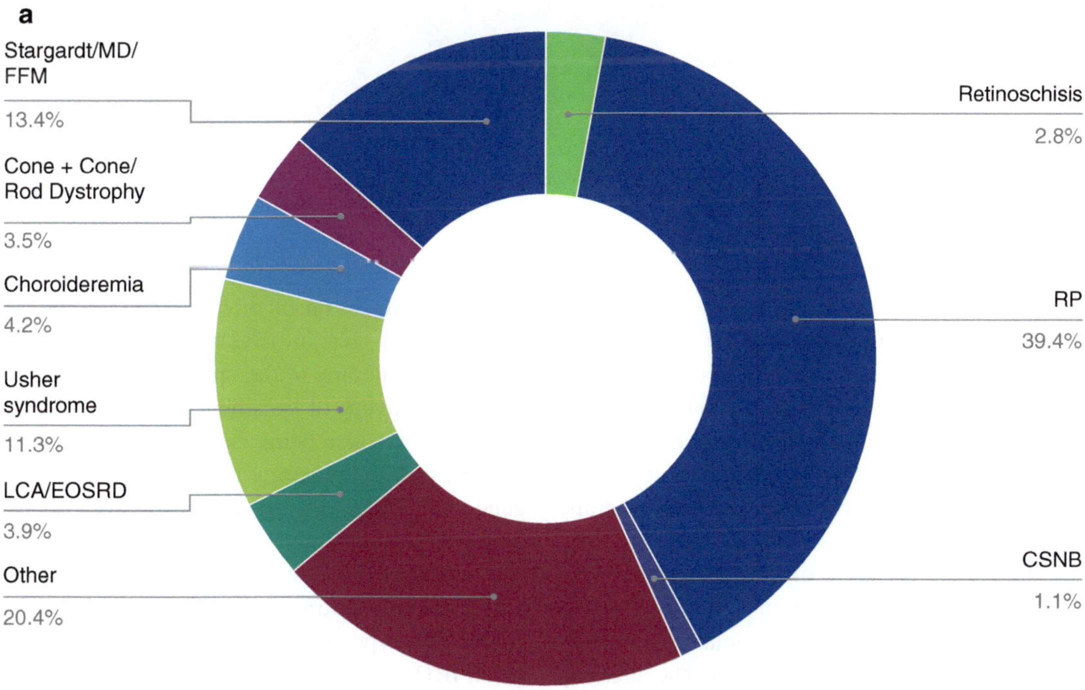

Fig. 3.3 Relative frequency of inherited retinal diseases (**a**) and associated genes. (**b**) Mutations in different genes can result in the same disease phenotype, but with varying degrees of expressivity. Similarly, different types of mutations within the same gene can lead to several phenotypes (adapted from Carrigan M, Duignan E, Malone CPG, et al. Panel-Based Population Next-Generation Sequencing for Inherited Retinal Degenerations. Sci Rep. 2016;(6):1–9.). MD, macular dystrophy; FFM, fundus flavimaculatus; LCA, Leber congenital amaurosis; EOSRD, early-onset severe retinal dystrophy; RP, retinitis pigmentosa; CSNB, congenital stationary night blindness

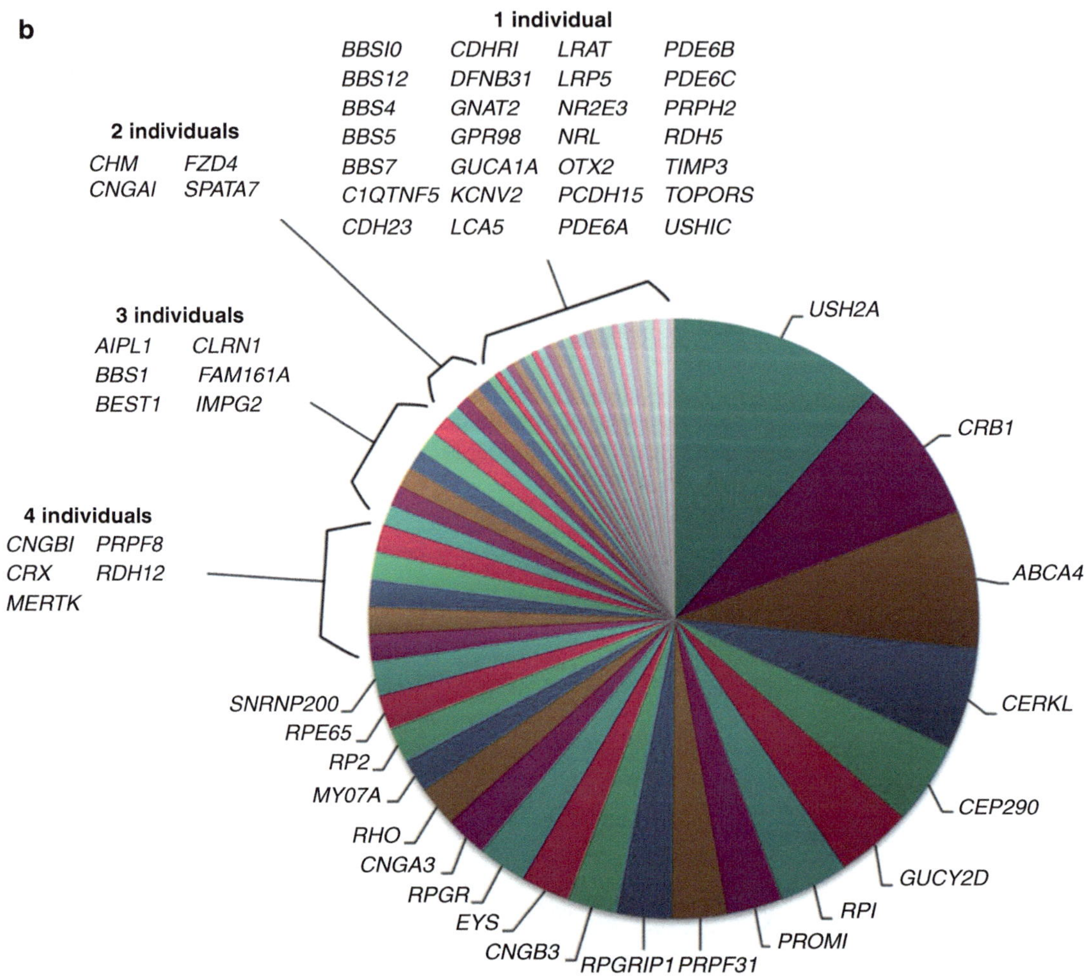

Fig. 3.3 (continued)

generation sequencing and whole genome sequencing) have allowed for more sophisticated molecular diagnoses of the IRD. Precise molecular diagnosis of the IRD is of critical importance for gene therapy, as the gene size, type of mutation (e.g., nonsense and missense), and autosomal inheritance pattern all dictate gene therapy options.

The classic principle of gene therapy for the IRD involves transfection of photoreceptor or RPE cells that carry defective genes with a normally functioning gene copy [105]. The anatomy of the eye and its immune privilege status makes IRD an ideal target for gene therapy [106]. The compartmentalized structures of the eye allow target cells to be reached rather easily with an intravitreal injection of therapy in the clinic, or more directly (but invasively) with a subretinal injection of therapy in the operating room. More recently, delivery of treatment via the suprachoroidal space is also being explored [105].

Types of gene therapy include gene addition, gene silencing, therapeutic oligonucleotides, clustered regularly interspaced short palindromic repeats (CRISPR) gene editing, prime editing and epigenetic editing. All are being explored for IRDs. The type of gene therapy selected for a given IRD often depends on the type of mutation associated with the IRD. For example, gene addition or replacement would be appropriate for an IRD with loss-of-function mutation, in which there is reduced or abolished protein function.

Conversely, gene silencing or gene replacement would be appropriate for an IRD associated with a gain-of-function mutation, in which there are deleterious effects due to enhanced or overexpressed protein function.

The success of gene therapy is immensely dependent on the type of vector used and the ability of the selected vector to navigate the biochemical architecture of target cells. The two major categories of vectors used for gene therapy are viral and non-viral vectors. The following are features of vectors that are considered for selection for gene therapy: (1) the maximum size of genetic payload that can be carried, (2) the ability to deliver the genetic material into nondividing versus dividing cells, (3) the ability to penetrate through cell membranes of target cells, (4) the degree of undesired integration of native viral DNA into the target cells, (5) the possibility of unintended insertional mutagenesis or off-target effects, and (6) the possibility of persistent transgenic expression and immunogenicity (7).

A combination of different gene therapies and vectors has shown promising results in animal models of IRD and human clinical trials of IRD. The latest advancements in gene therapy, such as prime editing and epigenetic editing, suggest extremely precise therapies can be delivered with minimally deleterious effects [107, 108]. In this portion of the chapter, a brief overview of the types of gene therapies and vectors is provided as introduction to the most up-to-date listing of gene therapy clinical trials subdivided by specific IRD being studied.

3.3.1 Types of Gene Therapy

In this chapter, we collectively refer to any modification of a cell genome as "gene therapy." This includes gene addition, gene silencing, and gene editing. An understanding of the distinction between these genomic modifications is necessary for understanding the latest IRD gene therapy treatments under investigation.

Prior to the development of gene editing techniques, there was no excision of mutant alleles. In diseased cells with a genetic mutation resulting in a loss-of-function of the coding proteins, normal genetic information can be inserted somewhere along the genomic sequence to produce functional proteins; this is sometimes referred to as "gene augmentation." [109] For diseased cells with genetic mutation resulting in abnormal coding of additional functioning protein, genetic code could be inserted into the genome to produce RNA interference molecules (small interfering RNAs or microRNAs) to "knockdown" translation of the mutant gene [110]. In contrast, gene editing allows for removal of the mutant gene in order to achieve a complete "knockout," or to exchange it for a functioning allele ("ablate and replace").

3.3.2 Vectors

Whatever the approach used for gene therapy, the genetic material is delivered into the target cells via a vector. There are two types of vectors available that have been explored for gene therapy research and clinical applications, viral and non-viral.

Most vectors used for IRD are viral vectors. Viruses are adept at entering cells because they have protein coats (capsids) that bind proteins on the cell surface to enter cells. The viral vectors include adenoviruses, adenovirus-associated viruses (AAV), alphaviruses, flaviviruses, herpes simplex viruses, measles viruses, rhabdoviruses, retroviruses, lentiviruses, Newcastle disease virus, poxviruses, and picornaviruses [111]. The most applied viral vectors in gene therapy, including the IRD, are summarized in Table 3.2. They include adenoviruses, AAV, and lentiviruses (LV).

Nonviral vectors, such as nanoparticles, or synthetic vectors have had limited use in IRD, but may be of future importance as a viable carrier system for gene editing which can involve transfer of larger amount of genetic material.

3.3.2.1 Adenovirus

Adenoviruses have the largest carrying capacity (up to 48 kb) among the viral vectors and can be transduced into several cell types regardless of

Table 3.2 Comparison of commonly used viral vectors (adapted) [5]

Vector type	Packaging capacity (kB)	Diameter (nm)	Genome type	Advantages	Disadvantages
AAV	<4.4	20–22	ssDNA	Large variety of target tissues, low immunogenicity on first injection	Low packaging capacity, pre-existing antibodies
AV	>8; up to 48	80–100	dsDNA	Large packaging capacity	Limited ability for long-term transfection, high immunogenicity
LV	<8.5	80–120	ssRNA	Large packaging capacity	Potential insertional mutagenesis

AAV, adeno-associated viral vector; AV, adenoviral vectors; LV, lentiviral vector

the cell cycle. They have a limited safety profile and a shorter persistence of genetic transduction, lasting months [106]. The limited safety profile is due to the undesired and variable viral genes of the vector backbone. These viral gene products trigger an immune response against the transduced cells. As such, adenoviral vectors are generally ineffective for pathologies in which long-lasting transgenic expression is needed, including IRD. Additionally, the laminar architecture of the retina appears to result in poorer transduction of photoreceptor cells when compared to RPE cells following subretinal administration [112]. Thus, adenoviral vectors may be more effective for gene therapy to correct RPE gene defects than retinal gene defects. Improvements to adenovirus vectors have been made to reduce toxicity and increase transgene expression, but adoption of these vectors for IRD still remains limited [113].

3.3.2.2 Adenovirus-Associated Virus

Adenovirus-associated viral vectors have been the most promising vectors to use for gene therapy for IRDs. Adenovirus-associated viruses (AAVs) require a helper virus (e.g., adenovirus) for replication. Thus, they intrinsically have minimal pathogenicity. Like adenoviruses, they can transduce mitotic and nonmitotic cells. The major limitation of AAV vectors is the small payload capacity (<4.4 kb) which limits their use to delivery of smaller genes with a short sequence. When used as a vector for gene editing techniques, the main components (e.g., Cas9 endonuclease for CRISPR) must be split into fragments to allow room for the wild-type gene. This splitting reduces the efficiency of delivery and editing of specific genes [114].

There are a variety of AAV serotypes that differ in the sequence of the capsid protein. The most studied and utilized is serotype 2 (AAV2). AAV2 has been hallmark vector studied for IRD treatment, and is the vector utilized by voretigene neparvovec (Luxturna). Hybrid AAV vectors, including mosaic or chimeric capsids, have been developed to optimize cell penetration and intracellular trafficking [106, 115–118]. Unfortunately, more than half the human population has had prior exposure to AAV2 and therefore carry neutralizing antibodies which may limit their usefulness as vectors.

3.3.2.3 Lentivirus

Lentiviruses (LVs) are a subtype of retrovirus. Whereas standard retroviruses can only infect mitotically active cell types, LVs are capable of infecting non-dividing and actively dividing cell types [119]. This ability, combined with a larger payload capacity compared to AAVs, make lentiviruses a viable vector choice in developing gene therapies for IRD. However, LV runs a much higher risk of insertional mutagenesis, and this must be considered carefully when developing gene therapies. Lentiviruses have a transgene cargo capacity of ~8.5 kb and are capable of infecting post-mitotic RPE cells and, to a lesser extent, differentiated photoreceptors [120, 121]. For IRDs, LV vectors have been used most extensively for *ABCA4* mutations (e.g., Stargardt disease gene therapy) since the gene is too large for AAVs [122]. Overall, LV vector for IRD is best suited for RPE targets, as this cell type is transduced sufficiently to show an effect. However, LVs can be used to promote regeneration of damaged photoreceptors via paracrine effects. Transducing the RPE cells to produce growth factors may indirectly promote photoreceptor cell regeneration [123].

3.3.2.4 Non-viral Vectors

In order to overcome the limitations of viral vectors, non-viral/synthetic vectors have been developed. They include nanoparticles of metal, polymer, lipid, liposomes, and naked DNA that are electroporated into cells [106, 124, 125]. These vectors can carry a larger genetic payload than viral vectors. Their lower risk of immune activation also makes repeated dosing possible [126]. Non-viral vectors are less expensive and generally easier to produce compared to viral vectors. Nanoparticle vectors are usually coated with an inert component, such as polyethylene glycol, the chains of which can be modified to target specific ligands or to co-deliver other molecular cargo [5].

Some disadvantages of synthetic vectors include toxicity, biologic incompatibility with certain cell types, and inefficient release of genetic payload. For example, the vitreous has been shown to limit the mobility of cationic liposome vectors [127]. Synthetic vectors continue to be researched and developed, particularly for the large molecular machinery needed for gene editing. The use of synthetic vectors for IRD remains limited, though there are reports of successful delivery of messenger RNA to the retina [128]. The major limitation of non-viral vectors in IRD is the transience of transduction when compared to the viral vectors [129].

3.3.3 Gene Editing

The most common gene editing technology being explored for gene therapy is CRISPR (Clustered Regularly Interspaced Short Palindromic Repeats). This gene editing technology is a repurposing of the adaptive immune system used by bacteria (originally discovered in *E. coli*) to detect and clear bacteriophages [130]. The CRISPR immune system takes foreign, viral RNA when initially encountered and incorporates it into a spacer region within the palindromic repeats. This allows the bacterium to develop immune memory of the bacteriophage's RNA products. When the bacteriophage next attempts to infect the bacterium, the RNA products it releases into the host cell are detected. The bacterium then transcribes CRISPR RNA (crRNA) from the appropriate CRISPR DNA spacer region, which joins with *cas* complex proteins (endonucleases and helicases). The crRNA allows the complex to home in on viral DNA and the *cas* proteins cleave and destroy it. Thus, a bacterium's CRISPR spacer regions contain a unique history of previous viral infections it has incorporated into its immune memory [131].

CRISPR gene editing technology hinges on replacing crRNA with guide RNA (gRNA) developed in the laboratory to target and manipulate genomic sequences (Fig. 3.4). Instead of crRNA for a viral target, gRNA complementary to a specific allele can be anchored to the *cas* protein complex (most commonly Cas9). The complex will travel to that specific allele and create a double-stranded break on either side of the sequence. The DNA strands are then reannealed by non-homologous-end-joining, thus "editing out" or "knocking out" the mutant allele. The Cas9 complex can be modified to do more than just delete a specific sequence of DNA. For example, it can be fused with a deaminase protein to change nucleotides, known as base editing [132]. It can also be modified to both ligate the gene sequence and replace it with a new genetic code through homologous recombination, typically for the functioning, wild-type allele.

The most recent gene editing technique is referred to as prime editing. Instead of causing double-stranded breaks, the Cas9 protein complex "nicks" a single strand of the DNA double helix, thus reducing the rate of unwanted mutagenesis. A new guide, called prime editing guide RNA (pegRNA), contains the RNA template (of a wild-type allele) for an attached reverse transcriptase enzyme to make a new DNA strand to insert at the nicked site [107]. The target site is left with one edited, and one unedited strand that is mismatched. The prime editor then nicks the unedited strand, and the cell uses its own DNA mismatch repair machinery to replace the nicked strand, using the incorporated, edited strand as a template.

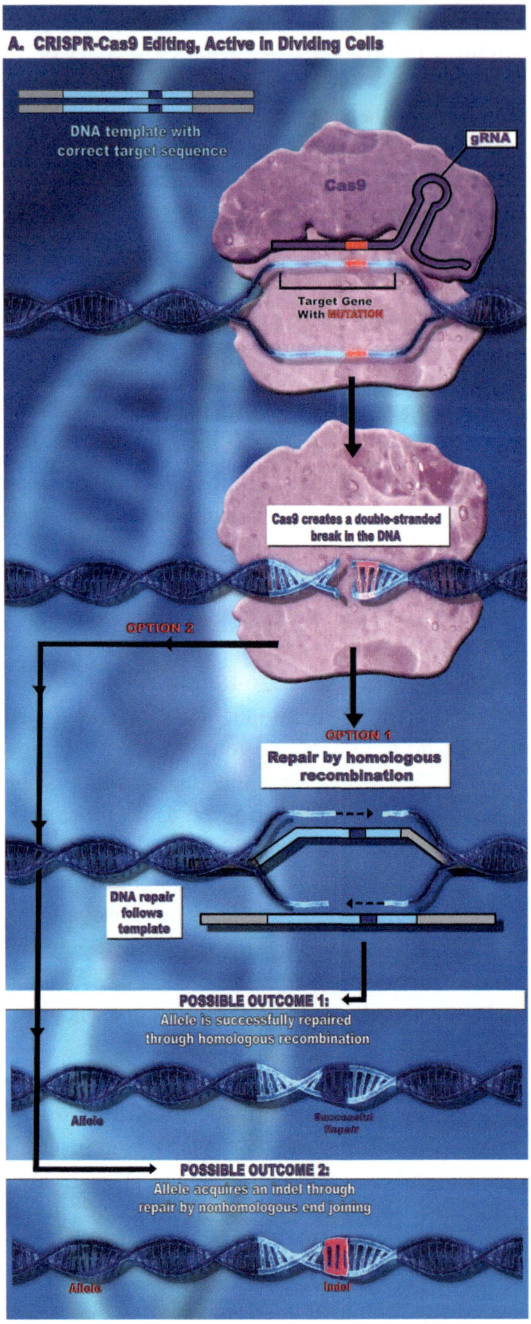

Fig. 3.4 Gene editing with the use of clustered regularly interspaced short palindromic repeats (CRISPR)–Cas9 through DNA-template-based homology-directed repair of a Cas9-induced double-stranded break

The development of these gene editing techniques is considered a pivotal breakthrough and will almost assuredly be the basis for IRD treatment in the future. Indeed, the first CRISPR treatment ever inserted directly into the human body occurred in March 2020, as part of a clinical trial to treat Lebers Congenital Amaurosis (LCA) [133].

3.3.4 Gene Therapy for Inherited Retinal Disease

There are a variety of current and completed clinical trials for gene therapy of the IRD (Table 3.3). This chapter is limited to the IRDs that are caused by single gene mutations that result in progressive worsening of vision with age. Gene therapy for common retinal degenerative conditions, such as AMD and diabetic retinopathy, is being explored given their high frequency in the population [134]. However, gene therapy for these common conditions remains challenging because of genotypic and phenotypic heterogeneity and multiple environmental risk factors that influence the expression of these common diseases. Although there are ongoing clinical trials for neovascular AMD delivering gene therapy for inhibition of vascular endothelial growth factor [134], there are no clinical trials to date using gene therapy to limit or reverse the retinal degeneration associated with AMD or diabetic retinopathy. Nonetheless, success in treating IRD using gene therapy may lead to research exploring gene therapy for more common retinal degenerative conditions.

3.3.5 History of Gene Therapy

The first gene therapy in a human was administered in 1990 to a 4-year-old girl with severe combined immunodeficiency (SCID). She was given an infusion of the wildtype adenosine deaminase (ADA) gene in a retroviral vector [135]. The treatment was not completely curative, but the proof-of-concept was established. With growing enthusiasm regarding gene therapy research, many new gene therapy clinical trials started thereafter.

Unfortunately, the first reported death from a gene therapy clinical trial occurred in 1999 [136].

An 18-year-old man, who suffered from a partial ornithine transcarbamoylase (OTC) deficiency, died after mounting a severe immune reaction to the adenoviral vector used to deliver the wildtype OTC gene. The FDA suspended the trial. Subsequently, gene therapy trials in the United States came under increased scrutiny. In 2000, the FDA and the National Institutes of Health enacted two new programs to improve patient protection: Gene Therapy Clinical Trial Monitoring Plan and the Gene Transfer Safety Symposia [137]. The overall momentum for gene therapy clinical trials was dampened thereafter, but research continued.

The retina became an attractive target for gene therapy due to the relative immune privilege state of the eye. Local ocular delivery of gene therapy may be associated with less risk for systemic immune reaction. The first published gene therapy study for the IRD was in a mouse model of RP in 1996 [138]. An adenoviral vector was delivered via a subretinal injection with the wild-type gene for phosphodiesterase. These researchers extended their work to Briard dogs with an *RPE65* mutation that causes LCA, a severe form of RP [139]. *RPE65* encodes a protein directly responsible for the generation of 11-*cis*-retinal in the phototransduction cycle. Without this functioning protein, Vitamin A cannot be converted to the chemical form required by photoreceptors, and there is a progressive loss of photoreceptors. Canines that received subretinal injection of wildtype *RPE65* in a recombinant adenovirus-associated vector (rAAV) showed improved visual function based on ERG and movement in an obstacle course when compared to control canines. Younger dogs, with less damaged retinas, demonstrated more recovery of visual function compared to older dogs.

These promising results led to the first IRD gene therapy clinical trials in human patients with LCA [140–142]. In these trials, individuals, who had LCA from a biallelic missense mutation of *RPE65*, received one subretinal injection of gene therapy. The gene therapy product consisted of a rAAV with wildtype complementary DNA for RPE65 under the control of a different promoter depending on the clinical trial. In the study using a human RPE65 promoter, the gene therapy was well tolerated but rescue of retinal function was not observed [140]. However, two other clinical trials using a stronger promoter such as the CBA promoter, showed improved visual function [141, 142]. A phase 1 dose-escalation study enrolled 12 participants, 8–44 years of age. No adverse effect or visual acuity improvement was noted, but sustained improvement in visual function based on dark-adapted full-field sensitivity testing (FST) was observed which appeared greater with earlier intervention [141, 143, 144]. Based on these results, a phase 3 study for LCA was started which used a multi-luminance mobility test (MLMT) developed to calibrate the ability of participants to navigate through a maze under dim light [145]. The phase 3 open-labeled study enrolled 31 participants with crossover at 1 year. The study showed improvement in MLMT and FST following gene therapy, especially in younger subjects. The RPE65 rAAV gene therapy product, marketed as voretigene neparvovec (Luxturna), was approved by the FDA in December 2017 for IRD associated with RPE65 mutation. It is the first FDA-approved gene therapy and the only FDA-approved therapy for IRD at the current time. Subsequently, it also was approved for use by the European Commission in November 2018. Follow-up studies have shown that the improvement in MLMT and FST had a sustained effect for up to 4 years [146, 147].

Many new gene therapy clinical trials for IRD have started since the success of RPE65 rAAV gene therapy (Table 3.3). Some of these ocular clinical trials are showing some promising results although they only account for less than 2% of all gene therapy clinical trials [148, 149].

3.3.6 Gene Therapy Clinical Trials

Figure 3.3 summarizes the relative frequency of IRDs and the genes that have been identified as associated with IRDs. Many IRDs are being investigated in clinical trials using gene therapy

Table 3.3 Current and completed gene therapy clinical trials for inherited retinal diseases listed on www.ClinicalTrials.gov

Identifier	Gene therapy	Sponsor	Clinical study phase	Therapy	Administration route	Start date	Recruitment status
Syndromic retinitis pigmentosa (AR)							
NCT03780257	USH2A gene (Usher type 2)	ProQR Therapeutics	I/II	QR-421 (antisense oligonucleotide for Usher syndrome 2A, exon 13)	Intravitreal	Dec. 2018	Recruiting
NCT01505062	MYO7A gene (Usher Type 1B	Sanofi	I/II	Lentiviral MYO7A (SAR421869/UshStat)	Subretinal	Jan. 2012	Terminated (Not stopped for safety reasons)
Non-syndromic retinitis pigmentosa (AR)							
NCT01482195 [6]	MERTK	Fowzan Alkuraya	I	rAAV2-VMD2-hMERTK	Subretinal	Nov. 2011	Recruiting
NCT03328130	PDE6B	Horama S.A.	I/II	AAV2/5-hPDE6B	Subretinal	Nov. 2017	Terminated (Not stopped for safety reasons)
Non-syndromic retinitis pigmentosa (any inheritance pattern)							
NCT03326336	Multiple	GenSight Biologics	I/II	rAAV2.7m8-CAG-ChrimsonR-tdTomato) combined with visual interface stimulating glasses	Intravitreal	Oct. 2018	Recruiting
Retinitis pigmentosa (AD)							
NCT04123626	RHO	ProQR Therapeutics	I/II	QR-1123 (antisense oligonucleotide) for mutant P23H mRNA	Intravitreal	Oct. 2019	Recruiting
Retinitis pigmentosa (X-linked)							
NCT03116113 [7]	RPGR	NightstaRx Ltd.	II/III	AAV8-RPGR	Subretinal	Apr. 2017	Recruiting
NCT03316560	RPGR	Applied Genetic Technologies Corp	I/II	rAAV2tYF-GRK1-RPGR	Subretinal	Oct. 2017	Recruiting
NCT03252847	RPGR	MeiraGTx UK II Ltd	I/II	AA2/5-RPGR	Subretinal	Aug. 2017	Active, not recruiting
Leber congenital amaurosis (AR)							
NCT00999609 [8]	RPE65	Spark Therapeutics	III	AAV2-hRPE65v2 (voretigene neparvovec-rzyl)	Subretinal	Oct. 2009	Active, not recruiting
NCT01496040	RPE65	Nantes University Hospital	I/II	rAAV2/4.hRPE65	Subretinal	Dec. 2011	Completed

NCT00643747	RPE65	University College, London	I/II	rAAV 2/2.hRPE65p.hRPE65	Subretinal	March. 2008	Completed
NCT02781480	RPE65	MeiraGTx UK II Ltd	I/II	AAV2/5-OPTIRPE65	Subretinal	May. 2016	Completed
NCT03872479 [9]	CEP290	Allergan and Editas Medicine, Inc.	I/II	CRISPR with AAV5 vector (AGN-151587, aka EDIT-101) to edit c.2991+1655A>G in intron 26 of the CEP290 gene	Subretinal	March. 2019	Active, not recruiting
Choroideremia (X-linked)							
NCT02341807	CHM	Spark Therapeutics	I/II	AAV2-hCHM	Subretinal	Jan. 2015	Active, not recruiting
NCT01461213 [10]	CHM	University of Oxford	I/II	rAAV2.REP1	Subretinal	Oct. 2011	Completed
NCT02077361	CHM	Ian M. MacDonald	I/II	rAAV2.REP1	Subretinal	Mar. 2014	Completed
NCT02553135	CHM	Byron Lam	I	rAAV2.REP1	Subretinal	Sep. 2015	Completed
NCT02671539	CHM	STZ Eyetrial	II	rAAV2.REP1	Subretinal	Feb. 2016	Active, not recruiting
NCT02407678	CHM	University of Oxford	II	rAAV2.REP1	Subretinal	Apr. 2015	Active, not recruiting
Achromatopsia							
NCT02599922	CNGB3	Applied Genetic Technologies Corp	I/II	rAAV2tYF-PR1.7-hCNGB3	Subretinal	Nov. 2015	Recruiting
NCT02935517	CNGA3	Applied Genetic Technologies Corp	I/II	AGTC-402 (CNGA3)	Subretinal	Oct. 2016	Recruiting
NCT02610582	CNGA3	STZ eyetrial	I/II	rAAV.hCNGA3	Subretinal	Nov. 2015	Active, not recruiting
NCT03758404	CNGA3	MeiraGTx UK II Ltd	I/II	AAV2/8-hG1.7p.coCNGA3	Subretinal	Nov. 2018	Recruiting
NCT03001310	CNGB3	MeiraGTx UK II Ltd	I/II	AAV2/8-hCARp.hCNGB3	Subretinal	Dec. 2016	Completed
Juvenile macular degeneration/Stargardt (AR)							
NCT01367444	ABCA4	Sanofi	I/II	Lentiviral ABCA4 (SAR422459)	Subretinal	June. 2011	Terminated (Not stopped for safety reasons)
Retinoschisis (X-linked)							
NCT02416622	RS1	Applied Genetic Technologies Corp	I/II	rAAV2tYF-CB-hRs1	Intravitreal	Apr. 2015	Active, not recruiting
NCT02317887 [11]	RS1	National Eye Institute	I/II	AAV-RS1, AKA AAV8-scRS/IRBPhRS	Intravitreal	Dec. 2014	Recruiting

(Table 3.3). The published results of these clinical trials are summarized for each IRD.

3.3.7 Retinitis Pigmentosa

Retinitis pigmentosa (RP) is one of the most recognized and frequently encountered IRD. It is characterized by progressive loss of rod photoreceptors leading to night blindness and progressive loss of peripheral vision. Retinitis pigmentosa has tremendous genetic heterogeneity, with over 100 associated genes identified [150]. Generally, RP is classified as non-syndromic (not affecting organs or tissues other than the retina), syndromic (affecting other neurosensory systems, often hearing), or systemic (affecting multiple tissues) [151]. The disease is then further classified based on its Mendelian inheritance pattern.

3.3.7.1 Syndromic Retinitis Pigmentosa

Usher syndrome, also called deafness-blindness syndrome, is one of the more well-characterized syndromic forms of RP. It is an autosomal recessive disorder. There are three different clinical types of Usher syndrome. Usher syndrome type I has the earliest onset and most severe vision and hearing loss. About half of these cases results from mutations in *MYO7A*. Other mutations, such as *USH1C*, *CDH23*, *PCDH15*, *USH1G*, or *CIB2,* also can cause type 1 Usher syndrome [152]. Usher syndrome type II has a later age of onset and is associated with less severe sensorineural impairment. Type II Usher syndrome is caused by one of three gene mutations, *ADGRV1*, *WHRN* (*DFNB31*), or *USH2A* [153]. Usher syndrome type III is the rarest form, occurring predominately in individuals of Ashkenazi Jewish and Finnish heritage. It is associated with *CLRN1* gene mutations and may manifest clinically at a later age than other types of Usher syndrome.

There is one active clinical trial for Usher syndrome type II that targets a specific mutation of *USH2A* in exon 13. It is an intravitreal injection of an antisense oligonucleotide for exon 13 of the *USH2A* gene. This is meant to prevent translation of the mutant exon 13 from the *USH2A* mRNA. This technique is called exon skipping and can be considered a "downstream" approach of gene silencing, since the mRNA antisense oligonucleotide blocks the mRNA from being translated rather than preventing transcription of the gene. Unpublished, interim findings indicate a single intravitreal injection is safe and well tolerated in patients [154].

The other major syndromic RP is Bardet-Biedl. There is no gene therapy clinical trial for this or other syndromic RP at the current time.

3.3.7.2 Non-syndromic Retinitis Pigmentosa

Autosomal Recessive Retinitis Pigmentosa

Two clinical trials are evaluating gene therapy for selected types of non-syndromic, autosomal recessive RP. One trial is targeting mutations of the *MERTK* gene (MER Proto-Oncogene, Tyrosine Kinase). This protein is part of the signaling network that regulates phagocytosis of shed photoreceptors by the RPE [155]. Impaired phagocytosis leads to an accumulation of debris within the RPE that is toxic to photoreceptors. The delivery of normal *MERTK* using an adenovirus vector in rats improved scotopic ERG and restored RPE phagocytosis [156]. Similar results were shown using a rAAV2 vector [157]. These results led to the phase I trial of subretinally administered *rAAV2-VMD2-hMERTK*, which demonstrated safety [6]. Three of six patients showed visual acuity gain which was lost after 2 years in two patients.

The other clinical trial for autosomal recessive RP targets the heterotetrameric phosphodiesterase (PDE) 6 complex, which consists of α, β, and two γ subunits [158]. The PDE6 complex hydrolyzes cGMP after activation of light-sensitive G protein-coupled receptors in both rods and cones. Approximately 8% of all diagnosed autosomal recessive RP is attributed to mutations in the PDE6 gene. Notably, *PDE6B* mutations can also lead to an autosomal dominant congenital stationary night blindness. Loss of full function of PDE6 activity causes rod-cone degeneration, though the exact mechanism remains unsolved [159, 160]. Some researchers suggest that PDE6 inactivity leads to high levels of calcium in rods, which cause apoptosis. The current gene therapy clinical trial uses AAV2/5-hPDE6B administered subretinally with results pending (Table 3.3).

Autosomal Dominant Retinitis Pigmentosa

While 22 different genes have been identified associated with autosomal dominant RP, mutations of rhodopsin (*RHO* gene) is the most common (30–40%) [158]. Rhodopsin is the first component of the visual transduction pathway and is activated by absorption of light. The P23H mutation within *RHO* causes rhodopsin misfolding, endoplasmic reticulum stress, and activates the unfolded protein response, leading to rod photoreceptor degeneration [161]. A clinical trial is investigating the use of an antisense oligonucleotide injected intravitreally to prevent translation of *RHO* mRNA with a P23H mutation. This approach was validated in a transgenic mouse preclinical study [162]. Since there is no modification at the DNA level, this treatment would not be durable or permanent. Patients would require repeated injections of the antisense oligonucleotide. A gene editing approach may lead to a more elegant and permanent treatment for patients with P23H *RHO* mutations.

X-Linked Retinitis Pigmentosa

About 10–15% of RP patients have X-Linked RP (XLRP). It is characterized by a severe phenotype in males and early age of onset [158]. Sometimes, females can manifest a milder phenotype due to genetic lyonization. Six gene loci responsible for XLRP have been mapped (*RP6, RP23, RP24, RP34, RP2*, and *RPGR*). However, almost 75% of cases of XLRP are due to *RPGR* mutations and 15% are due to *RP2* mutations. Retinitis pigmentosa GTPase regulator (*RPGR/RP3*) is expressed in rod photoreceptors and is essential for cell viability while retinitis pigmentosa 2 protein (*RP2*) codes for human cofactor C involved in beta-tubulin folding.

X-linked RP is an attractive target for gene therapy since most cases are caused by mutations in one of two different genes. The difficulty in using gene therapy for XLRP is the severity of disease even at younger age which may make therapy less successful. There are three clinical trials for XLRP (Table 3.3). The results of a phase I/II clinical trial were recently published [7]. Among 18 patients with XLRP from *RPGR* mutations given subretinal AAV8-*coRPGR* at three different doses, no adverse effect was noted except for steroid-responsive subretinal inflammation at higher doses. A dose-dependent response was observed, with higher-dose cohorts demonstrating increased retinal sensitivity and reversal of visual field loss that extended to 6 months of follow-up. These gains were not observed in the untreated, contralateral eye. A particularly interesting observation was the development of a new linear structure on optical coherence tomography retinal imaging in some eyes following gene therapy. The investigators hypothesized that this line may represent regeneration of photoreceptor outer segments. This structural change appeared to correlate with increased functional visual gain.

3.3.7.3 Leber Congenital Amaurosis

Leber congenital amaurosis (LCA) is usually an autosomal recessive disease and can be considered a more severe form of RP that occurs earlier in life. There have been at least 25 genes implicated in the development of LCA. *RPE65* is one of the most frequently mutated genes in LCA and the target of most current clinical trials [163]. As previously mentioned, voretigene neparvovec (Luxturna) was the first gene therapy to obtain FDA and European Commission approval. The results from a 4-year phase 1 follow-up and a 2-year phase 3 follow-up indicate a good safety profile and sustained improvement in visual function [8].

LCA remains ahead of the other IRD in terms of gene therapy development. The first gene editing clinical trial using CRISPR technology has been started for LCA [9]. The phase I/II study involves a subretinal injection to treat an LCA type 10 (LCA10) due to a *CEP290* mutation. *CEP290* localizes to the photoreceptor-connecting cilium and is required for outer segment regeneration and phototransduction [9]. The most common LCA10-causing mutation is IVS26—an adenine to guanine point mutation located within intron 26 (referred to as c.2991+1655A>G) that ultimately results in a premature stop codon. CRISPR technology is being used to edit c.2991+1655A>G in intron 26 of the *CEP290* gene.

3.3.8 Choroideremia

As an X-linked IRD, choroideremia results in nyctalopia and progressive visual field constriction in men. It affects about 1 in 50,000 individuals and is characterized by photoreceptor degeneration and RPE depigmentation [164]. It is caused by mutations in the *CHM* gene that encodes ras-associated blinding (Rab) escort protein 1, REP1 [165]. This mutation results in RPE cell death and photoreceptor degeneration. The first Phase I/II clinical trial with subretinal administration of the gene therapy product using a rAAV2 vector showed that 2 of 6 participants had 21 and 11 ETDRS letters improvement at 3.5 years [10]. More recently, results of additional Phase 2 clinical trials have been published using the same vector construct. No major safety concerns were noted beyond those associated with the surgical procedure [166–169]. The visual acuity outcomes were mixed among these relatively small studies. One study reported improved visual acuity in all 14 treated eyes [167]. Other studies showed some eyes with visual acuity gain and others with some vision loss [168, 169]. A larger phase 3 study is planned to further evaluate the safety and efficacy of this gene therapy.

3.3.9 Achromatopsia

Achromatopsia is a special form of cone dystrophy in which individuals have congenital color blindness, greatly decreased visual acuity, and photophobia in bright light. ERG shows a characteristic absence of measurable cone response. Mutations of the β-subunit of the cone cGMP-gated channel (*CNGB3*) are responsible for 50–70% of complete achromatopsia [170]. Mutations of the alpha-subunit (*CNGA3*) account for about 25% of the disease. Three active clinical trials target *CNGA3*, while two are targeting *CNGB3* with a subretinal injection of AAV vector. Though there are some interesting gene therapy results in mouse models, the preclinical findings are difficult to extrapolate to humans, as mice lack maculae [171]. Results of one gene therapy clinical trial targeting *CNGA3* showed a small benefit to visual function in terms of visual acuity and contrast sensitivity after subretinal administration [172]. The gene therapy was administered to 9 subjects using AAV vector and was well tolerated.

3.3.10 Stargardt Disease

Stargardt disease is commonly recessively inherited, and results in the accumulation of lipofuscin within the RPE. It is the most common juvenile macular dystrophy. Fundus examination reveals classic golden, "pisciform flecks" throughout the fundus, and fluorescein angiography shows a dark choroid, as the lipofuscin within the RPE blocks choroidal fluorescence. A mutation in ATP-binding cassette subfamily A, member 4 (*ABCA4*) is the most common cause of this dystrophy. Studies of LV gene therapy in a mouse model of Stargardt disease showed decreased lipofuscin accumulation [173]. An LV vector was chosen because the *ABCA4* gene (6.8 kb) is too large to be packaged in an AAV vector. There was a single clinical trial that investigated the use of a subretinal injection of LV vector to deliver *ABCA4*. However, in early 2020, the study sponsor terminated the study (not due to safety reasons). Given the large size of *ABCA4* gene, non-viral vectors or gene editing techniques would be reasonable alternative approaches for future study.

3.3.11 X-Linked Retinoschisis

X-linked retinoschisis (XLRS) is characterized by a schisis or splitting of the neurosensory retina. It results in decreased central visual acuity in boys and men. The causative gene is *RS1* which codes for retinoschisin protein. Retinoschisin protein is secreted principally in the outer retina, and its absence results in retinal cavities, reduced visual acuity, and susceptibility to retinal detachment [11]. *RS1* is required for normal function of the synapse between photoreceptor and bipolar cells [174].

A gene therapy product using an AAV vector and delivered intravitreally showed improvements in retinal morphology and electroretinogram (ERG) testing in mouse models [175, 176]. This led to two phase I/II clinical trials, one conducted at the National Eye Institute. The studies use different vector serotypes (AAV2 and AAV8), but both are delivered intravitreally. Interestingly, expression of the delivered gene is achieved in mice with XLRS but not wild-type mice after intravitreal delivery. It is hypothesized that XLRS pathology disrupts the inner limiting membrane barrier, allowing the viral vector to penetrate the retina and transduce target cells [174–176]. The initial clinical findings of the phase I/II trial using AAV8 vector showed well-tolerated treatment except for steroid responsive dose-dependent ocular inflammation [11]. One treated XLRS patient showed closure of the schisis cavities. Systemic antibodies to AAV8 were noted in a dose-related manner but no systemic antibody to *RS1* was detected [11].

3.4 Summary

There is no doubt that stem cell and gene therapy are both promising novel therapies for IRD. Although gene therapy addresses the genetic defect and may provide a more long-term therapeutic effect than stem cell therapy, stem cell therapy can be used to regenerate the damaged retina or RPE regardless of the underlying genetic defect. Thus, both modes of retinal regeneration may play an important role in treating vision loss associated with IRD.

The ongoing story of stem cell and gene therapy underscores the power of human ingenuity and scientific progress in translational research. Like most advancements in science, there will be both successes and setbacks. But those "Eureka!" moments, sprung from bench research have led to promising novel therapies. Whereas individuals with IRDs have lost their vision with no hope for recovery, both stem cell and gene therapies provide new hope and promise for these affected individuals by providing treatments that may restore the degenerating retina and preserve sight.

Acknowledgments The authors thank Paul Sieving, MD PhD for his invaluable input in preparation of the gene therapy section of the chapter. The authors also thank Kyle Nicolos, BA, for preparing some of the figures in this chapter. This work was partially supported by the Barbara A. & Alan M. Roth, MD Endowed Chair of Discovery, Education and Patient Care from University of California Davis (SSP).

References

1. Schwartz SD, Regillo CD, Lam BL, et al. Human embryonic stem cell-derived retinal pigment epithelium in patients with age-related macular degeneration and Stargardt's macular dystrophy: follow-up of two open-label phase 1/2 studies. Lancet (London, England). 2015;385:509–16.
2. Schwartz SD, Tan G, Hosseini H, Nagiel A. Subretinal transplantation of embryonic stem cell-derived retinal pigment epithelium for the treatment of macular degeneration: an assessment at 4 years. Invest Ophthalmol Vis Sci. 2016;57:ORSFc1–9.
3. Mehat MS, Sundaram V, Ripamonti C, et al. Transplantation of human embryonic stem cell-derived retinal pigment epithelial cells in macular degeneration. Ophthalmology. 2018;125:1765–75. Available at: https://doi.org/10.1016/j.ophtha.2018.04.037.
4. Park SS, Bauer G, Abedi M, et al. Intravitreal autologous bone marrow cd34+ cell therapy for ischemic and degenerative retinal disorders: preliminary phase 1 clinical trial findings. Invest Ophthalmol Vis Sci. 2015;56:81–9.
5. Wilbie D, Walther J, Mastrobattista E. Delivery aspects of CRISPR/Cas for in vivo genome editing. Acc Chem Res. 2019;52:1555–64.
6. Ghazi NG, Abboud EB, Nowilaty SR, et al. Treatment of retinitis pigmentosa due to MERTK mutations by ocular subretinal injection of adeno-associated virus gene vector: results of a phase I trial. Hum Genet. 2016;135:327–43.
7. Cehajic-Kapetanovic J, Xue K, Martinez-Fernandez de la Camara C, et al. Initial results from a first-in-human gene therapy trial on X-linked retinitis pigmentosa caused by mutations in RPGR. Nat Med. 2020;26:354–9.

8. Maguire AM, Russell S, Wellman JA, et al. Efficacy, safety, and durability of voretigene neparvovec-rzyl in RPE65 mutation-associated inherited retinal dystrophy. Ophthalmology. 2019;126:1273–85.
9. Maeder ML, Stefanidakis M, Wilson CJ, et al. Development of a gene-editing approach to restore vision loss in Leber congenital amaurosis type 10. Nat Med. 2019;25:229–33.
10. MacLaren RE, Groppe M, Barnard AR, et al. Retinal gene therapy in patients with choroideremia: initial findings from a phase 1/2 clinical trial. Lancet. 2014;383:1129–37.
11. Cukras C, Wiley HE, Jeffrey BG, et al. Retinal AAV8-RS1 gene therapy for X-linked retinoschisis: initial findings from a phase I/IIa trial by intravitreal delivery. Mol Ther J Am Soc Gene Ther. 2018;26:2282–94.
12. Idelson M, Alper R, Obolensky A, et al. Directed differentiation of human embryonic stem cells into functional retinal pigment epithelium cells. Cell Stem Cell. 2009;5:396–408. Available at: http://www.ncbi.nlm.nih.gov/pubmed/19796620. Accessed 5 May 2020.
13. Jin ZB, Gao ML, Deng WL, et al. Stemming retinal regeneration with pluripotent stem cells. Prog Retin Eye Res. 2019;69:38–56. Available at: https://doi.org/10.1016/j.preteyeres.2018.11.003.
14. Diniz B, Thomas P, Thomas B, et al. Subretinal implantation of retinal pigment epithelial cells derived from human embryonic stem cells: improved survival when implanted as a monolayer. Invest Ophthalmol Vis Sci. 2013;54:5087–96.
15. Xiang P, Wu KC, Zhu Y, et al. A novel Bruch's membrane-mimetic electrospun substrate scaffold for human retinal pigment epithelium cells. Biomaterials. 2014;35:9777–88.
16. Warnke PH, Alamein M, Skabo S, et al. Primordium of an artificial Bruch's membrane made of nanofibers for engineering of retinal pigment epithelium cell monolayers. Acta Biomater. 2013;9:9414–22. Available at: http://www.ncbi.nlm.nih.gov/pubmed/23917149 Accessed 5 May 2020.
17. Liu Z, Yu N, Holz FG, et al. Enhancement of retinal pigment epithelial culture characteristics and subretinal space tolerance of scaffolds with 200 nm fiber topography. Biomaterials. 2014;35:2837–50.
18. Kashani AH, Lebkowski JS, Rahhal FM, et al. A bioengineered retinal pigment epithelial monolayer for advanced, dry age-related macular degeneration. Sci Transl Med. 2018;10
19. Da Cruz L, Fynes K, Georgiadis O, et al. Phase 1 clinical study of an embryonic stem cell-derived retinal pigment epithelium patch in age related macular degeneration. Nat Biotechnol. 2018;36:1–10.
20. Mandai M, Watanabe A, Kurimoto Y, et al. Autologous induced stem-cell-derived retinal cells for macular degeneration. N Engl J Med. 2017;376:1038–46.
21. MacLaren RE, Pearson RA, MacNeil A, et al. Retinal repair by transplantation of photoreceptor precursors. Nature. 2006;444:203–7.
22. Pearson RA, Barber AC, Rizzi M, et al. Restoration of vision after transplantation of photoreceptors. Nature. 2012;485:99–103.
23. Lamba DA, Gust J, Reh TA. Transplantation of human embryonic stem cell-derived photoreceptors restores some visual function in Crx-deficient mice. Cell Stem Cell. 2009;4:73–9.
24. Liu Y, Chen SJ, Li SY, et al. Long-term safety of human retinal progenitor cell transplantation in retinitis pigmentosa patients. Stem Cell Res Ther. 2017;8:209.
25. Lamba DA, McUsic A, Hirata RK, et al. Generation, purification and transplantation of photoreceptors derived from human induced pluripotent stem cells. PLoS One. 2010;5:e8763. Available at: http://www.ncbi.nlm.nih.gov/pubmed/20098701. Accessed 5 May 2020.
26. Tucker BA, Park IH, Qi SD, et al. Transplantation of adult mouse iPS cell-derived photoreceptor precursors restores retinal structure and function in degenerative mice. PLoS One. 2011;6
27. Ortin-Martinez A, Tsai ELS, Nickerson PE, et al. A reinterpretation of cell transplantation: GFP transfer from donor to host photoreceptors. Stem Cells. 2017;35:932–9. Available at: http://doi.wiley.com/10.1002/stem.2552. Accessed 5 May 2020
28. Pearson RA, Gonzalez-Cordero A, West EL, et al. Donor and host photoreceptors engage in material transfer following transplantation of post-mitotic photoreceptor precursors. Nat Commun. 2016;7:1–15.
29. Singh MS, Balmer J, Barnard AR, et al. Transplanted photoreceptor precursors transfer proteins to host photoreceptors by a mechanism of cytoplasmic fusion. Nat Commun. 2016;7:1–5.
30. Waldron PV, Di Marco F, Kruczek K, et al. Transplanted donor- or stem cell-derived cone photoreceptors can both integrate and undergo material transfer in an environment-dependent manner. Stem Cell Rep. 2018;10:406–21.
31. Singh MS, Park SS, Albini TA, et al. Retinal stem cell transplantation: balancing safety and potential. Prog Retin Eye Res. 2020;75:100779. Available at: https://doi.org/10.1016/j.preteyeres.2019.100779.
32. Park SS, Moisseiev E, Bauer G, et al. Advances in bone marrow stem cell therapy for retinal dysfunction. Prog Retin Eye Res. 2017;56:148–65. Available at: https://doi.org/10.1016/j.preteyeres.2016.10.002
33. Nakano T, Ando S, Takata N, et al. Self-formation of optic cups and storable stratified neural retina from human ESCs. Cell Stem Cell. 2012;10:771–85.
34. Zhong X, Gutierrez C, Xue T, et al. Generation of three-dimensional retinal tissue with functional photoreceptors from human iPSCs. Nat Commun. 2014;5:4047.
35. Assawachananont J, Mandai M, Okamoto S, et al. Transplantation of embryonic and induced pluripotent stem cell-derived 3D retinal sheets into retinal degenerative mice. Stem Cell Rep. 2014;2:662–74.
36. Shirai H, Mandai M, Matsushita K, et al. Transplantation of human embryonic stem cell-

derived retinal tissue in two primate models of retinal degeneration. Proc Natl Acad Sci U S A. 2016;113:E81–90.
37. Cho MS, Kim SJ, Ku SY, et al. Generation of retinal pigment epithelial cells from human embryonic stem cell-derived spherical neural masses. Stem Cell Res. 2012;9:101–9.
38. Klimanskaya I, Hipp J, Rezai KA, et al. Derivation and comparative assessment of retinal pigment epithelium from human embryonic stem cells using transcriptomics. Cloning Stem Cells. 2004;6:217–45. Available at: http://www.ncbi.nlm.nih.gov/pubmed/15671670. Accessed 6 May 2020.
39. Carr AJ, Vugler A, Lawrence J, et al. Molecular characterization and functional analysis of phagocytosis by human embryonic stem cell-derived RPE cells using a novel human retinal assay. Mol Vis. 2009;15:283–95.
40. Hongisto H, Jylhä A, Nättinen J, et al. Comparative proteomic analysis of human embryonic stem cell-derived and primary human retinal pigment epithelium. Sci Rep. 2017;7
41. Lu B, Malcuit C, Wang S, et al. Long-term safety and function of RPE from human embryonic stem cells in preclinical models of macular degeneration. Stem Cells. 2009;27:2126–35. Available at: http://www.ncbi.nlm.nih.gov/pubmed/19521979. Accessed 5 May 2020.
42. Lund RD, Wang S, Klimanskaya I, et al. Human embryonic stem cell-derived cells rescue visual function in dystrophic RCS rats. Cloning Stem Cells. 2006;8:189–99. Available at: http://www.ncbi.nlm.nih.gov/pubmed/17009895. Accessed 6 May 2020.
43. Mcgill TJ, Bohana-Kashtan O, Stoddard JW, et al. Long-Term efficacy of GMP grade xeno-free hESC-derived rpe cells following transplantation. Sci Tech. 2017;6:17.
44. Lamba DA, Karl MO, Ware CB, Reh TA. Efficient generation of retinal progenitor cells from human embryonic stem cells. Proc Natl Acad Sci U S A. 2006;103:12769–74.
45. Chao JR, Lamba DA, Klesert TR, et al. Transplantation of human embryonic stem cell-derived retinal cells into the subretinal space of a non-human primate. Transl Vis Sci Technol. 2017;6:4.
46. Takahashi K, Yamanaka S. Induction of pluripotent stem cells from mouse embryonic and adult fibroblast cultures by defined factors. Cell. 2006;126:663–76.
47. Buchholz DE, Hikita ST, Rowland TJ, et al. Derivation of functional retinal pigmented epithelium from induced pluripotent stem cells. Stem Cells. 2009;27:2427–34.
48. Maeda T, Lee MJ, Palczewska G, et al. Retinal pigmented epithelial cells obtained from human induced pluripotent stem cells possess functional visual cycle enzymes in vitro and in vivo. J Biol Chem. 2013;288:34484–93.
49. Iwasaki Y, Sugita S, Mandai M, et al. Differentiation/purification protocol for retinal pigment epithelium from mouse induced pluripotent stem cells as a research tool. PLoS One. 2016;11
50. Kamao H, Mandai M, Okamoto S, et al. Characterization of human induced pluripotent stem cell-derived retinal pigment epithelium cell sheets aiming for clinical application. Stem Cell Rep. 2014;2:205–18. Available at: http://www.ncbi.nlm.nih.gov/pubmed/24527394. Accessed 5 May 2020.
51. Kamao H, Mandai M, Ohashi W, et al. Evaluation of the surgical device and procedure for extracellular matrix-scaffold-supported human iPSC-derived retinal pigment epithelium cell sheet transplantation. Invest Ophthalmol Vis Sci. 2017;58:211–20.
52. Yoshihara M, Hayashizaki Y, Murakawa Y. Genomic instability of iPSCs: challenges towards their clinical applications. Stem Cell Rev Rep. 2017;13:7–16.
53. Mandai M, Fujii M, Hashiguchi T, et al. iPSC-derived retina transplants improve vision in rd1 end-stage retinal-degeneration mice. Stem Cell Rep. 2017;8:69–83. Available at: https://doi.org/10.1016/j.stemcr.2016.12.008. Accessed 4 May 2020
54. Jin ZB, Okamoto S, Osakada F, et al. Modeling retinal degeneration using patient-specific induced pluripotent stem cells. PLoS One. 2011;6
55. Sugita S, Iwasaki Y, Makabe K, et al. Lack of T cell response to iPSC-derived retinal pigment epithelial cells from HLA homozygous donors. Stem Cell Rep. 2016;7:619–34.
56. Sugita S, Iwasaki Y, Makabe K, et al. Successful transplantation of retinal pigment epithelial cells from MHC homozygote iPSCs in MHC-matched models. Stem Cell Rep. 2016;7:635–48.
57. Klassen HJ, Ng TF, Kurimoto Y, et al. Multipotent retinal progenitors express developmental markers, differentiate into retinal neurons, and preserve light-mediated behavior. Invest Ophthalmol Vis Sci. 2004;45:4167–73.
58. Radtke ND, Aramant RB, Petry HM, et al. Vision improvement in retinal degeneration patients by implantation of retina together with retinal pigment epithelium. Am J Ophthalmol. 2008;146:172–82.
59. Baranov PY, Tucker BA, Young MJ. Low-oxygen culture conditions extend the multipotent properties of human retinal progenitor cells. Tissue Eng Part A. 2014;20:1465–75.
60. Luo J, Baranov P, Patel S, et al. Human retinal progenitor cell transplantation preserves vision. J Biol Chem. 2014;289:6362–71.
61. Siqueira RC, Messias A, Voltarelli JC, et al. Intravitreal injection of autologous bone marrow-derived mononuclear cells for hereditary retinal dystrophy: a phase 1 trial. Retina. 2011;31:1207–14.
62. Cotrim CC, Toscano L, Messias A, et al. Intravitreal use of bone marrow mononuclear fraction containing CD34(+) stem cells in patients with atrophic age-related macular degeneration. Clin Ophthalmol. 2017;11:931–8.
63. Siqueira RC, Messias A, Messias K, et al. Quality of life in patients with retinitis pigmentosa submit-

ted to intravitreal use of bone marrow-derived stem cells (reticell -clinical trial). Stem Cell Res Ther. 2015;6:1–5.
64. Mackie AR, Losordo DW. CD34-positive stem cells: in the treatment of heart and vascular disease in human beings. Texas Hear Inst J. 2011;38:474–85.
65. Pang WW, Price EA, Sahoo D, et al. Human bone marrow hematopoietic stem cells are increased in frequency and myeloid-biased with age. Proc Natl Acad Sci U S A. 2011;108:20012–7.
66. Asahara T, Murohara T, Sullivan A, et al. Isolation of putative progenitor endothelial cells for angiogenesis. Science. 1997;275:964–7.
67. Yazdanyar A, Zhang P, McBride Z, et al. Intravitreal injection of human CD34+ bone marrow stem cells in a murine model of diabetic retinopathy. Exp Eye Res. 2020;190:107865.
68. Park SS, Caballero S, Bauer G, et al. Long-term effects of intravitreal injection of GMP-grade bone-marrow-derived CD34 + cells in NOD-SCID mice with acute ischemia-reperfusion injury. Invest Ophthalmol Vis Sci. 2012;53:986–94.
69. Otani A, Dorrell MI, Kinder K, et al. Rescue of retinal degeneration by intravitreally injected adult bone marrow-derived lineage-negative hematopoietic stem cells. J Clin Invest. 2004;114:765–74.
70. Moisseiev E, Smit-McBride Z, Oltjen S, et al. Intravitreal administration of human bone marrow CD34+ stem cells in a murine model of retinal degeneration. Invest Ophthalmol Vis Sci. 2016;57:4125–35.
71. Ding DC, Shyu WC, Lin SZ. Mesenchymal stem cells. Cell Transplant. 2011;20:5–14. Available at: http://journals.sagepub.com/doi/full/10.3727/096368910X. Accessed 10 May 2020
72. Caplan AI, Dennis JE. Mesenchymal stem cells as trophic mediators. J Cell Biochem. 2006;98:1076–84.
73. Johnson TV, Bull ND, Hunt DP, et al. Neuroprotective effects of intravitreal mesenchymal stem cell transplantation in experimental glaucoma. Invest Ophthalmol Vis Sci. 2010;51:2051–9.
74. Tzameret A, Sher I, Belkin M, et al. Transplantation of human bone marrow mesenchymal stem cells as a thin subretinal layer ameliorates retinal degeneration in a rat model of retinal dystrophy. Exp Eye Res. 2014;118:135–44.
75. Bara JJ, Richards RG, Alini M, Stoddart MJ. Concise review: bone marrow-derived mesenchymal stem cells change phenotype following in vitro culture: implications for basic research and the clinic. Stem Cells. 2014;32:1713–23.
76. Bernardo ME, Fibbe WE. Mesenchymal stromal cells: sensors and switchers of inflammation. Cell Stem Cell. 2013;13:392–402.
77. Tassoni A, Gutteridge A, Barber AC, et al. Molecular mechanisms mediating retinal reactive gliosis following bone marrow mesenchymal stem cell transplantation. Stem Cells. 2015;33:3006–16.
78. Satarian L, Nourinia R, Safi S, et al. Intravitreal injection of bone marrow mesenchymal stem cells in patients with advanced retinitis pigmentosa: a safety study. J Ophthalmic Vis Res. 2017;12:58–64.
79. Eiraku M, Takata N, Ishibashi H, et al. Self-organizing optic-cup morphogenesis in three-dimensional culture. Nature. 2011;472:51–6.
80. Maekawa Y, Onishi A, Matsushita K, et al. Optimized culture system to induce neurite outgrowth from retinal ganglion cells in three-dimensional retinal aggregates differentiated from mouse and human embryonic stem cells. Curr Eye Res. 2016;41:558–68.
81. Kuwahara A, Ozone C, Nakano T, et al. Generation of a ciliary margin-like stem cell niche from self-organizing human retinal tissue. Nat Commun. 2015;6:1–15.
82. Völkner M, Zschätzsch M, Rostovskaya M, et al. Retinal organoids from pluripotent stem cells efficiently recapitulate retinogenesis. Stem Cell Rep. 2016;6:525–38.
83. Wahlin KJ, Maruotti JA, Sripathi SR, et al. Photoreceptor outer segment-like structures in long-term 3D retinas from human pluripotent stem cells. Sci Rep. 2017;7:1–15.
84. Achberger K, Haderspeck JC, Kleger A, Liebau S. Stem cell-based retina models. Adv Drug Deliv Rev. 2019;140:33–50.
85. Llonch S, Carido M, Ader M. Organoid technology for retinal repair. Dev Biol. 2018;433:132–43. Available at: https://doi.org/10.1016/j.ydbio.2017.09.028.
86. DiStefano T, Chen HY, Panebianco C, et al. Accelerated and improved differentiation of retinal organoids from pluripotent stem cells in rotating-wall vessel bioreactors. Stem Cell Rep. 2018;10:300–13.
87. Achberger K, Probst C, Haderspeck JC, et al. Merging organoid and organ-on-a-chip technology to generate complex multi-layer tissue models in a human retina-on-a-chip platform. Elife. 2019;8:1–26.
88. Megaw R, Abu-Arafeh H, Jungnickel M, et al. Gelsolin dysfunction causes photoreceptor loss in induced pluripotent cell and animal retinitis pigmentosa models. Nat Commun. 2017;8:1–9. Available at: https://doi.org/10.1038/s41467-017-00111-8
89. Deng WL, Gao ML, Lei XL, et al. Gene correction reverses ciliopathy and photoreceptor loss in iPSC-derived retinal organoids from retinitis pigmentosa patients. Stem Cell Rep. 2018;10:1267–81.
90. Parfitt DA, Lane A, Ramsden CM, et al. Identification and correction of mechanisms underlying inherited blindness in human iPSC-derived optic cups. Cell Stem Cell. 2016;18:769–81.
91. Reichman S, Slembrouck A, Gagliardi G, et al. Generation of storable retinal organoids and retinal pigmented epithelium from adherent human iPS cells in xeno-free and feeder-free conditions. Stem Cells. 2017;35:1176–88. Available at: http://

doi.wiley.com/10.1002/stem.2586. Accessed 9 May 2020
92. Kuroda T, Yasuda S, Kusakawa S, et al. Highly sensitive in vitro methods for detection of residual undifferentiated cells in retinal pigment epithelial cells derived from human iPS cells. PLoS One. 2012;7:e37342. Available at: https://dx.plos.org/10.1371/journal.pone.0037342. Accessed 9 May 2020
93. Kanemura H, Go MJ, Shikamura M, et al. Tumorigenicity studies of induced pluripotent stem cell (iPSC)-derived retinal pigment epithelium (RPE) for the treatment of age-related macular degeneration. PLoS One. 2014;9:e85336. Available at: https://dx.plos.org/10.1371/journal.pone.0085336. Accessed 9 May 2020
94. Drukker M, Katz G, Urbach A, et al. Characterization of the expression of MHC proteins in human embryonic stem cells. Proc Natl Acad Sci U S A. 2002;99:9864–9.
95. Boyd AS, Rodrigues NP, Lui KO, et al. Concise review: immune recognition of induced pluripotent stem cells. Stem Cells. 2012;30:797–803.
96. Kruse V, Hamann C, Monecke S, et al. Human induced pluripotent stem cells are targets for allogeneic and autologous natural killer (NK) cells and killing is partly mediated by the activating NK receptor DNAM-1. PLoS One. 2015;10
97. Taylor CJ, Bolton EM, Pocock S, et al. Banking on human embryonic stem cells: estimating the number of donor cell lines needed for HLA matching. Lancet. 2005;366:2019–25.
98. Nakajima F, Tokunaga K, Nakatsuji N. Human leukocyte antigen matching estimations in a hypothetical bank of human embryonic stem cell lines in the Japanese population for use in cell transplantation therapy. Stem Cells. 2007;25:983–5.
99. Kuriyan AE, Albini TA, Townsend JH, et al. Vision loss after intravitreal injection of autologous "stem cells" for AMD. N Engl J Med. 2017;376:1047–53.
100. Rong AJ, Lam BL, Ansari ZA, Albini TA. Vision loss secondary to autologous adipose stem cell injections: a rising problem. JAMA Ophthalmol. 2018;136:97–9.
101. Saraf SS, Cunningham MA, Kuriyan AE, et al. Bilateral retinal detachments after intravitreal injection of adipose-derived "stem cells" in a patient with exudative macular degeneration. Ophthalmic Surg Lasers Imaging Retina. 2017;48:772–5.
102. Leung EH, Flynn HWJ, Albini TA, Medina CA. Retinal detachment after subretinal stem cell transplantation. Ophthalmic Surg Lasers Imaging Retina. 2016;47:600–1.
103. Rao RC, Dedania VS, Johnson MW. Stem cells for retinal disease: a perspective on the promise and perils. Am J Ophthalmol. 2017;179:32–8. Available at: https://doi.org/10.1016/j.ajo.2017.04.007
104. RetNet—Retinal Information Network [Internet] [cited 5 Apr 2020]. Available from: https://sph.uth.edu/retnet/
105. Yiu G, Chung SH, Mollhoff IN, et al. Suprachoroidal and subretinal injections of AAV using transscleral microneedles for retinal gene delivery in nonhuman primates. Mol Ther Methods Clin Dev. 2020;16:179–91.
106. Ziccardi L, Cordeddu V, Gaddini L, et al. Gene therapy in retinal dystrophies. Int J Mol Sci. 2019;20:5722.
107. Anzalone AV, Randolph PB, Davis JR, et al. Search-and-replace genome editing without double-strand breaks or donor DNA. Nature. 2019;576:149–57.
108. Nuñez JK, Chen J, Pommier GC, et al. Genome-wide programmable transcriptional memory by CRISPR-based epigenome editing. Cell. 2021;184(9):2503–2519.e17. https://doi.org/10.1016/j.cell.2021.03.025.
109. Xu CL, Ruan MZC, Mahajan VB, Tsang SH. Viral delivery systems for CRISPR. Viruses. 2019;11:28. https://doi.org/10.3390/v11010028.
110. Jiang L, Zhang H, Dizhoor AM, et al. Long-term RNA interference gene therapy in a dominant retinitis pigmentosa mouse model. Proc Natl Acad Sci USA. 2011;108:18476–81.
111. Lundstrom K. Viral vectors in gene therapy. Diseases. 2018;6:42.
112. Li T, Adamian M, Roof DJ, et al. In vivo transfer of a reporter gene to the retina mediated by an adenoviral vector. Invest Ophthalmol Vis Sci. 1994;35:2543–9.
113. Wen S, Graf S, Massey PG, Dichek DA. Improved vascular gene transfer with a helper-dependent adenoviral vector. Circulation. 2004;110:1484–91.
114. Zetsche B, Volz SE, Zhang F. A split-Cas9 architecture for inducible genome editing and transcription modulation. Nat Biotechnol. 2015;33:139–42.
115. Bowles DE, Rabinowitz JE, Samulski RJ. Marker rescue of adeno-associated virus (AAV) capsid mutants: a novel approach for chimeric AAV production. J Virol. 2003;77:423–32.
116. Gigout L, Rebollo P, Clement N, et al. Altering AAV tropism with mosaic viral capsids. Mol Ther. 2005;11:856–65.
117. Hauck B, Chen L, Xiao W. Generation and characterization of chimeric recombinant AAV vectors. Mol Ther. 2003;7:419–25.
118. Muzyczka N, Warrington KH Jr. Custom adeno-associated virus capsids: the next generation of recombinant vectors with novel tropism. Hum Gene Ther. 2005;16:408–16.
119. Addgene: techniques featured in Addgene's newsletter [Internet] [cited 25 Apr 2020]. Available from: https://www.addgene.org/newsletter/techniques/
120. Cashman SM, Sadowski SL, Morris DJ, Frederick J, Kumar-Singh R. Intercellular trafficking of adenovirus-delivered HSV VP22 from the retinal pigment epithelium to the photoreceptors—implications

for gene therapy. Mol Ther J Am Soc Gene Ther. 2002;6:813–23.
121. Saenz DT, Loewen N, Peretz M, et al. Unintegrated lentivirus DNA persistence and accessibility to expression in nondividing cells: analysis with class I integrase mutants. J Virol. 2004;78:2906–20.
122. Han Z, Conley SM, Naash MI. Gene therapy for Stargardt disease associated with ABCA4 gene. In: Ash JD, Grimm C, Hollyfield JG, Anderson RE, LaVail MM, Bowes Rickman C, editors. Retinal degenerative diseases (Advances in experimental medicine and biology, vol. 801) [Internet]. New York: Springer; 2014 [cited 25 Apr 2020]. p. 719–24. Available from: http://link.springer.com/10.1007/978-1-4614-3209-8_90
123. van Adel BA, Kostic C, Déglon N, Ball AK, Arsenijevic Y. Delivery of ciliary neurotrophic factor via lentiviral-mediated transfer protects axotomized retinal ganglion cells for an extended period of time. Hum Gene Ther. 2003;14:103–15.
124. Nishi T, Yoshizato K, Yamashiro S, et al. High-efficiency in vivo gene transfer using intraarterial plasmid DNA injection following in vivo electroporation. Cancer Res. 1996;56:1050–5.
125. Dezawa M, Takano M, Negishi H, Mo X, Oshitari T, Sawada H. Gene transfer into retinal ganglion cells by in vivo electroporation: a new approach. Micron Oxf Engl. 2002;33:1–6.
126. Finn JD, Smith AR, Patel MC, et al. A single administration of CRISPR/Cas9 lipid nanoparticles achieves robust and persistent in vivo genome editing. Cell Rep. 2018;22:2227–35.
127. Peeters L, Sanders NN, Braeckmans K, et al. Vitreous: a barrier to nonviral ocular gene therapy. Invest Ophthalmol Vis Sci. 2005;46:3553–61.
128. Patel S, Ryals RC, Weller KK, Pennesi ME, Sahay G. Lipid nanoparticles for delivery of messenger RNA to the back of the eye. J Control Release. 2019;303:91–100.
129. Conley SM, Cai X, Naash MI. Nonviral ocular gene therapy: assessment and future directions. Curr Opin Mol Ther. 2008;10:456–63.
130. Rath D, Amlinger L, Rath A, Lundgren M. The CRISPR-Cas immune system: biology, mechanisms and applications. Biochimie. 2015;117:119–28.
131. Jinek M, Chylinski K, Fonfara I, Hauer M, Doudna JA, Charpentier E. A programmable dual-RNA-guided DNA endonuclease in adaptive bacterial immunity. Science. 2012;337:816–21.
132. Rees HA, Liu DR. Base editing: precision chemistry on the genome and transcriptome of living cells. Nat Rev Genet. 2018;19:770–88.
133. Ledford H. CRISPR treatment inserted directly into the body for first time. Nature. 2020;579:185.
134. Constable IJ, Lai C-M, Magno AL, et al. Gene therapy in neovascular age-related macular degeneration: three-year follow-up of a phase 1 randomized dose escalation trial. Am J Ophthalmol. 2017;177:150–8.
135. Blaese RM, Culver KW, Miller AD, et al. T Lymphocyte-directed gene therapy for ADA SCID: initial trial results after 4 years. Science. 1995;270:475–80.
136. Wilson JM. Lessons learned from the gene therapy trial for ornithine transcarbamylase deficiency. Mol Genet Metab. 2009;96:151–7.
137. Sibbald B. Death but one unintended consequence of gene-therapy trial. Can Med Assoc J. 2001;164:1612.
138. Bennett J, Tanabe T, Sun D, et al. Photoreceptor cell rescue in retinal degeneration (rd) mice by in vivo gene therapy. Nat Med. 1996;2:649–54.
139. Acland GM, Aguirre GD, Ray J, et al. Gene therapy restores vision in a canine model of childhood blindness. Nat Genet. 2001;28:92–5.
140. Bainbridge JWB, Smith AJ, Barker SS, et al. Effect of gene therapy on visual function in Leber's congenital amaurosis. N Engl J Med. 2008;358:2231–9.
141. Hauswirth WW, Aleman TS, Kaushal S, et al. Treatment of Leber congenital amaurosis due to *RPE65* mutations by ocular subretinal injection of adeno-associated virus gene vector: short-term results of a phase I trial. Hum Gene Ther. 2008;19:979–90.
142. Maguire AM, Simonelli F, Pierce EA, et al. Safety and efficacy of gene transfer for Leber's congenital amaurosis. N Engl J Med. 2008;358:2240–8.
143. Maguire AM, High KA, Auricchio A, et al. Age-dependent effects of RPE65 gene therapy for Leber's congenital amaurosis: a phase 1 dose-escalation trial. Lancet. 2009;374:1597–605.
144. Cideciyan AV, Aleman TS, Boye SL, et al. Human gene therapy for RPE65 isomerase deficiency activates the retinoid cycle of vision but with slow rod kinetics. Proc Natl Acad Sci USA. 2008;105:15112–7.
145. Russell S, Bennett J, Wellman JA, et al. Efficacy and safety of voretigene neparvovec (AAV2-hRPE65v2) in patients with RPE65 -mediated inherited retinal dystrophy: a randomised, controlled, open-label, phase 3 trial. Lancet. 2017;390:849–60.
146. Testa F, Maguire AM, et al. Three-year follow-up after unilateral subretinal delivery of adeno-associated virus in patients with Leber congenital amaurosis type 2. Ophthalmology. 2013;120:1283–91.
147. Bainbridge JWB, Mehat MS, Sundaram V, et al. Long-term effect of gene therapy on Leber's congenital amaurosis. N Engl J Med. 2015;372:1887–97.
148. Ginn SL, Alexander IE, Edelstein ML, Abedi MR, Wixon J. Gene therapy clinical trials worldwide to 2012—an update: gene therapy clinical trials worldwide to 2012—an update. J Gene Med. 2013;15:65–77.
149. Samiy N. Gene therapy for retinal diseases. J Ophthalmic Vis Res. 2014;9:506–9.
150. Galan A, Chizzolini M, Milan E, Sebastiani A, Costagliola C, Parmeggiani F. Good epidemiologic practice in retinitis pigmentosa: from phenotyping to biobanking. Curr Genomics. 2011;12:260–6.
151. Fahim AT, Daiger SP, Weleber RG. nonsyndromic retinitis pigmentosa overview. In: Adam MP, Ardinger HH, Pagon RA, Wallace SE, Bean LJ,

Stephens K, et al., editors. GeneReviews® [Internet]. Seattle, WA: University of Washington; 1993 [cited 26 Apr 2020]. Available from: http://www.ncbi.nlm.nih.gov/books/NBK1417/
152. Lentz J, Keats BJ. Usher syndrome type I. In: Adam MP, Ardinger HH, Pagon RA, Wallace SE, Bean LJ, Stephens K, et al., editors. GeneReviews® [Internet]. Seattle, WA: University of Washington; 1993 [cited 26 Apr 2020]. Available from: http://www.ncbi.nlm.nih.gov/books/NBK1265/
153. Lentz J, Keats B. Usher syndrome type II. In: Adam MP, Ardinger HH, Pagon RA, Wallace SE, Bean LJ, Stephens K, et al., editors. GeneReviews® [Internet]. Seattle, WA: University of Washington; 1993 [cited 26 Apr 2020]. Available from: http://www.ncbi.nlm.nih.gov/books/NBK1341/
154. Read about QR-421a for Usher syndrome type 2 [Internet]. ProQR Therapeutics [cited 28 Apr 2020]. Available from: https://www.proqr.com/qr-421a-for-usher-syndrome-type-2/
155. Feng W, Yasumura D, Matthes MT, LaVail MM, Vollrath D. Mertk triggers uptake of photoreceptor outer segments during phagocytosis by cultured retinal pigment epithelial cells. J Biol Chem. 2002;277:17016–22.
156. Vollrath D, Feng W, Duncan JL, et al. Correction of the retinal dystrophy phenotype of the RCS rat by viral gene transfer of Mertk. Proc Natl Acad Sci USA. 2001;98:12584–9.
157. Conlon TJ, Deng W-T, Erger K, et al. Preclinical potency and safety studies of an AAV2-mediated gene therapy vector for the treatment of *MERTK* associated retinitis pigmentosa. Hum Gene Ther Clin Dev. 2013;24:23–8.
158. Ferrari S, Di Iorio E, Barbaro V, Ponzin D, Sorrentino FS, Parmeggiani F. Retinitis pigmentosa: genes and disease mechanisms. Curr Genomics. 2011;12:238–49.
159. Tsang SH, Tsui I, Chou CL, et al. A novel mutation and phenotypes in phosphodiesterase 6 deficiency. Am J Ophthalmol. 2008;146:780–8.
160. Dvir L, Srour G, Abu-Ras R, Miller B, Shalev SA, Ben-Yosef T. Autosomal-recessive early-onset retinitis pigmentosa caused by a mutation in PDE6G, the gene encoding the gamma subunit of rod cGMP phosphodiesterase. Am J Hum Genet. 2010;87:258–64.
161. Gorbatyuk MS, Knox T, LaVail MM, et al. Restoration of visual function in P23H rhodopsin transgenic rats by gene delivery of BiP/Grp78. Proc Natl Acad Sci USA. 2010;107:5961–6.
162. Chadderton N, Millington-Ward S, Palfi A, et al. Improved retinal function in a mouse model of dominant retinitis pigmentosa following AAV-delivered gene therapy. Mol Ther. 2009;17:593–9.
163. Kumaran N, Moore AT, Weleber RG, Michaelides M. Leber congenital amaurosis/early-onset severe retinal dystrophy: clinical features, molecular genetics and therapeutic interventions. Br J Ophthalmol. 2017;101:1147–54.
164. Coussa RG, Traboulsi EI. Choroideremia: a review of general findings and pathogenesis. Ophthalmic Genet. 2012;33:57–65.
165. Seabrea MC, Brown MS, Goldstein JL. Retinal degeneration in choroideremia: deficiency of rab geranylgeranyl transferase. Science. 1993;259:377–81.
166. Fischer MD, Ochakovski GA, Beier B, et al. Efficacy and safety of retinal gene therapy using adeno-associated virus vector for patients with choroideremia: a randomized clinical trial. JAMA Ophthalmol. 2019;137:1247–54.
167. Xue K, Jolly JK, Barnard AR, et al. Beneficial effects in vision in patients undergoing retinal gene therapy for choroideremia. Nat Med. 2018;24:1507–12.
168. Dimopoulos IS, Hoang SC, Radziwon A, et al. Two-year results after AAV2-mediated gene therapy for choroideremia: the Alberta experience. Am J Ophthalmol. 2018;193:130–42.
169. Lam BL, Davis JL, Gregori NZ, et al. Chroideremia gene therapy phase 2 clinical trial: 24-month results. Am J Ophthalmol. 2019;197:65–73.
170. Wissinger B, Gamer D, Jägle H, et al. CNGA3 mutations in hereditary cone photoreceptor disorders. Am J Hum Genet. 2001;69:722–37.
171. Mühlfriedel R, Tanimoto N, Schön C, et al. AAV-mediated gene supplementation therapy in achromatopsia type 2: preclinical data on therapeutic time window and long-term effects. Front Neurosci. 2017;11:292.
172. Fischer MD, Michalakis S, Wilhelm B, et al. Safety and vision outcome of subretinal gene therapy targeting cone photoreceptors in achromatopsia: a nonrandomized controlled trial. JAMA Ophthalmol. 2020;e201032.
173. Kong J, Kim S-R, Binley K, et al. Correction of the disease phenotype in the mouse model of Stargardt disease by lentiviral gene therapy. Gene Ther. 2008;15:1311–20.
174. Ou J, Vivaysasarathy C, Ziccardi L, et al. Synaptic pathology and therapeutic repair in adult retinoschisis mouse by AAV-*RS1* transfer. J Clin Invest. 2015;125:2891–903.
175. Min SH, Molday LL, Seeliger MW, et al. Prolonged recovery of retinal structure/function after gene therapy in an Rs1h-deficient mouse model of x-linked juvenile retinoschisis. Mol Ther J Am Soc Gene Ther. 2005;12:644–51.
176. Bush RA, Zeng Y, Colosi P, et al. Preclinical dose-escalation study of intravitreal AAV-RS1 gene therapy in a mouse model of X-linked retinoschisis: dose-dependent expression and improved retinal structure and function. Hum Gene Ther. 2016;27:376–89.

4 Retinitis Pigmentosa

Hyeong-Gon Yu

4.1 Introduction

Retinitis pigmentosa (RP) is a serious disease characterized by progressive degeneration of retina and usually ends up with bilateral blindness. RP is the most common inherited retinal disease. Recent advance in genetic research has greatly improved our knowledge about RP. Since the first identification of causal gene Rhodopsin, more than 60 causal genes and 3000 disease causing mutations have been reported until now [1]. And imaging technology such as a high-resolution spectral domain optical coherence tomography (OCT) revealed new aspects of RP [2]. In RP patients, the vision-specific quality of life cannot be explained only by visual acuity or field, and both are related to the visual function [3].

The prevalence of typical nonsyndromic RP is approximately 1:3000–1:5000 worldwide. The prevalence was 1:5200 in Maine, United States, and birth incidence was calculated to be 1:3500 [4]. A relatively lower prevalence of 1:7000 was reported in Switzerland [5]. The registration for RP revealed the prevalence of 1:3943 in Denmark [6]. The prevalence in southern China was 1:4000 [7]. Excluding epidemiologic study obtained from a small-sized cohort, the prevalence of RP looks similar among the ethnicities.

The purpose of this chapter is to review the knowledges that have piled until now about retinitis pigmentosa. The relative rarity and slow progression of disease make it difficult to reveal the nature of disease. However, advances in imaging technologies, cutting-edge genetic analysis, and gene modifying techniques enable to progress. Herein, we tried to comprehend the knowledges about nonsyndromic retinitis pigmentosa.

4.2 Clinical Findings

4.2.1 Fundus Finding

Retinitis pigmentosa (RP) is the most common inherited retinal disorder. It is characterized by rod dysfunction followed by involvement of cone function. Eventually both rod and cone functions become severely impaired. Clinical symptoms include night blindness, progressive visual field constriction, and gradual visual loss. Retina appearance shows pale waxy optic disk, attenuation of arteriole, depigmentation, and retinal degeneration. Degeneration, mottling, and granularity of the retinal pigment epithelium (RPE) and bony spicule shaped intraretinal pigmentation

H.-G Yu (✉)
Department of Ophthalmology, Seoul National University College of Medicine, Seoul, Korea

Retinal Degeneration Research Laboratory, Seoul National University Hospital Biomedical Research Institute, Seoul, Korea

Interdisciplinary Programs: Stem Cell Biology, Seoul National University College of Medicine, Seoul, Korea
e-mail: hgonyu@snu.ac.kr

H.-G. Yu (ed.), *Inherited Retinal Disease*, https://doi.org/10.1007/978-981-16-7337-5_4

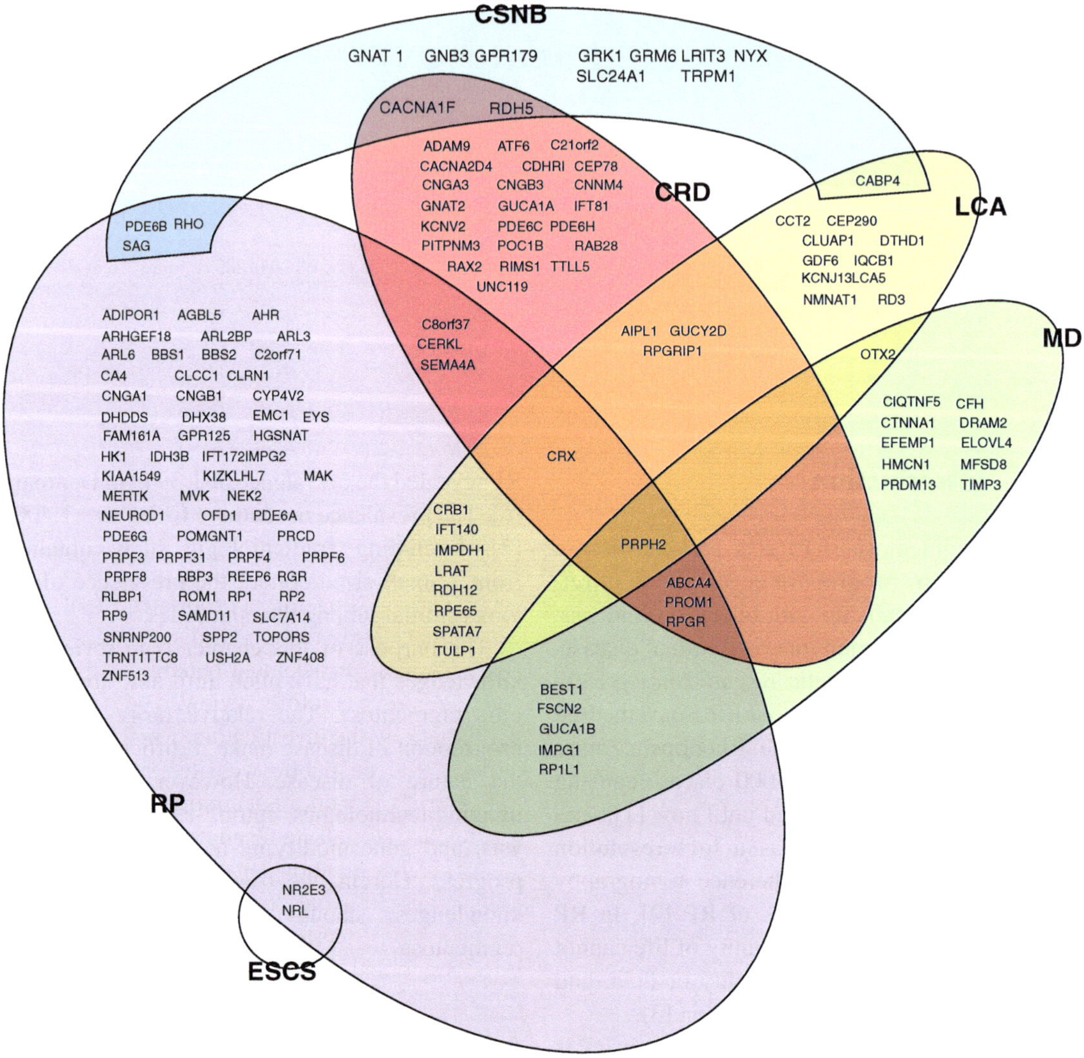

Fig. 4.1 Venn diagram presenting causal genes of multiple inherited retinal disorders. CRD, cone-rod dystrophy; CSNB, congenital stationary night blindness; ESCS, enhanced S-cone syndrome; LCA, Leber congenital amaurosis; MD, macular dystrophy; RP, retinitis pigmentosa

appear initially and distinctly from mid-peripheral area. Although bony spicule seems to typical finding, not all patients develop bony pigmentation. Some develop dust-like pigmentation or nummular hyperpigmentation. Bone spicules consist of RPE derived cells that detach from Bruch membrane [8]. And degree of pigmentations does not reflect disease severity. Macular abnormality usually occurs at an advanced stage and is more frequently observed in autosomal-recessive RP. Macular appearance variably expressed as to causal gene, type of genetic alteration, different individual of the family having same mutation, or even in different eye of patient. RP occurs mostly alone in eye but appears as syndromic form in 20–30% of cases. Retinitis pigmentosa is a highly variable disorder; some patients develop symptomatic visual loss in childhood whereas others remain asymptomatic until mid-adulthood. RP is one of IRDs, in which clinical symptoms and causal genes overlap (Fig. 4.1).

4.2.2 Prevalence

Typical nonsyndromic RP prevalence is approximately 1:3000–1:5000 worldwide. The prevalence was 1:5200 in Maine, United States, and birth incidence was calculated to be 1:3500 [9]. Relatively lower prevalence of 1:7000 was reported in Switzerland [5]. The registration for RP revealed the prevalence of 1:3943 in Denmark [6]. The prevalence in southern China was 1:4000 [7].

4.2.3 Inheritance

RP is inherited as an autosomal-dominant (AD, about 30–40% of cases), autosomal-recessive (AR, 50–60%), or X-linked (XR, 5–15%) trait if sporadic cases are assumed to be AR [10]. The proportions of AD, AR, X-linked recessive, and simplex cases were reported to be 11%, 33.1%, 7.7%, and 48.3%, respectively, in China [11]. In a study of Japanese RP patients, AD, AR, X-linked recessive, and simplex cases were 16.9%, 25.2%, 1.6%, and 56.3%, respectively [12]. Cohort study including 302 Korean RP patients, the most common inheritance pattern was sporadic (182 patients, 60.3%), followed by ARRP (55 patients, 18.2%), ADRP (38 patients, 12.6%), and an unknown pattern (27 patients, 8.9%) [13].

4.3 Clinical Testing

4.3.1 Electroretinogram

Standard electroretinogram (ERG) is essential for differential diagnoses of inherited retinal disorder and helpful for monitoring of disease progression. Abnormality of ERG can be detected before nyctalopia or fundus abnormality develops. In RP patients, mixed rod and cone ERG shows subnormal a wave and isolated rod response is reduced severely or barely detected in scoptopic condition. Cone response can be also impaired in early stage but usually occur after rod dysfunction. In photopic condition, bright flash response decreased and the amplitude of 30 Hz flicker reduced and delayed [14]. Oscillatory potentials may also be reduced in RP patients [15]. Rate of decline in full field ERG ranges from 9 to 11% annually [16]. Central cone function decrease is estimated to be 4–7% per year, which is slower than total ERG activity decay [17, 18]. In advanced phase, ERG response may become undetectable. Multifocal ERG can elicit response and be helpful in this circumstance [19]. Moreover, multifocal ERG amplitude later can be delayed even in patients having normal looking retina that it has potential to predict visual field decline.

4.3.2 Visual Field

Progressive visual field constriction is typical finding in RP. Therefore, visual field test has been widely used to be index of disease progression. Visual field loss is usually symmetric, initially starts from scotoma of mid periphery to gradually form ring shape scotoma. And ring shape scotoma expands inside and outside. Sometimes concentric visual field loss without annular scotoma or arcuate pattern may develop [20]. Kinetic visual field test is widely used. Annual peripheral visual field loss is reported to be 2–12% [21, 22]. For central visual field examination, static automatic perimetry is used. Microperimetry measures retinal sensitivity while matching to specific macular location accurately that it is adequate for evaluating macular function with retinal degeneration.

4.3.3 Optical Coherence Tomography

Optical coherence tomography is a well-established method to examine retina structural. This non-invasive imaging technique provides detailed morphologic abnormality in situ. Spectral domain OCT increased our understanding of the structural change in retinal disease. Thus, OCT enables to infer insight into the pathology and predict the prognosis of RP patients. Here we try to summarize knowledges about morphologic changes and related retinal function as well.

4.3.3.1 Outer Retina

The earliest histopathologic change in the rods is shortening of their outer segments (OS) [23]. This is also reflected as spectral domain optical coherence tomography (OCT) finding. Photoreceptors reside between outer plexiform layer and retinal pigment epithelium (RPE). Total retinal thickness as well as OS thickness of photoreceptor decreased even when inner retina thickness is not affected and central vision is preserved [24]. OS of photoreceptor is located between inner segment ellipsoid (ISE) band to retinal pigment epithelium in OCT. Therefore, integrity of three hyperreflective bands in this region reflects photoreceptor change in RP. Central structure is preserved longer than peripheral structure that length of these bands is constricting as RP progresses. Preserved length of band was the longest in the ELM, followed by the ISE and IZ line. This finding suggests that retinal layer may become disorganized first at the IZ, followed by the ISE and finally the ELM [25]. Retinal layer thickness was also observed at transition zone between healthy and diseased retina. The structural changes followed an orderly progression from a thinning of the OS layer, to a thinning of the outer nuclear layer (ONL) plus outer plexiform layer (OPL), to a loss of the OS, to an ONL plus OPL reduced to an asymptotically small level [26].

Photoreceptor layer, especially outer segment structure, is impaired earlier. Because photoreceptor is the first cell which captures and reacts to photon, loss of photoreceptor or its function can directly impair visual function. Decrease of photoreceptor outer segment thickness correlated with central vision decline [27]. Remaining thickness of photoreceptor is also correlated with multifocal electroretinogram amplitude and visual field sensitivity [28]. The thicknesses of the OS and ONL were significantly and positively correlated with the retinal sensitivities measured by Humphrey visual field 10-2 analysis [29]. Structures related to outer segment, ISE and EZ bands, are more closely related to vision. Integrity of ISE and EZ directly affects visual function [30]. And preserved ISE extent is correlated with visual field area [2, 31]. Overall progression of visual function in RP has been reported. Visual field loss has been reported to be about 5% annually [20, 32]. Amplitude of electroretinogram decreased 16–19% annually [33]. As psychophysical test is well correlated to outer retinal structure integrity, macular structure of SD-OCT may reflect the progression of this functional study in RP [30]. Preserved ISE length decreases 7–9% annually in X-linked inheritance RP, which is known having fastest progression. And that was 3–4% in autosomal-dominant RP [34, 35]. ISE length of 7% (248 μm) is calculated as 13% of area, which corresponds to visual field area constriction. Besides good correlation with functional study, obtaining OCT image requires less acquisition time and accompanies less discomfort than visual field and electroretinogram test. ISE length can be an optimal surrogate biomarker of RP progression.

4.3.3.2 Inner Retina

The majority of studies showed that inner retina is relatively stable while outer retinal change is distinct in RP. Postmortem morphometric studies have revealed that retinal ganglion cells are relatively preserved compared to outer nuclear cells in eyes with RP. Although number of ganglion cells was reduced, that was less profound than outer nuclear cell loss [36–38]. Studies in animal models of RP also support inner retinal preservation. Findings from an RP mouse model showed that retinal ganglion cells were resistant to degeneration, and that they retained their fine structures well after photoreceptor death [39]. Inner nuclear layer (INL) and inner plexiform layer (IPL) were thickened in a mouse model of Leber's congenital amaurosis (LCA) [40].

Relative preservation or thickening of inner retina is also observed in vivo OCT study [26, 41, 42]. Several human studies suggested inner retinal thickening in RP patients. Thickening of the inner retinal layers, including the RNFL and the GCIPL, was detected on OCT images obtained from LCA patients [40]. Based on the findings of IPL thickening and Müller glial cell hypertrophy in a mouse model having the same mutation as human LCA patients, the authors suggested that Müller glial cell activation in neuronal injury may be responsible for IPL thickening. Mid-inner retinal (ganglion cell layer to outer plexiform layer) thickening was also observed [43]. Inner retinal layer thickening, especially of the inner nuclear layer, was observed in regions with outer nuclear layer thinning in RP patients having certain Rho mutations [44].

The ganglion cell layer is also preserved longer in OCT study. Ganglion cell inner plexiform layer (GCIPL) thickness is not different in RP patients compared to normal control [24]. Centrally located GCIPL was preserved when foveal multifocal ERG is detectable [41]. When compared to healthy control, GCIPL was thicker in less advanced RP and not different in more advanced RP [42].

Regarding the RNFL, there is discrepancy in thickness results. Several groups have reported a relative thickening of the peripapillary RNFL, but others have reported both thinning and thickening of the peripapillary RNFL [45, 46]. Regional difference of RNFL thickness has been reported. RNFL was thicker in temporal quadrant and thinner in nasal quadrant [47]. Macular RNFL was thicker in RP [42]. Glial cell proliferation within the RNFL or neuronal remodeling and migration into the RNFL can contribute to RNFL thickening [47].

Inner retinal thickness is also reported to be associated with visual function but it is not as strong and consistent as outer retinal integrity. Inner nuclear layer (INL) was negatively correlated with visual field sensitivity but this relation was weaker than OS or ONL. And the thickness of the RNFL was not correlated with the sensitivity [29]. GCIPL also showed negative correlation with visual acuity but not with visual field extent [42].

4.3.3.3 Choroid

Degeneration of RPE and choroidal vessel layer is observed in RP patients. Histopathological studies have showed RPE and choriocapillaris degeneration localized to the areas of clinically apparent atrophy in RP. Previous cross-sectional studies revealed decreased choroidal thickness in RP patients than that in controls [48–50]. Moreover, choroid morphology is alternated in RP. The thickest point of choroid was not subfoveal as healthy eyes and exaggerated nasal thinning was observed in two thirds of patients. And large choroidal vessel layer is affected more than small choroidal vessel layer [51]. Although choroidal thickness decreases in RP, the correlation with visual acuity, retinal thickness as well as disease duration is not consistent. Changes in choroidal thickness can occur secondary to retinal degeneration. A decreased demand for oxygen and nutrients might result in choroidal thinning [52]. Alternatively, decrease in trophic factors due to RPE degeneration could lead to choroidal thinning [53]. The exact mechanism underlying changes in choroidal thickness in RP should be elucidated in further studies.

4.3.3.4 Macular Abnormality

Macular abnormality including cystoid macular edema (CME) and epiretinal membrane is frequently observed in RP. CME is prevalent in 20–50% and mostly around 20% of RP [54–56]. OCT is sensitive for detecting CME of RP that CME was detected in 32% of patients who showed no cystic change in fundus [57]. Moreover, central macular thickness (CMT) was normal range in 32% of patients who showed CME because of gradual retinal thinning in RP [58]. Therefore, one should carefully observe macular morphology not just judge by CMT to find CME in RP. In RP eyes, macular edema showed little dye accumulation in FA and different fluid accumulation in OCT. Cystoid spaces were found mainly in the inner nuclear layer, but sometimes in the outer nuclear layer, outer plexiform layer, and the ganglion cell layer. On the contrary, diabetic macular edema predominantly located in the outer plexiform layer [59]. Retinal atrophy and the destruction of retinal are supposed to contribute macular edema formation of RP based on the OCT feature [60]. However, the mechanism of CME in RP in incompletely understood until now. CME is reported to be associated with autosomal dominant and female gender [55]. Visual impact of CME is not clear if it present or absent. Severe CME is correlated with ISE integrity and visual acuity is worse in unilateral CME eye. Therefore, severe CME seemed to be a predictor of worse visual outcome [61].

Vitreomacular interface disease is also prevalent in RP. Epiretinal membrane has been presented as second most frequent macular abnormality in RP with an incidence ranged 15–20% [54, 55, 62]. And vitreomacular traction (VMT) and lamellar followed in 13.6% and 5.8%, respectively. Longitudinal analysis revealed significant loss of vision was observed only in ERM [62].

Summarizing retinal degeneration in RP, outer retinal is the structure which impaired early. Integrity of inner retinal tends to be preserved longer than outer retina. Inner retinal layer change seems to follow outer retinal loss. Visual function showed more robust and direct correlation with outer retina integrity. RPE and choroid are also degenerated to become thinned. OCT provides clues about pathology in vivo. In addition to animal model data, OCT images increase our understanding about RP.

4.3.4 Optical Coherence Tomography Angiography

Optical coherence tomography angiography is a recently developed non-invasive imaging technique utilizing motion contrast imaging of blood flow to visualize three-dimensional angiogram of retina and choroid without the need for fluorescent dye injection. Although RP is not primary vascular disease, multiple studies have reported that retinal and choriocapillaris microvasculatures are affected in RP. Meta-analysis about OCTA findings revealed that superficial and deep vessel density were significantly lower in foveal and parafoveal zones of RP patients compared to controls [63]. Outcomes about foveal vascularity were inconsistent. Toto et al. and Koyanagi et al. reported that superficial and deep plexus vascular density was not different in foveal area [64, 65]. Rezaei et al. reported that superficial retinal layer plexus was affected in end stage eyes [66]. Multiple studies also compared choriocapillaris flow between RP patients and control. Although lower choriocapillaris flow density and higher flow voids were observed in RP eyes, meta-analysis revealed there was no statistically significant difference between RP patients and control [63, 65, 67]. For FAZ area, the deep FAZ was significantly larger in RP patients than in controls, whereas there was no significant difference in the superficial FAZ in the two groups.

Association between visual acuity and OCTA parameters was also analyzed. Visual acuity was significantly associated with flow density of parafoveal superficial and deep retina and flow density of foveal superficial retina [64, 67]. And superficial FAZ was reported to be associated with visual acuity [64, 68]. Superficial and deep capillary plexus vessel densities were correlated to multifocal electroretinogram values and ganglion cell complex layer thickness [65]. One study reported that FAZ and flow area were smaller in RP patients having normal visual acuity. Authors also showed flow areas of superficial retinal layer was associated with the length of ISE, ELM, and visual field perimeter area and suggested that OCTA measured flow area gradually reduced with RP progression [69]. Jauregui et al. observed OCTA progression over time and revealed that perfusion density decreased by 2.42% per year at the superficial capillary plexus and FAZ area increased by 0.078 and 0.152 mm^2 at superficial and deep capillary plexus [70].

4.3.5 Fundus Autofluorescence

Fundus autofluorescence (FAF) can reveal abnormality of RPE. Short wave (SW)-FAF using blue or green light detects emission from lipofuscin of RPE while near-infrared (NIR)-FAF shows signal from melanin or fluorophore of RPE and choroid [71, 72]. As FAF reflects degree of degeneration, FAF is increasingly used for monitoring of disease progression in RP. Round or ellipsoid ring shape abnormal autofluorescence, which is not visible in fundus examination, is observed in 50–60% of patients [73]. This ring can be observed in both SW-AF and NIR-AF. This ring is usually symmetric in both eyes and located usually from 3 to 20° [74]. This ring indicates transition zone between preserved and degenerated outer retina. Relatively normal retina is observed within the ring and severely degenerated retina is located outside the ring. SD-OCT revealed that ISE and ELM are lost and outer nuclear layer is thinned outside the ring [75]. Hyperfluorescent ring corresponds to loss of outer segment and lipofuscin creation. AF within the ring is iso-fluorescent compared to normal retinal fluorescence [76]. The ring progressively constricts and the speed of constriction varies widely. The speed tends to be faster in large rings. Inner border of the ring corresponds to the preserved area of cone function. On the contrary, rod dysfunction spreads throughout the entire retina even including the fovea [77]. Eventually, the ring may disperse, and this phenomenon is correlated with a widespread loss of sensitivity and visual acuity [77, 78]. Microperimetry reveals that retinal sensitivity is relatively preserved in the ring and reduced or undetectable outside the ring [79]. In addition, other abnormal autofluorescent pattern other than hyperfluorescent ring can be observed. In wide field AF, patchy area hypofluorescence is sometimes observed at mid-periphery and this is related to peripheral visual defect [80]. Case having abnormal hyperfluorescence at central macula is related to central visual loss [78].

4.3.6 Fluorescein Angiography

Fluorescein angiogram (FA) is not widely used in RP. However, FA has several benefits. FA shows chorioretinal atrophy better than conventional fundus image. Vessel attenuation and fluorescein leakage are often observed. Extend of cystoid macular edema is well visualized in FA. Choroidal neovascularization is seldom found in FA.

4.3.7 Adaptive Optics

Adaptive optics device was developed to correct the aberrations using wave-front sensors and deformable mirrors. Scanning laser ophthalmoscopy (SLO) adopting adaptive optics allows microscopic detection of photoreceptors. Several studies have reported a decrease of cone density or increased cone spacing using AOSLO in RP patients. Foveal cone density was reduced up to 38% before visual acuity and macular structure were affected in both patients with RP and Usher syndrome [81]. Another study also showed that up to 62% reduction on peak cone density in patients having normal visual acuity and retinal sensitivity [82]. Retinal mosaicism can be visualized by AOSLO. Female carriers of X-linked RP having RPGR mutation showed a mosaic pattern of cone disruption using AOSLO, who had no visual symptom and normal retinal thickness [83].

4.4 Genetics of Nonsyndromic RP

Until now 84 genes and 7 candidate loci are known to be related to RP. Autosomal-dominant RP (adRP) includes 25 genes, autosomal-recessive RP (arRP) includes 55 genes, and X-linked RP (xlRP) includes 3 genes. In addition, 5 genes are cause of both adRP and arRP. These genes play an essential role and synthesize structural protein in neurosensory retina and RPE. Mutation in specific pathway impairs or destroys entire visual pathway. Theoretically, genes sharing common pathway is expected to express similar phenotype. However, genetic heterogeneity modifies activity of pathway that influences common pathway variably and makes clinical heterogeneity. Herein, we try to review the important pathways that affected in RP and to define the related genes. Phototransduction cascade (10 RP genes related), the visual cycle (7 RP genes), ciliary structure and transport (35 RP genes), and the interphotoreceptor matrix (1 RP gene) are described below. These genes and other 38 RP genes are listed in Table 4.1. Estimated

Table 4.1 Overview of the genes associated with nonsyndromic RP

Gene	Protein	Involved in	Function	Inheritance	Reference
ABCA4	ATP-binding cassette protein A4	Visual cycle	Photoreceptor disk membrane flippase for all-trans-retinal	AR	[84]
ADIPOR1	Adiponectin receptor protein 1	Retinal metabolism	Uptake and retention of DHA in photoreceptor and RPE	AD	[85, 86]
AGBL5	ATP/GTP binding protein-like 5	Ciliary structure and transport	Posttranslational modification of tubulin, a central component of microtubules	AR	[87]
AHR	Aryl hydrocarbon receptor	Retinal homeostasis	Transcription factor involved in response to toxins and ligands including halogenated aromatic hydrocarbons	AR	[88]
ARHGEF18	Rho/Rac guanine nucleotide exchange factor 18	Cell–cell adhesion, Retinal development	Epithelial cell tight-junction formation and apicobasal polarity determination	AR	[89, 90]
ARL2BP	ADP-ribosylation factor-like 2 binding protein	Ciliary transport	PR ciliary doublet formation and axonemal elongation, which are required for PR maintenance and function	AR	[91, 92]
ARL3	ADP-ribosylation factor-like GTPase 3	Ciliary structure and transport	Ciliogenesis, regulates the trafficking of specific kinesins to cilia tips, interacts with RP2	AD	[93, 94]
ARL6	ADP-ribosylation factor-like 6	Ciliary transport	Recruits BBSome to membrane	AR	[95, 96]
BBS1	BBS1 protein	Ciliary transport	BBSome component, involved in ciliary transport.	AR	[97]
BBS2	BBS2 protein	Ciliary transport	BBSome component, involved in ciliary transport.	AR	[97]
BEST1	Bestrophin 1	Retinal homeostasis	Predominantly expressed in RPE, Anion channel and a regulator of intracellular calcium signaling	AR, AD	[97]
C2orf71	Chromosome 2 open reading frame 71	Ciliary structure and transport, Retinal development	Regulates the actin-driven expansion of the ciliary membrane at the initiation of new outer segment disk formation	AR	[98, 99]
C8orf37	Chromosome 8 open reading frame 37	Retinal homeostasis	Participates in the secretory pathway of OS membrane proteins in the photoreceptor and maintains the homeostasis of these proteins	AR	[100]
CA4	Carbonic anhydrase IV	Retinal homeostasis	Membrane-anchored enzyme found in retinal choriocapillaris; involved in pH regulation of retina and choriocapillaris	AD	[100]
CERKL	Ceramide kinase-like	Retinal homeostasis	Regulation of vesicle formation, autophagy and OS phagocytosis	AR	[101]
CLCC1	CLCC1 (Chloride Channel CLIC Like 1)	Retinal homeostasis	Functions as an intracellular chloride channel, maintaining retinal integrity	AR	[102]
CLRN1	Clarin 1	Ciliary structure	Protein localizes to the plasma membrane of the connecting cilium	AR	[103, 104]

CNGA1	Rod cGMP-gated cation channel α-subunit	Phototransduction	α-subunit of the cGMP-gated cation channel that enables sodium, calcium, and magnesium influx in photoreceptor cells	AR	[105]
CNGB1	Rod cGMP-gated cation channel β-subunit	Phototransduction	β-subunit of the cGMP-gated cation channel that enables sodium, calcium, and magnesium influx in photoreceptor cells	AR	[106, 107]
CRB1	Crumbs homolog 1	Cell–cell adhesion, retinal development	Localizes to the Muller glial cell and photoreceptor, apoptosis during retinal development, present at adherens junction	AR, AD	[108, 109]
CRX	Cone-rod otx-like photoreceptor homeobox transcription factor	Gene transcription	Functions with rod and cone transcription factors to coordinately control photoreceptor gene expression	AD	[110]
CYP4V2	Cytochrome P450 4V2	Retinal metabolism	Hydroxylating the omega-3 poly unsaturated fatty acid, including DHA and EPA	AR	[111]
DHDDS	Dehydrodolichyl diphosphate synthase	Phototransduction	Essential enzyme for dolichol synthesis permitting global N-linked glycosylation, which is required for rhodopsin	AR	[112, 113]
DHX38	DEAH (Asp-Glu-Ala-His) box polypeptide 38	DEAH (Asp-Glu-Ala-His) box polypeptide 38	DHX38 encodes for pre-mRNA splicing factor PRP16, which is important in catalyzing pre-mRNA splicing	AR	[114]
EMC1	Endoplasmatic reticulum membrane protein complex subunit 1	Unknown	Subunit of the endoplasmic reticulum protein complex; possibly involved in protein folding and/or processing.	AR	[115]
EYS	Eyes shut/spacemaker (Drosophila) homolog	Ciliary transport Interphotoreceptor matrix	Ciliary transportation role, maintenance of photoreceptor morphology and visual function	AR	[116, 117]
FAM161A	Family with sequence similarity 161 member A	Ciliary structure and transport, Retinal development	Molecular delivery into the outer segment cilium; microtubule stabilization; interaction with ciliopathy protein Cep290 and lebercilin	AR	[118–120]
FSCN2	Retinal fascin homolog 2	Ciliary structure	crosslinks and bundle F-actin filaments	AD	[121]
GPR125	G-protein-coupled receptor 125 (ADGRA3)	Unknown	Unknown	AR	[115]
GUCA1B	Guanylate cyclase activating protein 1B	Phototransduction	Up-regulates cGMP synthesis by activating retinal membrane guanylate cyclase in low Ca	AD	[122]
HGSNAT	Heparan-alpha-glucosaminide *N*-acetyltransferase	Retinal homeostasis	Catalyzes transmembrane acetylation of the terminal glucosamine residues of heparan sulfate	AR	[123]
HK1	Hexokinase 1	Retinal metabolism	Glucose is converted to glucose 6 phosphate by hexokinase; first step in glucose metabolism	AD	[123]

(continued)

Table 4.1 (continued)

Gene	Protein	Involved in	Function	Inheritance	Reference
IDH3B	NAD(+)-specific isocitrate dehydrogenase 3 beta	Retinal metabolism	Subunit of heterotetramer IDH3, catalyzes conversion of isocitrate to α-ketogluterate in the citric acid cycle in mitochondria.	AR	[124]
IFT140	Intraflagellar transport 140 (Chlamydomonas) homolog	Ciliary transport, retinal development	Subunit of IFT-A complex, development and the maintenance of outer segments and has a specific role in opsin transport across the connecting cilium	AR	[125, 126]
IFT172	Intraflagellar transport 172	Ciliary transport, Retinal development	Subunit of IFT-B complex, involved in transition of anterograde to retrograde transport, involved in ciliogenesis	AR	[127]
IMPDH1	Inosine-5′ monophosphate dehydrogenase type I	Nucleotide synthesis	Catalyzes the synthesis of xanthine monophosphate from inosine-5′-monophosphate with reduction of nicotinamide adenine dinucleotide	AD	[128]
IMPG1	Interphotoreceptor matrix proteoglycan 1	Interphotoreceptor matrix	Proteoglycan that binds chondroitin sulfate and hyaluronan, plays a role in the organization of the IPM and may promote the growth and maintenance of the photoreceptor outer segment	AD	[129]
IMPG2	Interphotoreceptor matrix proteoglycan 2	Interphotoreceptor matrix	Proteoglycan that binds chondroitin sulfate and hyaluronan, plays a role in the organization of the IPM and may promote the growth and maintenance of the photoreceptor outer segment	AR	[130]
KIAA1549	KIAA1549 protein	Unknown	Found in the connecting cilium of the mouse retina	AR	[131]
KIZ	Kizuna centrosomal protein	Ciliary structure	Localizes to basal body of connecting cilium	AR	[132]
KLHL7	Kelch-like 7 protein	Retinal homeostasis	Participates as an adaptor and/or chaperone in the ubiquitin-proteasome protein-degradation pathway	AD	[133]
LRAT	Lecithin retinol acetyltransferase	Visual cycle	Esterifies all-trans-retinol into all-trans-retinol retinyl ester	AR	[134]
MAK	Male germ-cell associated kinase	Ciliary structure	Regulates retinal photoreceptor ciliary length and subcompartmentalization	AR	[135]
MERTK	Mer tyrosine kinase proto-oncogene	Retinal homeostasis	Photoreceptor outer segment internalization prior to phagocytosis	AR	[135]
MVK	Mevalonate kinase	Retinal homeostasis	Enzyme catalyzing the transformation of mevalonic acid into phosphomevalonate	AR	[136]
NEK2	NIMA related kinase 2	Retinal development	Regulation of cell cycle progression through localization to the centrosomes and interaction with microtubules.	AR	[137]
NEUROD1	Neuronal differentiation 1	Gene transcription	E box-containing promoter sequences to serve as a transcription activator, thus specifically regulating gene expression.	AR	[138]
NR2E3	Nuclear receptor subfamily 2	Gene transcription	Dual regulatory role in the terminal differentiation and in the maintenance of the rod phenotype	AR	[139]
NRL	Neural retina leucine zipper	Gene transcription	Acts through NR2E3 to inhibit cone photoreceptor fate and promote rod photoreceptor fate	AR, AD	[140]

OFD1	Oral-facial-digital syndrome 1 protein	Ciliary transport, retinal development, retinal homeostasis	Controlling photoreceptor cilium length and number. Neuroprotective function by protecting the photoreceptor from oxidative stress and apoptosis	XL	[141]
PDE6A	Rod cGMP-phosphodiesterase α-subunit	Phototransduction	Rod cGMP-phosphodiesterase hydrolyses cGMP to 5′-GMP	AR	[142]
PDE6B	Rod cGMP-phosphodiesterase β-subunit	Phototransduction	Rod cGMP-phosphodiesterase hydrolyses cGMP to 5′-GMP	AR	[142]
PDE6G	Rod cGMP-phosphodiesterase γ-subunit	Phototransduction	Inhibitory subunit of cGMP phosphodiester	AR	[142]
POMGNT1	O-linked mannose N-acetylglucosaminyl-transferase 1 (beta 1,2-)	Ciliary structure and transport	Specifically expressed in photoreceptor basal body	AR	[143]
PRCD	Progressive rod-cone degeneration protein	Ciliary structure (OS [disk] morphology)	Evaginating membranes of new disks tightly apposed to each other, which is essential for the high fidelity of photoreceptor disk morphogenesis and photoreceptor survival	AR	[144]
PROM1	Prominin 1	Ciliary structure (OS disk morphology)	Generates membrane curvature and tethers disk edge in support of disk stacking stability	AR	[145]
PRPF3	Precursor-mRNA processing factor 3	RNA splicing	Member of the U4/U6-U5 tri-snRNP particle complex (spliceosome)	AD	[146]
PRPF31	Precursor-mRNA processing factor 31	RNA splicing	Member of the U4/U6-U5 tri-snRNP particle complex (spliceosome)	AD	[146]
PRPF4	Precursor-mRNA processing factor 4	RNA splicing	Member of the U4/U6-U5 tri-snRNP particle complex (spliceosome)	AD	[146]
PRPF6	Precursor-mRNA processing factor 6	RNA splicing	Member of the U4/U6-U5 tri-snRNP particle complex (spliceosome)	AD	[147]
PRPF8	Precursor-mRNA processing factor 8	RNA splicing	Member of the U4/U6-U5 tri-snRNP particle complex (spliceosome)	AD	[147]
PRPH2	Peripherin-2	Ciliary structure (OS [disk] morphology)	Helps outer segment disk rim formation and supposed to be related to disk stabilization and shedding	AD, digenic	[147]
RBP3	Retinol binding protein 3	Visual (retinoid) cycle	Binds and transports retinoids in the interphotoreceptor matrix between the RPE and photoreceptors.	AR	[148]
RDH12	Retinol dehydrogenase 12	Visual (retinoid) cycle	Reduction of all-trans-retinal to all-trans-retinol	AD	[149]

(continued)

Table 4.1 (continued)

Gene	Protein	Involved in	Function	Inheritance	Reference
REEP6	Receptor accessory protein	Retinal homeostasis	Rod photoreceptor ER homoeostasis and trafficking of essential phototransduction proteins	AR	[150]
RGR	RPE-vitamin A G-protein-coupled receptor	Visual (retinoid) cycle	Binds all-trans retinal which light converts to 11-cis retinal in the RPE	AR	[151]
RHO	Rhodopsin	Phototransduction	G-protein-coupled photon receptor; activation of transducin after photoactivation.	AD, AR	[152]
RLBP1	Cellular retinaldehyde-binding protein (CRALBP)	Visual (retinoid) cycle	Transport recovered 11-cis-retinal into photoreceptor matrix space	AR	[153]
ROM1	Rod outer segment protein 1	Ciliary structure (OS disk morphology)	Assembles with Peripherin2. Essential for photoreceptor disk morphogenesis	AD, digenic	[154]
RP1	Retinitis pigmentosa 1, axonemal microtubule-associated protein	Ciliary structure	Associated with axonemal microtubules at the IS-OS junction, link nascent OS disk to the axoneme to render morphogenesis and stacking	AR, AD	[155]
RP1L1	Retinitis pigmentosa 1-like protein 1	Ciliary structure and transport	Interacts with RP1, affects photosensitivity and OS morphogenesis of rod photoreceptors	AR	[156]
RP2	Plasma membrane associated protein	Ciliary transport	Regulates the trafficking of specific kinesins to cilia tips	XL	[157]
RP9	PIM1-kinase associated protein 1	RNA splicing	Localizes to the nuclear splicing factor compartment. Splicing of the FSCN2 and BBS2 gene	AD	[157]
RPE65	Vitamin A trans-cis isomerase	Visual (retinoid) cycle	Isomerization of all-trans-retinylester to 11-cis-retinol	AR	[158]
RPGR	Retinitis pigmentosa GTPase regulator	Ciliary transport	Plays a role in the ciliary gate, which controls access of both membrane and soluble proteins to the photoreceptor outer segment	XL	[159]
SAG	Arrestin	Phototransduction	Phosphorylase metarhodopsin II (activated rhodopsin) to stop the activation of transducin	AR	[160]
SAMD11	Sterile alpha motif domain containing 11	Gene transcription	Three nuclear layers of the human retina. CRX-mediated transcriptional regulation in the retina	AR	[161]
SEMA4A	Semaphorin 4A (semaphorin B)	Retinal development	Protecting cell against oxidative stress. Involved in sorting of retinoid-binding proteins in the retinoid cycle	AD	[161]
SLC7A14	Solute carrier family 7 member 14	Retinal development	Transporter protein. Speculated to play important role in retinal development	AR	[162]
SNRNP200	Small nuclear ribonucleoprotein 200 kDa (U5)	RNA splicing	Member of the U4/U6-U5 tri-snRNP particle complex (spliceosome).	AD	[163]

SPATA7	Spermatogenesis-associated protein 7	Ciliary transport	Maintain distal connecting cilium via interacting with RPGR and RPGRIP1	AR	[164]
SPP2	Secreted phosphoprotein 2	Unknown	Unknown	AD	[165]
TOPORS	Topoisomerase I binding arginine/serine rich protein	Ciliary structure or transport, Photoreceptor development	Localizes to the basal body of the connecting cilium, may play a key role in regulating primary cilia-dependent photoreceptor development and function	AD	[166]
TRNT1	CCA adding tRNA nucleotidyl transferase 1	Retinal homeostasis	tRNA processing. Defect in autophagy may result in retinal cell degeneration	AR	[167]
TTC8	Tetratricopeptide repeat domain 8	Ciliary transport	BBSome component, involved in ciliary transport.	AR	[168]
TULP1	Tubby-like protein 1	Ciliary transport	Transport of newly synthesized proteins destined for the outer segment compartment of photoreceptor	AR	[169]
USH2A	Usherin	Ciliary structure and transport	Localizes to photoreceptor calyceal process and periciliary membrane. Intracellular trafficking, movement of phototransduction proteins and lipids to the OS	AR	[170]
ZNF408	Zinc finger protein 408	Retinal development	DNA binding protein that interacts with other proteins	AR	[171]
ZNF513	Zinc finger protein 513	Retinal development	Regulation of photoreceptor-specific genes in retinal development and photoreceptor maintenance	AR	[172]

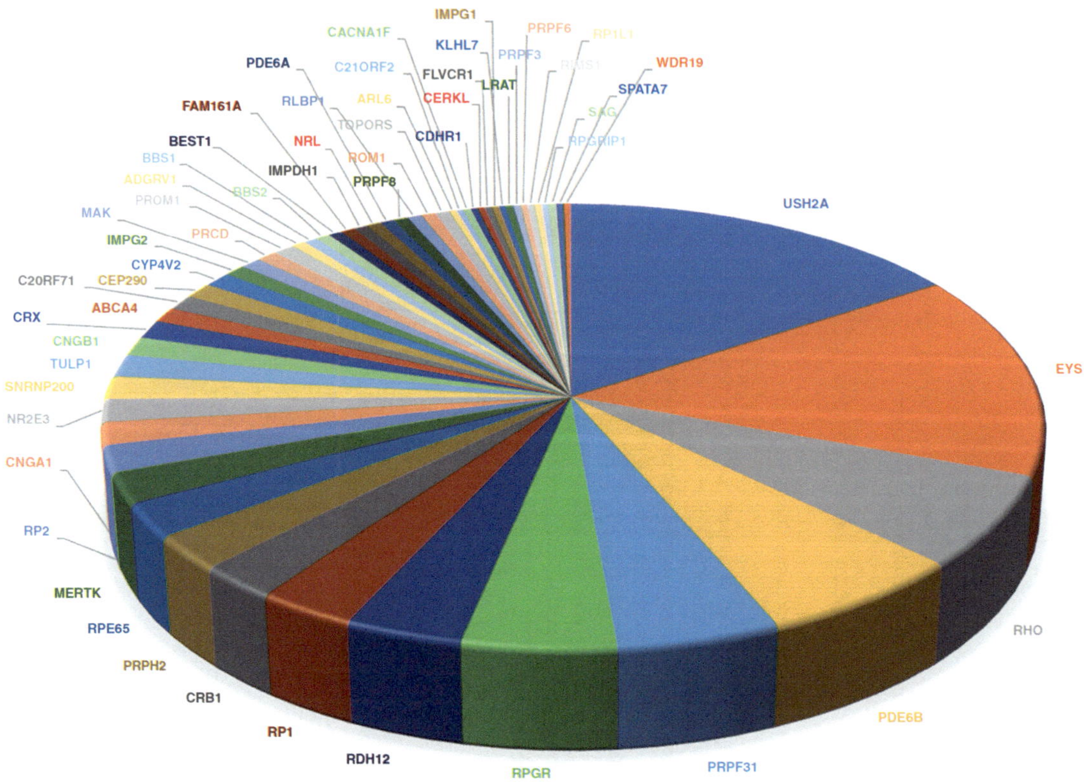

Fig. 4.2 Causal genes contribute to nonsyndromic retinitis pigmentosa. This graph is summarization of nine unbiased next generation sequencing studies about retinitis pigmentosa

relative contribution of genes to nonsyndromic retinitis pigmentosa is depicted in Fig. 4.2.

4.4.1 Phototransduction Cascade

Phototransduction cascade refers electron transport chain elicited by photon driven excitation of opsin molecule. Eventually, this cascade transmits electric signal to visual cortex via optic nerve. This is generally similar in both rod and cone cell except for the different sensitivity to dim or bright light.

Rhodopsin (coded by *RHO* gene) is comprised of apolipoprotein opsin and chromophore 11 cis retinal. After capturing photon, 11 cis retinal is converted to all-trans-retinal isomer and this process transforms structure of rhodopsin into photoactive metarhodopsin II [173]. Metarhodopsin II activates G protein transducin (encoded by *GNAT1*), which then activates cyclic guanosine monophosphate (cGMP) phosphodiesterase (subunits are encoded by *PDE6A, PDE6B,* and *PDE6G*), which then hydrolyzes cGMP into 5′-GMP [142]. This lowers concentration of intracellular cGMP and closes cGMP-gated cation channel (encoded by *CNGA1* and *CNGB1*). This, in turn, lowers intracellular calcium concentration and hyperpolarize that lowers glutamate concentration at synapse. After phototransduction completion, this system returns to before photoactivation state. (1) Attachment of rhodopsin kinase to arrestin phosphorylase metarhodopsin II, then deactivates transducin [174], (2) converting all-trans-retinal to 11-cis-retinal by dissociation from photopigment via visual cycle, (3) GTPase accelerating protein (RGS9) deactivates transducin and photodiesterase (subunits encoded by *PDE6A, PDE6B,* and *PDE6G*) [175], and (4) guanylate cyclase (encoded by *GUCY2D*) normalizes intracellular cGMP [176, 177]. All-trans-retinal dissociates from opsin, then 11-cis-retinal adheres to opsin to re-generate rhodopsin. After that it dissociates from arrestin. Rhodopsin is depolarized by protein phosphatase 2A. Rhodopsin is usually non phosphorylated state in dark circumstances

Most of molecules in rod cell are not so different from those of cone cell. There are two differences between rod and cone. Cone cell has three different opsins, which have specific for certain range of wavelength although these are not as sensitive as opsin of rod. As cone opsin has faster kinetics than rod opsin, it is rarely saturated. Although difference from faster kinetics is not known, it is suggested that fast response of cone cell allows rapid recovery time. It seems based on fast phosphorylation of activated cone pigment, fast dissociation from all-trans-retinal, fast inactivation of transducin [178, 179]. While hydrolyzation of transducin attached GTP is rate limiting reaction, concentration of GTPase accelerating complex is ten times more abundant in cone cell.

4.4.2 Visual Cycle

Vitamin A derivative, 11-cis-retinal, is main component of visual cycle. Vitamin A (all-trans-retinol), ingested as food, is absorbed via gut and runs through blood vessel, then converted to 11-cis-retinal in the RPE. Visual cycle is a process involved in regeneration of 11-cis-retinal from all-trans-retinal, which occurs simultaneously with phototransduction.

After photoactivation, all-trans-retinal released from activated photopigment enters into lumen of outer segment, then reacts with phosphatidylethanolamine and generates N-retinylidene-phosphatidylethanolamine. Via the flippase activity of the ABC (ATP-binding cassette) transporter ABCR (encoded by the *ABCA4*), all-trans-retinal is released into the cytoplasm of the photoreceptor, where it is reduced to all-trans-retinol by the enzyme all-trans-retinal dehydrogenase (encoded by the *RDH8, RDH12*, and *RDH14*) [149]. All-trans-retinol moves to subretinal space and binds to interphotoreceptor retinoid-binding protein (IRBP, encoded by *RBP3*). Then it is transported into RP cell and binds to cellular retinol binding protein (encoded by *CRBP1*), then is re-isomerized via cascade associated with lecithin-retinol acyltransferase (LRAT), RPE65 (retinoid isomerohydrolase), retinal G coupled receptor (RGR), and 11-cis-retinol dehydrogenase (encoded by *RDH5 and RDH11*). Recovered 11-cis retinal is transported into interphotoreceptor matrix space via cellular retinaldehyde-binding protein (CRALBP, encoded by *RLBP1*), then returned to photoreceptor cytoplasm by IRBP. 11-cis-retinal attached to opsin and generates new rhodopsin molecule. This process, known as canonical visual cycle, catalyzes re-isomerization of retinal in rod cell [180–182]. Recent work revealed cone cell has second non-canonical visual cycle in addition to above mentioned canonical visual cycle. This works between Muller cell and outer segment. This cycle, in which not all the protein is revealed, regenerates 11-cis-retinal 20-fold faster. This process starts after cone-specific opsin is photobleached and all-trans-retinal is released into cytoplasm, then all-trans-retinal is reduced to all-trans-retinol by retinol dehydrogenase (encoded by *RDH8* and *RDH14*) and the cone-specific retSDR1 (encoded by *DHRS3*). All-trans-retinol binds to IRBP and is transported to Muller cell where dihydroceramide desaturase1 (DES1, encoded by *DEGS1*) catalyzes direct isomerization of all-trans-retinol that produces 11 cis retinol, 9-cis-retinol, and 13-cis-retinol. Isomerization catalyzed by DES1 is reversible that 11-cis-retinol is vulnerable to re-isomerization. Cone cells utilize two different strategies to reduce the risk of re-isomerization. First, 11-cis-retinol is esterified by multifunctional O-acyltransferase (encoded by *MEAT and AWAT2*) and converted to 11-cis-retinyl-ester. Secondly, newly produced 11-cis-retinol is captured by CRALBP. Hydrolyzation of 11-cis-retinyl ester occurs only when CRALBP is available to bind to 11-cis retinol. Thus, this mechanism prevents re-isomerization of 11-cis-retinol. 11-cis-retinol is transported to interphotoreceptor matrix when bound to CRALBP. Then, it binds to IRBP and moved to cone outer segment. 11-cis-retinol is oxidized to form 11-cis-retinal and binds to opsin to produce new photopigment. Final oxidization reaction occurs only in cone cell.

4.4.3 Ciliary Transport

Cilium is hair-like microtubule-based projections, which extends through mammalian cells with variable shape and size. Cilia are classified as motile cilia and non-motile primary cilia. Motile cilium predominantly serves to move fluid across membrane surface, for example, mucus on surface of lung epithelium and cerebrospinal fluid in the ventricles of the brain [183]. On the contrary, primary cilia lack the central microtubule pair of the motile cilium, exist in vast majority of non-motile eukaryotic cells, and serve as "antenna" in most sensory organ [184]. As cilia found on almost all cells in the human body, mutation in genes encoding cilia protein can result in syndromic disorder called ciliopathy, which affects multiple organs.

Photoreceptor cells contain a highly specific sensory cilium, which consists of distinct subcompartments: connecting cilium, basal body, axoneme, and the ciliary membrane. Until now mutation of more than 30 cilia protein coding genes is related to nonsyndromic retinal disease [185]. As outer segments lack the machinery for protein synthesis, all of its components should be synthesized and pre-assembled in the inner segment and transported. Specialized trafficking system for protein along the ciliary axoneme has been termed intraflagellar transport (IFT) and this is integral to the cilium's structure and function [186]. IFT is a bidirectional transportation system that moves cargos from base to tip (antegrade movement: IFT-B complex with kinesin-2 motor complex) or tip to base (retrograde movement: dynein 2-driven IFT-A complexes) using microtubule-based motile molecules. This system is able to move thousands of molecules such as rhodopsin or arrestin within several seconds. Although participating in IFT of opposite direction, separation of complex A and B leads to defective ciliary transport, suggesting that cooperative interaction between IFT complexes [187].

Many genes causing RP are related to multiple proteins associated with ciliary transport. For example ARL3 and RP2 mediate localization of specific kinesins at the tip [188]. IFT is mediated by IFT proteins (IFT140 and IFT172), which form two complexes (complex A and B) attached to cargo transportation system [189]. BBSome complex plays adaptor role between cargo and IFT complex. BBSome consists of eight protein subunits and mutation in BBSome compartments make can Bardet–Biedl syndrome [190]. However, genes of four subunits of BBSome (BBS1, BBS2, BBS9, and TTC8) and that encoding ARL6 (protein recruits the BBSome complex to the protein membrane) are related to nonsyndromic RP [191].

Ciliary trafficking is regulated by specified ciliary structures, called "ciliary gate." This structure forms general barrier to the periciliary particle diffusion and regulates cargo transportation into the structurally isolated outer segment. Soluble proteins that are not associated with the membrane can enter the cilium by passive diffusion or active transport. Function of ciliary gate is mediated by distal appendage (also referred as transition fibers when associated with ciliary membrane) and transition zone [192]. Transition fibers execute size-dependent entry and exit of soluble protein. Y-links and protein meshwork in transition zone have been proposed to act as a molecular sieve-like barrier [193]. Connecting cilium of photoreceptor is analogous to transition zone of prototypical cilium. Many ciliopathy proteins such as CEP290 localizes to transition zone and serves as hub to connect the important protein complexes including MKS module (CC2D2A/MKS1,3/TCTNs/TMEMs/B9D1,2) and NPHP module (RPGRIP/RPGRIP1L/NPHP1/NPHP4) [194]. These modules interact with nearby transition zone component (ex BBSome complex) and complex contains protein-like RPGR. *RPGR* gene is presumed to contribute 70–90% of X-linked RP and 10–20% of RP [159]. SPATA7 (Spermatogenesis-associated protein7) is suggested to maintain distal connecting cilium via interacting with RPGR and RPGRIP1 (RPGR interacting protein 1) [195]. Defect in RPGR/

RPGRIP1/SPATA7 complex leads to mislocalization of specific opsin that these proteins are believed to play an important role in transporting this specific opsin [196].

4.4.4 Outer Segment Structure

Outer segment of photoreceptor refers specialized compartment consisting of stacked intracellular disks (rod cell) or lamellae (cone cell). Proteins participate in outer segment disk development or orientation are responsible for some subtypes of nonsyndromic RP.

Outer segment disk morphogenesis takes two steps. Growth of the ciliary membrane creates an evagination with an upper surface at an axonemal microtubule, and disk internalization begins by expansion of the rim region that anchors evaginations to the axoneme [197]. F-actin microfilament located at basal axonemal microtubule is required for evagination of new disks. Retinal fascin homolog2 (encoded by *FSCN2*) crosslinks and bundles F-actin filaments. Peripherin-2 (encoded by *PRPH2*) is always accompanied by the appearance of an enclosing plasma membrane in both rods and cones. PRPH2 helps outer segment disk rim formation and supposed to be related to disk stabilization and shedding [145]. Photoreceptor cilia has an ability to release massive amount of ectosome, which is suppressed and morphed into disks by PRPH [198]. Rod outer segment protein 1 (ROM1) assembles with Peripherin 2 and modifies its function [154]. Although inherited defects in ROM1 do not by themselves cause monogenic disease, ROM1 can act as a modifier gene for peripherin associated disease [199]. Prominin 1 (encoded by *PROM1*) that located at the U-shaped disk edge is required for OS disk edge formation and maintenance. Prominin 1 serves to generate membrane curvature and tether disk edge in support of disk stacking stability [145]. Protocadherin 21 (also known as photoreceptor-specific cadherin, encoded by *CDHR1*) localized at the basal OS only along the edges of open disk, also participates in disk morphogenesis cooperatively with PROM1 [200]. Photoreceptor-specific protein RP1 is associated with axonemal microtubules at the IS-OS junction and supposed to link nascent OS disk to the axoneme to render morphogenesis and stacking [155]. RP1 acts cooperatively with RP1L1 which resides in similar site and is also related to outer segment formation [201].

4.4.5 Interphotoreceptor Matrix

Interphotoreceptor matrix (IPM) fills subretinal space between the photoreceptor cells and the RPE. Known functional role of IPM includes retinal adhesion to the RPE, providing receptors for growth factor presentation, retinoid metabolism, cytoskeleton arrangement, and the transport regulation of oxygen and nutrients to the photoreceptor cells [202]. Therefore, defects in gene constitutes IPM may cause IRD. Moreover, extracellular matrix containing IPM may play an important role in progressive retinal degenerative disorders [203].

Interphotoreceptor matrix consists of proteins and carbohydrates secreted by RPE. Major components of IPM include glycosaminoglycan, proteoglycan, hyaluronic acid, collagen, elastin fiber, fibronectin, fibrillin, laminin, and fibulin. Hyaluronic acid polymer forms large polysaccharides that produce mesh network. This is linked to Muller cell via CD44 and to RPE via RHAMM (receptor for hyaluronic acid mediated motility)-type binding motifs. And SPACR, SPACRCAN, PEDF, and IRBP are also connected to hyaluronic network via RHAMM-binding motifs [204].

Mutation in four genes (*IMPG2, RBP3, EYS,* and *IMPG1*), encoding proteins constitute hyaluronan network, is associated with nonsyndromic RP [205–208]. SPACRCAN (encoded by *IMPG2*) is a chondroitin sulfate proteoglycan and SPACR (encoded by *IMPG1*) is a glycoprotein. They are closely associated with regulating hyaluronan during normal ocular development and aging [209]. IRBP (encoded by *RBP*), primary soluble protein in interphotoreceptor matrix, plays an important role in visual cycle.

EYS gene (encoding Drosophila eyes shut protein) is the largest gene expressed in human retina. The resulting protein, having multiple sites bind to glycosaminoglycan chain, is an extracellular protein in drosophila. However, this protein can localize to subcellular compartment in the cytoplasm and to the axoneme of the connecting cilium in human [210]. Inhibiting EYS expression results in outer segment protein mislocalization, which suggests ciliary transportation role of EYS [211]. And EYS seems to be important for the maintenance of photoreceptor morphology and visual function [212].

4.5 Management and Treatment of RP

4.5.1 Counseling

Great advances in genetic sequencing provided large knowledges about genetics and so as in RP. Genetic diagnosis becomes routine examination these days. Gene panel is usually used and even whole exome or genome sequencing is available. Detection rate of genetic diagnosis is reported up to 60–80%. Concurrent familial genetic testing (Trio study) is recommended. Proper guideline of ocular and genetic examination for non-symptomatic children has not been suggested. Although genetic diagnosis supports clinical diagnosis and provides additional information, phenotype prediction based on genetic diagnosis is still limited. Understanding the underlying genetic profile and other modifiers that can influence the phenotype will help provide a more reliable clinical prognosis.

4.5.2 Management of Complications

One of the common complications of RP is lens opacities, especially posterior capsular opacity. Pruette et al. reported that lens opacity or pseudophakia was observed in 46.4% of 384 eyes in American RP patients [213]. Among lens opacities, 80% was posterior polar cataract, 10% was nuclear sclerosis, and 20% was both nuclear sclerosis and posterior polar opacity. Although older age group showed higher prevalence of lens opacities, 10.3% of patients younger than 20 showed cataract. In the study, lens opacity was more prevalent in AD inheritance group. Fishman et al. observed posterior subcapsular cataract (PSC) in 53% out of 338 American RP patients whose average age was 38.7 years [214]. PSC was more prevalent in X-linked group while it was relatively uncommon in AD group. Berson et al. also reported that lens opacities in RP were most prevalent in X-linked inheritance as 72% [215].

Cataract extraction is generally recommended in RP because subjective visual gain is considerable in RP patients. Objective visual gain following cataract surgery depends on the amount of residual macular function. Likelihood of visual recovery is highest in patients whose integrity of foveal ellipsoid zone is intact [216]. Complications associated with cataract surgery are reported to be relatively high in RP, which include zonular insufficiency (19%), posterior capsular opacification (44–45%), and anterior capsular opacification (10–38%). Excessive inflammation after in RP is sometimes suggested to cause higher rate of complication but it is not proved. Acceleration of RP progression following cataract surgery is not evidenced yet.

Large randomized controlled study for effective treatment of CME in RP has not been performed yet. Recently introduced meta-analysis suggested oral and topical carbonic anhydrase inhibitors (CAIs) as first line treatment [217]. However effect on visual function was inconsistent across studies in spite of definite reduction of macular edema [218]. Rebound after cessation of treatment was reported in about 42% of cases. However, resuming the treatment after discontinuation also showed favorable effect [219]. In case of inefficacy of CAIs intravitreal steroid can be an alternative treatment. Recent comparative study showed better visual outcome in dexamethasone implant group than oral acetazolamide group [220]. Intravitreal anti-VEGF agent showed inconsistent effect overall. Moreover, VEGF level was not increased in RP, while other retinal vascular diseases using anti-VEGF shows substantial increase [221].

While epiretinal membrane is commonly found in RP, its surgical treatment is usually not addressed. Ikeda et al reported long-term outcome of vitrectomy for epiretinal membrane in RP. They showed favorable morphological improvement without deleterious change. However visual benefit was limited [222]. Cautions should be addressed because of this limited effect and possible deleterious damage following surgery.

4.5.3 Treatment Based on Specific Genetic Abnormality

Most of genes whose mutation causing RP are expressed in photoreceptors or RPE. Therefore, these target cells should be intact if genetic alteration specific treatment takes effect. This means gene-specific treatment is effective in early stage when retinal cells minimally impaired. Gene augmentation therapy introduces wild type of cDNA sequence into target cell that generating healthy protein. Viral and non-viral vectors are tried. In RP, viral vectors such as Adeno-associated virus (AAV) is largely used as to insert genetic cargo into intravitreal or subretinal space of the eye. Gene augmentation therapy refers gene product supplementation and does not impact dominant-negative genetic mutations. Therefore, this method is limited to autosomal-recessive inherited genetic mutations, which makes "loss of function" mechanism. This treatment was first tried in LCA patient having biallelic RPE65 gene mutation at 2008. And Luxturna (voretigene neparvovec-rzyl) was recently FDA approved, which is the first gene therapy in RP. Hopeful result in RPE65 gene accelerates the research and clinical trial of other genes of RP and IRDs including RP associated with MERTK, PDE6A, RPGR, choroideremia, CNGA achromatopsia, Stargardt disease, and so on. In spite successful report of these trials, gene augmentation therapy is facing several challenges. First, long-lasting maintenance of one-time administration of a therapeutic vector is unclear. Second, cargo capacity of currently used is insufficient for certain genes causing IRDS (Ex, EYS, USH2A). Control of expressivity, relative scarcity of patients having target gene, plentiful amount of cost of the highly individualized forms, risk of collateral damage associated with subretinal gene delivery, and ineffectiveness for dominant-negative mutation are also problematic.

In disease caused by dominant-negative mutation (gain of function mutation) a combined approach is often warranted. Both gene suppression and replacement therapies are utilized. An AAV is initially delivered an RNA interference (RNAi) based gene suppressor to down-regulate to inactivate target. Then a separate AAV-vector to deliver functional replacement of gene is introduced. Additionally, direct gene editing using CRISPR (clustered regularly interspaced short palindromic repeats)-CaS is currently raising expectations. CRISPR technology, derived from a natural bacterial host defense system against bacteriophage, is able to cut and remove target cell's genome and add the desired functional gene with precision [223].

Another approach using anti sense oligonucleotides (AONs), which is versatile RNA molecule binding specific target site of pre-mRNA. This binding suppresses abnormal splicing resulted from mutation [224]. Pharmacologic therapy using small molecule has also been tried to treat RP having mutation of certain gene. Mutation in the LRAT and RPE65 gene disrupts the visual cycle converting all-trans-retinal into 11-cis-retinal. Administration of 9-cis-retinyl acetate showed improvement of vision [134].

4.5.4 Treatment Not Associated with Specific Genetic Abnormality

Several nutritional supplements have been recommended in RP. High dose Vitamin A slowed progression of cone dysfunction on ERG. Beta carotene, a dimerized form of vitamin A has shown b waves on ERG with no change of visual acuity. Blood concentration of clinical trials failed to show beneficial effect of docosahexaenoic acid (DHA) although blood concentration of DHA was positively correlated with slower progression in RP. Lutein supplements have modest effect on slowing extinction of visual field sensitivity. However, only limited evidence for beneficial effect of these nutritional supplements exist until now that additional well designed studies on combined supplements strategies may achieve more robust conclusions [225, 226].

Cell replacement therapy indicates introducing retinal progenitor cell or stem cell derived from non-ocular origin such embryonic stem cell (ESC) or induced pluripotent stem cell (iPSC) into intravitreal or subretinal space. Individual cell type has its own strengthness and weakness. Retinal progenitor cell (RPC) is easy to handle and do not need immunosuppressant but hard to harvest enough cells. In contrast, stem cell usually requires complicated process. Because iPSC is originated from patient, immune reaction is not concern but correcting genetic abnormality of iPSC is prerequisite. However, this highly individualized treatment takes tremendous costs. Therefore storage tissue bank of HLA matched iPSC is suggested as alternative modality of individualized treatment [227]. Although cell replacement therapy is starting, it is supposed to provide great opportunity of treatment option for RP.

Another treatment option for advanced RP is electronic retinal implant. Currently two products are available, which are Argus II and Alpha AMS. Inner retinal function should be guaranteed to use this device as they stimulate inner retina. Argus is epiretinal device, which directly stimulates inner retina, connected to small camera attached to glasses. On the contrary, Alpha AMS consists of photosensitive photodiode array implanted sub-retinally, which stimulate bipolar cells. Retinal implants restore vision in terms of improving daily performance. Although this strategy shows affirmative result, side effects, durability of device, and low resolution are problems to overcome.

Optogenetic technology is also being tried to treat RP. Originally these tools were developed and used in neuroscience. In order to restore vision optogenetic is used to express light sensitive proteins in subpopulation of retinal neurons which have no intrinsic light sensitivity. This allows to start phototransduction where native photoreceptors or other crucial retinal elements are damaged. As photosensitive receptor, two kinds of optogenetic effectors are employed, ion channels and G-protein-coupled receptors (GPCRs). Ion channel is fast responder but less sensitive, which requires intense light, while GPCRs are sensitive but have slower kinetics. Currently two clinical trials are underway, both of which use ion channel and channel rhodopsin. And viral transduction via AAV is the method to express photosensitive proteins.

Several kinds of growth factors have been known to slow down the photoreceptor degeneration, which include brain-derived neurotrophic factor (BNDF), basic fibroblast growth factor (bFGF), ciliary neurotrophic factor (CNDF), glial cell-derived neurotrophic factor (GDNF), nerve growth factor (NGF), and rod-derived cone variability factor (rdVCF). Some of these molecules were effective in animal model. Further studies are required to prove clinical benefit of treatment based on growth factor supply.

References

1. RetNet—Retinal Information Network. https://sph.uth.edu/retnet/. Accessed 9 Feb 2016
2. Yoon CK, Yu HG. The structure-function relationship between macular morphology and visual function analyzed by optical coherence tomography in retinitis pigmentosa. J Ophthalmol. 2013;2013:821460.
3. Seo JH, Yu HG, Lee BJ. Assessment of functional vision score and vision-specific quality of life in individuals with retinitis pigmentosa. Korean J Ophthalmol. 2009;23:164–8.
4. van Huet RA, Estrada-Cuzcano A, Banin E, Rotenstreich Y, Hipp S, Kohl S, Hoyng CB, den Hollander AI, Collin RW, Klevering BJ. Clinical characteristics of rod and cone photoreceptor dystrophies in patients with mutations in the C8orf37 gene. Invest Ophthalmol Vis Sci. 2013;54:4683–90.
5. Ammann F, Klein D, Franceschetti A. Genetic and epidemiological investigations on pigmentary degeneration of the retina and allied disorders in Switzerland. J Neurol Sci. 1965;2:183–96.
6. Haim M. Epidemiology of retinitis pigmentosa in Denmark. Acta Ophthalmol Scand Suppl. 2002;1–34.
7. You QS, Xu L, Xing Y, et al. Prevalence of retinitis pigmentosa in North China: the Beijing Eye Public Health Care Project. Acta Ophthalmol. 2013;91:499–500.
8. Li ZY, Possin DE, Milam AH. Histopathology of bone spicule pigmentation in retinitis pigmentosa. Ophthalmology. 1995;102:805–16.

9. Bunker CH, Berson EL, Bromley WC, Hayes RP, Roderick TH. Prevalence of retinitis pigmentosa in Maine. Am J Ophthalmol. 1984;97:357–65.
10. Hartong DT, Berson EL, Dryja TP. Retinitis pigmentosa. Lancet. 2006;368:1795–809.
11. Hu D-N. Genetic aspects of retinitis pigmentosa in China. Am J Med Genet. 1982;12:51–6.
12. Hayakawa M, Fujiki K, Kanai A, et al. Multicenter genetic study of retinitis pigmentosa in Japan: I. Genetic heterogeneity in typical retinitis pigmentosa. Jpn J Ophthalmol. 1997;41:1–6.
13. Kim KJ, Kim C, Bok J, et al. Spectrum of rhodopsin mutations in Korean patients with retinitis pigmentosa. Mol Vis. 2011;17:844–53.
14. Berson EL. Retinitis pigmentosa and allied diseases: applications of electroretinographic testing. Int Ophthalmol. 1981;4:7–22.
15. Wachtmeister L. Oscillatory potentials in the retina: what do they reveal. Prog Retin Eye Res. 1998;17:485–521.
16. Berson EL. Retinitis pigmentosa. The Friedenwald Lecture. Invest Ophthalmol Vis Sci. 1993;34:1659–76.
17. Falsini B, Galli-Resta L, Fadda A, Ziccardi L, Piccardi M, Iarossi G, Resta G. Long-term decline of central cone function in retinitis pigmentosa evaluated by focal electroretinogram. Invest Ophthalmol Vis Sci. 2012;53:7701–9.
18. Nagy D, Schönfisch B, Zrenner E, Jägle H. Long-term follow-up of retinitis pigmentosa patients with multifocal electroretinography. Investig Ophthalmol Vis Sci. 2008;49:4664–71.
19. Messias K, Jägle H, Saran R, Ruppert ADP, Siqueira R, Jorge R, Messias A. Psychophysically determined full-field stimulus thresholds (FST) in retinitis pigmentosa: relationships with electroretinography and visual field outcomes. Doc Ophthalmol. 2013;127:123–9.
20. Grover S, Fishman GA, Brown J Jr. Patterns of visual field progression in patients with retinitis pigmentosa. Ophthalmology. 1998;105:1069–75.
21. Sandberg MA, Rosner B, Weigel-DiFranco C, Dryja TP, Berson EL. Disease course of patients with X-linked retinitis pigmentosa due to RPGR gene mutations. Investig Ophthalmol Vis Sci. 2007;48:1298–304.
22. Hafler BP, Comander J, Weigel DiFranco C, Place EM, Pierce EA. Course of ocular function in PRPF31 retinitis pigmentosa. Semin Ophthalmol. 2016;31:49–52.
23. Milam AH, Li ZY, Fariss RN. Histopathology of the human retina in retinitis pigmentosa. Prog Retin Eye Res. 1998;17:175–205.
24. Hood DC, Lin CE, Lazow MA, Locke KG, Zhang X, Birch DG. Thickness of receptor and post-receptor retinal layers in patients with retinitis pigmentosa measured with frequency-domain optical coherence tomography. Invest Ophthalmol Vis Sci. 2009;50:2328–36.
25. Hagiwara A, Mitamura Y, Kumagai K, Baba T, Yamamoto S. Photoreceptor impairment on optical coherence tomographic images in patients with retinitis pigmentosa. Br J Ophthalmol. 2013;97:237–8.
26. Hood DC, Lazow MA, Locke KG, Greenstein VC, Birch DG. The transition zone between healthy and diseased retina in patients with retinitis pigmentosa. Investig Ophthalmol Vis Sci. 2011;52:101–8.
27. Witkin AJ, Ko TH, Fujimoto JG, Chan A, Drexler W, Schuman JS, Reichel E, Duker JS. Ultra-high resolution optical coherence tomography assessment of photoreceptors in retinitis pigmentosa and related diseases. Am J Ophthalmol. 2006;142:945–52.
28. Wen Y, Klein M, Hood DC, Birch DG. Relationships among multifocal electroretinogram amplitude, visual field sensitivity, and SD-OCT receptor layer thicknesses in patients with retinitis pigmentosa. Invest Ophthalmol Vis Sci. 2012;53:833–40.
29. Sayo A, Ueno S, Kominami T, Okado S, Inooka D, Komori S, Terasaki H. Significant relationship of visual field sensitivity in central 10° to thickness of retinal layers in retinitis pigmentosa. Investig Ophthalmol Vis Sci. 2018;59:3469–75.
30. Hara A, Nakazawa M, Saito M, Suzuki Y. The qualitative assessment of optical coherence tomography and the central retinal sensitivity in patients with retinitis pigmentosa. PLoS One. 2020;15:1–15.
31. Fischer MD, Fleischhauer JC, Gillies MC, Sutter FK, Helbig H, Barthelmes D. A new method to monitor visual field defects caused by photoreceptor degeneration by quantitative optical coherence tomography. Investig Opthalmology Vis Sci. 2008;49:3617.
32. Grover S, Fishman GA, Anderson RJ, Alexander KR, Derlacki DJ. Rate of visual field loss in retinitis pigmentosa. Ophthalmology. 1997;104:460–5.
33. Berson EL, Sandberg MA, Rosner B, Birch DG, Hanson AH. Natural course of retinitis pigmentosa over a three-year interval. Am J Ophthalmol. 1985;99:240–51.
34. Birch DG, Locke KGI, Wen Y, Locke KGI, Hoffman DR, Hood DC. Spectral-domain optical coherence tomography measures of outer segment layer progression in patients with X-linked retinitis pigmentosa. JAMA Ophthalmol. 2013;131:1143–50.
35. Cai CX, Locke KG, Ramachandran R, Birch DG, Hood DC. A comparison of progressive loss of the ellipsoid zone (EZ) band in autosomal dominant and x-linked retinitis pigmentosa. Invest Ophthalmol Vis Sci. 2014;55:7417–22.
36. Stone JL, Barlow WE, Humayun MS, de Juan Jr E, Milam AH. Morphometric analysis of macular photoreceptors and ganglion cells in retinas with retinitis pigmentosa. Arch Ophthalmol. 1992;110:1634–9.
37. Santos A, Humayun MS, de Juan Jr E, Greenburg RJ, Marsh MJ, Klock IB, Milam AH. Preservation of the inner retina in retinitis pigmentosa. A morphometric analysis. Arch Ophthalmol. 1997;115:511–5.
38. Humayun MS, Prince M, de Juan Jr E, Barron Y, Moskowitz M, Klock IB, Milam AH. Morphometric analysis of the extramacular retina from postmortem eyes with retinitis pigmentosa. Invest Ophthalmol Vis Sci. 1999;40:143–8.

39. Lin B, Peng EB. Retinal ganglion cells are resistant to photoreceptor loss in retinal degeneration. PLoS One. 2013;8:e68084.
40. Cideciyan AV, Aleman TS, Jacobson SG, et al. Centrosomal-ciliary gene CEP290/NPHP6 mutations result in blindness with unexpected sparing of photoreceptors and visual brain: implications for therapy of Leber congenital amaurosis. Hum Mutat. 2007;28:1074–83.
41. Vamos R, Tatrai E, Nemeth J, Holder GE, DeBuc DC, Somfai GM. The structure and function of the macula in patients with advanced retinitis pigmentosa. Invest Ophthalmol Vis Sci. 2011;52: 8425–32.
42. Yoon CK, Yu HG. Ganglion cell-inner plexiform layer and retinal nerve fibre layer changes within the macula in retinitis pigmentosa: a spectral domain optical coherence tomography study. Acta Ophthalmol. 2018;96:e180–8.
43. Wolsley CJ, Silvestri G, O'Neill J, Saunders KJ, Anderson RS. The association between multifocal electroretinograms and OCT retinal thickness in retinitis pigmentosa patients with good visual acuity. Eye. 2009;23:1524–31.
44. Aleman TS, Cideciyan AV, Sumaroka A, et al. Retinal laminar architecture in human retinitis pigmentosa caused by Rhodopsin gene mutations. Invest Ophthalmol Vis Sci. 2008;49:1580–90.
45. Oishi A, Otani A, Sasahara M, Kurimoto M, Nakamura H, Kojima H, Yoshimura N. Retinal nerve fiber layer thickness in patients with retinitis pigmentosa. Eye. 2009;23:561–6.
46. Anastasakis A, Genead MA, McAnany JJ, Fishman GA. Evaluation of retinal nerve fiber layer thickness in patients with retinitis pigmentosa using spectral-domain optical coherence tomography. Retina. 2012;32:358–63.
47. Ilhan C, Citirik M. Glial proliferation and atrophy: two poles of optic disc in patients with retinitis pigmentosa. J Curr Ophthalmol. 2019;31:416–21.
48. Ayton LN, Guymer RH, Luu CD. Choroidal thickness profiles in retinitis pigmentosa. Clin Exp Ophthalmol. 2013;41:396–403.
49. Dhoot DS, Huo S, Yuan A, Xu D, Srivistava S, Ehlers JP, Traboulsi E, Kaiser PK. Evaluation of choroidal thickness in retinitis pigmentosa using enhanced depth imaging optical coherence tomography. Br J Ophthalmol. 2013;97:66–9.
50. Sodi A, Lenzetti C, Murro V, Caporossi O, Mucciolo DP, Bacherini D, Cipollini F, Passerini I, Virgili G, Rizzo S. EDI-OCT evaluation of choroidal thickness in retinitis pigmentosa. Eur J Ophthalmol. 2018;28:52–7.
51. Adhi M, Regatieri CV, Branchini LA, Zhang JY, Alwassia AA, Duker JS. Analysis of the morphology and vascular layers of the choroid in retinitis pigmentosa using spectral-domain OCT. Ophthalmic Surg Lasers Imaging Retin. 2013;44:252–9.
52. Yu DY, Cringle SJ. Retinal degeneration and local oxygen metabolism. Exp Eye Res. 2005;80:745–51.
53. Saint-Geniez M, Kurihara T, Sekiyama E, Maldonado AE, D'Amore PA. An essential role for RPE-derived soluble VEGF in the maintenance of the choriocapillaris. Proc Natl Acad Sci U S A. 2009;106:18751–6.
54. Liew G, Strong S, Bradley P, Severn P, Moore AT, Webster AR, Mitchell P, Kifley A, Michaelides M. Prevalence of cystoid macular oedema, epiretinal membrane and cataract in retinitis pigmentosa. Br J Ophthalmol. 2019;103:1163–6.
55. Testa F, Rossi S, Colucci R, Gallo B, Di Iorio V, della Corte M, Azzolini C, Melillo P, Simonelli F. Macular abnormalities in Italian patients with retinitis pigmentosa. Br J Ophthalmol. 2014;98:946–50.
56. Hajali M, Fishman GA, Anderson RJ. The prevalence of cystoid macular oedema in retinitis pigmentosa patients determined by optical coherence tomography. Br J Ophthalmol. 2008;92:1065–8.
57. Hajali M, Fishman GA. The prevalence of cystoid macular oedema on optical coherence tomography in retinitis pigmentosa patients without cystic changes on fundus examination. Eye. 2009;23:915–9.
58. Gorovoy IR, Gallagher DS, Eller AW, Mayercik VA, Friberg TR, Schuman JS. Cystoid macular edema in retinitis pigmentosa patients without associated macular thickening. Semin Ophthalmol. 2013;28: 79–83.
59. Makiyama Y, Oishi A, Otani A, Ogino K. Prevalence and spatial distribution of cystoid spaces in retinitis pigmentosa. Retina. 2014;34:981–8.
60. Liu G, Liu X, Li H, Du Q, Wang F. Optical coherence tomographic analysis of retina in retinitis pigmentosa patients. Ophthalmic Res. 2016;56:111–22.
61. Kim YJ, Joe SG, Lee DH, Lee JY, Kim JG, Yoon YH. Correlations between spectral-domain OCT measurements and visual acuity in cystoid macular edema associated with retinitis pigmentosa. Invest Ophthalmol Vis Sci. 2013;54:1303–9.
62. Fragiotta S, Rossi T, Carnevale C, Cutini A, Tricarico S, Casillo L, Scuderi G, Vingolo EM. Vitreo-macular interface disorders in retinitis pigmentosa. Graefes Arch Clin Exp Ophthalmol. 2019;257:2137–46.
63. Ling L, Gao F, Zhang Q, He T, Zhao Y, Xing Y, Yu Y, Ji K. Optical coherence tomography angiography assessed retinal and choroidal microvasculature features in patients with retinitis pigmentosa: a meta-analysis. Biomed Res Int. 2019; https://doi.org/10.1155/2019/6723917.
64. Koyanagi Y, Murakami Y, Funatsu J, et al. Optical coherence tomography angiography of the macular microvasculature changes in retinitis pigmentosa. Acta Ophthalmol. 2018;96:e59–67.
65. Toto L, Borrelli E, Mastropasqua R, Senatore A, Di Antonio L, Di Nicola M, Carpineto P, Mastropasqua L. Macular features in retinitis pigmentosa: correlations among ganglion cell complex thickness, capillary density, and macular function. Investig Ophthalmol Vis Sci. 2016;57:6360–6.
66. Rezaei KA, Zhang Q, Chen CL, Chao J, Wang RK. Retinal and choroidal vascular features in patients with retinitis pigmentosa imaged by OCT

based microangiography. Graefes Arch Clin Exp Ophthalmol. 2017;255:1287–95.
67. Alnawaiseh M, Schubert F, Heiduschka P, Eter N. Optical coherence tomography angiography in patients with retinitis pigmentosa. Retina. 2019;39:210–7.
68. Wang XN, Zhao Q, Li DJ, et al. Quantitative evaluation of primary retinitis pigmentosa patients using colour Doppler flow imaging and optical coherence tomography angiography. Acta Ophthalmol. 2019;97:e993–7.
69. Takagi S, Hirami Y, Takahashi M, Fujihara M, Mandai M, Miyakoshi C, Tomita G, Kurimoto Y. Optical coherence tomography angiography in patients with retinitis pigmentosa who have normal visual acuity. Acta Ophthalmol. 2018;96: e636–42.
70. Jauregui R, Park KS, Duong JK, Mahajan VB, Tsang SH. Quantitative progression of retinitis pigmentosa by optical coherence tomography angiography. Sci Rep. 2018;8:1–7.
71. Delori FC, Dorey CK, Staurenghi G, Arend O, Goger DG, Weiter JJ. In vivo fluorescence of the ocular fundus exhibits retinal pigment epithelium lipofuscin characteristics. Investig Ophthalmol Vis Sci. 1995;36:718–29.
72. Keilhauer CN, Delori FC. Near-infrared autofluorescence imaging of the fundus: visualization of ocular melanin. Investig Ophthalmol Vis Sci. 2006;47:3556–64.
73. Lois N, Forrester JV. Fundus autofluorescence. Philadelphia, PA: Wolters Kluwer Health; 2015.
74. Sujirakul T, Davis R, Erol D, Zhang L, Schillizzi G, Royo-Dujardin L, Shen S, Tsang S. Bilateral concordance of the fundus hyperautofluorescent ring in typical retinitis pigmentosa patients. Ophthalmic Genet. 2015;36:113–22.
75. Lima LH, Cella W, Greenstein VC, Wang NK, Busuioc M, Smith RT, Yannuzzi LA, Tsang SH. Structural assessment of hyperautofluorescent ring in patients with retinitis pigmentosa. Retina. 2009;29:1025–31.
76. Schuerch K, Woods RL, Lee W, Duncker T, Delori FC, Allikmets R, Tsang SH, Sparrow JR. Quantifying fundus autofluorescence in patients with retinitis pigmentosa. Investig Ophthalmol Vis Sci. 2017;58:1843–55.
77. Robson AG, Lenassi E, Saihan Z, Luong VA, Fitzke FW, Holder GE, Webster AR. Comparison of fundus autofluorescence with photopic and scotopic fine matrix mapping in patients with retinitis pigmentosa: 4- to 8-year follow-up. Invest Ophthalmol Vis Sci. 2012;53:6187–95.
78. Wakabayashi T, Sawa M, Gomi F, Tsujikawa M. Correlation of fundus autofluorescence with photoreceptor morphology and functional changes in eyes with retinitis pigmentosa. Acta Ophthalmol. 2010;88:177–83.
79. Duncker T, Tabacaru MR, Lee W, Tsang SH, Sparrow JR, Greenstein VC. Comparison of near-infrared and short-wavelength autofluorescence in retinitis pigmentosa. Investig Ophthalmol Vis Sci. 2013;54:585–91.
80. Oishi A, Ogino K, Makiyama Y, Nakagawa S, Kurimoto M, Yoshimura N. Wide-field fundus autofluorescence imaging of retinitis pigmentosa. Ophthalmology. 2013;120:1827–34.
81. Sun LW, Johnson RD, Langlo CS, et al. Assessing photoreceptor structure in retinitis pigmentosa and usher syndrome. Investig Ophthalmol Vis Sci. 2016;57:2428–42.
82. Ratnam K, Carroll J, Porco TC, Duncan JL, Roorda A. Relationship between foveal cone structure and clinical measures of visual function in patients with inherited retinal degenerations. Investig Ophthalmol Vis Sci. 2013;54:5836–47.
83. Pyo Park S, Hwan Hong I, Tsang SH, Chang S. Cellular imaging demonstrates genetic mosaicism in heterozygous carriers of an X-linked ciliopathy gene. Eur J Hum Genet. 2013; https://doi.org/10.1038/ejhg.2013.21.
84. Sun H, Nathans J. Mechanistic studies of ABCR, the ABC transporter in photoreceptor outer segments responsible for autosomal recessive Stargardt disease. J Bioenerg Biomembr. 2001;33(6):523–30. https://doi.org/10.1023/A:1012883306823.
85. Rice DS, Calandria JM, Gordon WC, Jun B, Zhou Y, Gelfman CM, et al. Adiponectin receptor 1 conserves docosahexaenoic acid and promotes photoreceptor cell survival. Nat Commun. 2015;6:6228. https://doi.org/10.1038/ncomms7228.
86. Zhao G, Xu M, Zhao M, Dai X, Kong W, Gerald M, et al. ADIPOR1 is mutated in syndromic retinitis pigmentosa. Hum Mutat. 2013;82:34–44. https://doi.org/10.1038/ki.2012.40.Activation.
87. Astuti GDN, Arno G, Hull S, Pierrache L, Venselaar H, Carss K, et al. Mutations in AGBL5, encoding a-tubulin deglutamylase, are associated with autosomal recessive retinitis pigmentosa. Investig Ophthalmol Vis Sci. 2016;57:6180–7. https://doi.org/10.1167/iovs.16-20148.
88. Zhou Y, Li S, Huang L, Yang Y, Zhang L, Yang M, et al. A splicing mutation in aryl hydrocarbon receptor associated with retinitis pigmentosa. Hum Mol Genet. 2018;27:2563–72. https://doi.org/10.1093/hmg/ddy165.
89. Arno G, Carss KJ, Hull S, Zihni C, Robson AG, Fiorentino A, et al. Biallelic mutation of ARHGEF18, involved in the determination of epithelial apicobasal polarity, causes adult-onset retinal degeneration. Am J Hum Genet. 2017;100:334–42. https://doi.org/10.1016/j.ajhg.2016.12.014.
90. Loosli F. ArhGEF18 regulated Rho signaling in vertebrate retina development. Small GTPases. 2013;4(4):242–6. https://doi.org/10.4161/sgtp.27061.
91. Davidson AE, Schwarz N, Zelinger L, Stern-Schneider G, Shoemark A, Spitzbarth B, et al. Mutations in ARL2BP, encoding ADP-ribosylation-factor-like 2 binding protein, cause autosomal-

recessive retinitis pigmentosa. Am J Hum Genet. 2013;93:321–9. https://doi.org/10.1016/j.ajhg.2013.06.003.
92. Moye AR, Singh R, Kimler VA, Dilan TL, Munezero D, Saravanan T, et al. ARL2BP, a protein linked to retinitis pigmentosa, is needed for normal photoreceptor cilia doublets and outer segment structure. Mol Biol Cell. 2018;29:1590–8. https://doi.org/10.1091/mbc.E18-01-0040.
93. Hanke-Gogokhia C, Wu Z, Gerstner CD, Frederick JM, Zhang H, Baehr W. Arf-like protein 3 (ARL3) regulates protein trafficking and ciliogenesis in mouse photoreceptors. J Biol Chem. 2016;291:7142–55. https://doi.org/10.1074/jbc.M115.710954.
94. May-Simera H, Nagel-Wolfrum K, Wolfrum U. Cilia - the sensory antennae in the eye. Prog Retin Eye Res. 2017;60:144–80. https://doi.org/10.1016/j.preteyeres.2017.05.001.
95. Chou HT, Apelt L, Farrell DP, White SR, Woodsmith J, Svetlov V, et al. The molecular architecture of native BBSome obtained by an integrated structural approach. Structure. 2019;27:1384–1394.e4. https://doi.org/10.1016/j.str.2019.06.006.
96. Mouraõ A, Nager AR, Nachury MV, Lorentzen E. Structural basis for membrane targeting of the BBSome by ARL6. Nat Struct Mol Biol. 2014;21:1035–41. https://doi.org/10.1038/nsmb.2920.
97. Wingfield JL, Lechtreck KF, Lorentzen E. Trafficking of ciliary membrane proteins by the intraflagellar transport/BBSome machinery. Essays Biochem. Portland Press Ltd. 2018;62(6):753–63. https://doi.org/10.1042/EBC20180030.
98. Corral-Serrano JC, Lamers IJC, Van Reeuwijk J, Duijkers L, Hoogendoorn ADM, Yildirim A, et al. PCARE and WASF3 regulate ciliary F-actin assembly that is required for the initiation of photoreceptor outer segment disk formation. Proc Natl Acad Sci U S A. 2020;117:9922–31. https://doi.org/10.1073/pnas.1903125117.
99. Gerth-Kahlert C, Tiwari A, Hanson JVM, Batmanabane V, Traboulsi E, Pennesi ME, et al. C2orf71 mutations as a frequent cause of autosomal-recessive retinitis pigmentosa: clinical analysis and presentation of 8 novel mutations. Investig Ophthalmol Vis Sci. 2017;58:3840–50. https://doi.org/10.1167/iovs.17-21597.
100. Sharif AS, Yu D, Loertscher S, Austin R, Nguyen K, Mathur PD, et al. C8ORF37 is required for photoreceptor outer segment disc morphogenesis by maintaining outer segment membrane protein homeostasis. J Neurosci. 2018;38:3160–76. https://doi.org/10.1523/JNEUROSCI.2964-17.2018.
101. Domènech EB, Andrés R, López-Iniesta MJ, Mirra S, García-Arroyo R, Milla S, et al. A new Cerkl mouse model generated by CRISPR-Cas9 Shows progressive retinal degeneration and altered morphological and electrophysiological phenotype. Invest Ophthalmol Vis Sci. 2020;61:14. https://doi.org/10.1167/iovs.61.8.14.
102. Li L, Jiao X, D'Atri I, Ono F, Nelson R, Chan CC, et al. Mutation in the intracellular chloride channel CLCC1 associated with autosomal recessive retinitis pigmentosa. PLoS Genet. 2018;14:1–29. https://doi.org/10.1371/journal.pgen.1007504.
103. Khan MI, Kersten FFJ, Azam M, Collin RWJ, Hussain A, Shah STA, et al. CLRN1 mutations cause nonsyndromic retinitis pigmentosa. Ophthalmology. 2011;118:1444–8. https://doi.org/10.1016/j.ophtha.2010.10.047.
104. Zallocchi M, Meehan DT, Delimont D, Askew C, Garige S, Gratton MA, et al. Localization and expression of clarin-1, the Clrn1 gene product, in auditory hair cells and photoreceptors. Hear Res. 2009;255:109–20. https://doi.org/10.1016/j.heares.2009.06.006.
105. Dhallan RS, Macke JP, Eddy RL, Shows TB, Reed RR, Yau KW, et al. Human rod photoreceptor cGMP-gated channel: amino acid sequence, gene structure, and functional expression. J Neurosci. 1992;12:3248–56. https://doi.org/10.1523/jneurosci.12-08-03248.1992.
106. Batra-Safferling R, Abarca-Heidemann K, Körschen HG, Tziatzios C, Stoldt M, Budyak I, et al. Glutamic acid-rich proteins of rod photoreceptors are natively unfolded. J Biol Chem. 2006;281:1449–60. https://doi.org/10.1074/jbc.M505012200.
107. Poetsch A, Molday LL, Molday RS. The cGMP-gated channel and related glutamic acid-rich proteins interact with Peripherin-2 at the rim region of rod photoreceptor disc membranes. J Biol Chem. 2001;276:48009–16. https://doi.org/10.1074/jbc.M108941200.
108. Alves CH, Pellissier LP, Wijnholds J. The CRB1 and adherens junction complex proteins in retinal development and maintenance. Prog Retin Eye Res. 2014;40:35–52. https://doi.org/10.1016/j.preteyeres.2014.01.001.
109. Quinn PM, Pellissier LP, Wijnholds J. The CRB1 complex: following the trail of crumbs to a feasible gene therapy strategy. Front Neurosci. 2017;11:175. https://doi.org/10.3389/fnins.2017.00175.
110. Tran NM, Chen S. Mechanisms of blindness: animal models provide insight into distinct CRX-associated retinopathies. Dev Dyn. 2014;243:1153–66. https://doi.org/10.1002/dvdy.24151.
111. Wang Y, Guo L, Cai SP, Dai M, Yang Q, Yu W, et al. Exome sequencing identifies compound heterozygous mutations in CYP4V2 in a pedigree with retinitis pigmentosa. PLoS One. 2012;7:1–7. https://doi.org/10.1371/journal.pone.0033673.
112. Edani BH, Grabińska KA, Zhang R, Park EJ, Siciliano B, Surmacz L, et al. Structural elucidation of the *cis* -prenyltransferase NgBR/DHDDS complex reveals insights in regulation of protein glycosylation. Proc Natl Acad Sci. 2020;117:20794–802. https://doi.org/10.1073/pnas.2008381117.
113. Zuchner S, Dallman J, Wen R, Beecham G, Naj A, Farooq A, et al. Whole-exome sequencing links a variant in DHDDS to retinitis pigmentosa. Am J Hum

Genet. 2011;88:201–6. https://doi.org/10.1016/j.ajhg.2011.01.001.
114. Latif Z, Chakchouk I, Schrauwen I, Lee K, Santos-Cortez RLP, Abbe I, et al. Confirmation of the role of DHX38 in the etiology of early-onset retinitis pigmentosa. Investig Ophthalmol Vis Sci. 2018;59:4552–7. https://doi.org/10.1167/iovs.18-23849.
115. Abu-Safieh L, Alrashed M, Anazi S, Alkuraya H, Khan AO, Al-Owain M, et al. Autozygome-guided exome sequencing in retinal dystrophy patients reveals pathogenetic mutations and novel candidate disease genes. Genome Res. 2013;23:236–47. https://doi.org/10.1101/gr.144105.112.
116. Lu Z, Hu X, Liu F, Soares DC, Liu X, Yu S, et al. Ablation of EYS in zebrafish causes mislocalisation of outer segment proteins, F-actin disruption and cone-rod dystrophy. Sci Rep. 2017;7:46098. https://doi.org/10.1038/srep46098.
117. Messchaert M, Dona M, Broekman S, Peters TA, Corral-Serrano JC, Slijkerman RWN, et al. Eyes shut homolog is important for the maintenance of photoreceptor morphology and visual function in zebrafish. PLoS One. 2018;13:1–16. https://doi.org/10.1371/journal.pone.0200789.
118. Di Gioia SA, SJF L, Kostic C, Bandah-rozenfeld D, Hetterschijt L, Sharon D, et al. FAM161a, associated with retinitis pigmentosa, is a component of the cilia-basal body complex and interacts with proteins involved in ciliopathies. Hum Mol Genet. 2012;21:5174–84. https://doi.org/10.1093/hmg/dds368.
119. Karlstetter M, Sorusch N, Caramoy A, Dannhausen K, Aslanidis A, Fauser S, et al. Disruption of the retinitis pigmentosa 28 gene Fam161a in mice affects photoreceptor ciliary structure and leads to progressive retinal degeneration. Hum Mol Genet. 2014;23(19):5197–210. https://doi.org/10.1093/hmg/ddu242.
120. Zach F, Grassmann F, Langmann T, Sorusch N, Wolfrum U, Stöhr H. The retinitis pigmentosa 28 protein FAM161A is a novel ciliary protein involved in intermolecular protein interaction and microtubule association. Hum Mol Genet. 2012;21:4573–86. https://doi.org/10.1093/hmg/dds268.
121. Lin-Jones J, Burnside B. Retina-specific protein fascin 2 is an actin cross-linker associated with actin bundles in photoreceptor inner segments and calycal processes. Investig Ophthalmol Vis Sci. 2007;48:1380–8. https://doi.org/10.1167/iovs.06-0763.
122. Vinberg F, Peshenko IV, Chen J, Dizhoor AM, Kefalov VJ. Guanylate cyclase–activating protein 2 contributes to phototransduction and light adaptation in mouse cone photoreceptors. J Biol Chem. 2018;293:7457–65. https://doi.org/10.1074/jbc.RA117.001574.
123. Haer-Wigman L, Newman H, Leibu R, Bax NM, Baris HN, Rizel L, et al. Non-syndromic retinitis pigmentosa due to mutations in the mucopolysaccharidosis type IIIC gene, heparan-alpha-glucosaminide N-acetyltransferase (HGSNAT). Hum Mol Genet. 2015;24:3742–51. https://doi.org/10.1093/hmg/ddv118.
124. Hartong DT, Dange M, McGee TL, Berson EL, Dryja TP, Colman RF. Insights from retinitis pigmentosa into the roles of isocitrate dehydrogenases in the Krebs cycle. Nat Genet. 2008;40:1230–4. https://doi.org/10.1038/ng.223.
125. Hull S, Owen N, Islam F, Tracey-White D, Plagnol V, Holder GE, et al. Nonsyndromic retinal dystrophy due to bi-allelic mutations in the ciliary transport gene *IFT140*. Investig Opthalmology Vis Sci. 2016;57:1053. https://doi.org/10.1167/iovs.15-17976.
126. Crouse JA, Lopes VS, Sanagustin JT, Keady BT, Williams DS, Pazour GJ. Distinct functions for IFT140 and IFT20 in opsin transport. Cytoskeleton. 2014;71:302–10. https://doi.org/10.1002/cm.21173.
127. Taschner M, Weber K, Mourão A, Vetter M, Awasthi M, Stiegler M, et al. Intraflagellar transport proteins 172, 80, 57, 54, 38, and 20 form a stable tubulin-binding IFT -B2 complex. EMBO J. 2016;35:773–90. https://doi.org/10.15252/embj.201593164.
128. Bennett LD, Klein M, John FT, Radojevic B, Jones K, Birch DG. Disease progression in patients with autosomal dominant retinitis pigmentosa due to a mutation in inosine monophosphate dehydrogenase 1 (IMPDH1). Transl Vis Sci Technol. 2020;9:14. https://doi.org/10.1167/tvst.9.5.14.
129. Olivier G, Corton M, Intartaglia D, Verbakel SK, Dhaenens M, Sergouniotis PI, et al. Pathogenic variants in IMPG1 cause autosomal dominant and autosomal recessive retinitis pigmentosa. J Med Genet. 2020;1:1–9. https://doi.org/10.1136/jmedgenet-2020-107150.
130. Bandah-Rozenfeld D, Collin RW, Banin E, van den Born LI, Coene KL, Siemiatkowska AM, et al. Mutations in IMPG2, encoding interphotoreceptor matrix proteoglycan 2, cause autosomal-recessive retinitis pigmentosa. Am J Hum Genet. 2010;87:199–208. https://doi.org/10.1016/j.ajhg.2010.07.004.
131. De Bruijn SE, Verbakel SK, De Vrieze E, Kremer H, Cremers FPM, Hoyng CB, et al. Homozygous variants in KIAA1549, encoding a ciliary protein, are associated with autosomal recessive retinitis pigmentosa. J Med Genet. 2018;55:705–12. https://doi.org/10.1136/jmedgenet-2018-105364.
132. El SS, Méjécase C, Bertelli M, Terray A, Michiels C, Condroyer C, et al. Further insights into the ciliary gene and protein KIZ and its murine ortholog PLK1S1 mutated in rod-cone dystrophy. Genes (Basel). 2017;8:1–19. https://doi.org/10.3390/genes8100277.
133. Friedman JS, Ray JW, Waseem N, Johnson K, Brooks MJ, Hugosson T, et al. Mutations in a BTB-Kelch protein, KLHL7, cause autosomal-dominant retinitis pigmentosa. Am J Hum Genet. 2009;84:792–800. https://doi.org/10.1016/j.ajhg.2009.05.007.

134. Sears AE, Palczewski K. Lecithin:retinol acyltransferase: a key enzyme involved in the retinoid (visual) cycle. Biochemistry. 2016;55:3082–91.
135. Omori Y, Chaya T, Katoh K, Kajimura N, Sato S, Muraoka K, et al. Negative regulation of ciliary length by ciliary male germ cell-associated kinase (Mak) is required for retinal photoreceptor survival. Proc Natl Acad Sci U S A. 2010;107:22671–6. https://doi.org/10.1073/pnas.1009437108.
136. Roosing S, Collin RWJ, den Hollander AI, Cremers FPM, Siemiatkowska AM. Prenylation defects in inherited retinal diseases. J Med Genet. 2014;51:143–51. https://doi.org/10.1136/jmedgenet-2013-102138.
137. Nishiguchi KM, Tearle RG, Liu YP, Oh EC, Miyake N, Benaglio P, et al. Whole genome sequencing in patients with retinitis pigmentosa reveals pathogenic DNA structural changes and NEK2 as a new disease gene. Proc Natl Acad Sci U S A. 2013;110:16139–44. https://doi.org/10.1073/pnas.1308243110.
138. Wang F, Li H, Xu M, Li H, Zhao L, Yang L, et al. A homozygous missense mutation in NEUROD1 is associated with nonsyndromic autosomal recessive retinitis pigmentosa. Investig Ophthalmol Vis Sci. 2015;56:150–5. https://doi.org/10.1167/iovs.14-15382.
139. Coppieters F, Leroy BP, Beysen D, Hellemans J, De Bosscher K, Haegeman G, et al. Recurrent mutation in the first zinc finger of the orphan nuclear receptor NR2E3 causes autosomal dominant retinitis pigmentosa. Am J Hum Genet. 2007;81:147–57. https://doi.org/10.1086/518426.
140. Moore SM, Skowronska-Krawczyk D, Chao DL. Targeting of the NRL pathway as a therapeutic strategy to treat retinitis pigmentosa. J Clin Med. 2020;9:2224. https://doi.org/10.3390/jcm9072224.
141. Wang J, Chen X, Wang F, Zhang J, Li P, Li Z, et al. OFD1, as a ciliary protein, exhibits neuroprotective function in photoreceptor degeneration models. PLoS One. 2016;11:1–18. https://doi.org/10.1371/journal.pone.0155860.
142. Stryer L. Cyclic GMP cascade of vision. Annu Rev Neurosci. 1986;9:87–119.
143. Xu M, Yamada T, Sun Z, Eblimit A, Lopez I, Wang F, et al. Mutations in POMGNT1 cause non-syndromic retinitis pigmentosa. Hum Mol Genet. 2016;25:1479–88. https://doi.org/10.1093/hmg/ddw022.
144. Spencer WJ, Ding JD, Lewis TR, Yu C, Phan S, Pearring JN, et al. PRCD is essential for high-fidelity photoreceptor disc formation. Proc Natl Acad Sci U S A. 2019;116:13087–96. https://doi.org/10.1073/pnas.1906421116.
145. Goldberg AFX, Moritz OL, Williams DS. Molecular basis for photoreceptor outer segment architecture. Prog Retin Eye Res. 2016; https://doi.org/10.1016/j.preteyeres.2016.05.003.
146. Růžičková Š, Staněk D. Mutations in spliceosomal proteins and retina degeneration. RNA Biol. 2017;14:544–52. https://doi.org/10.1080/15476286.2016.1191735.
147. Tanackovic G, Ransijn A, Thibault P, Abou Elela S, Klinck R, Berson EL, et al. PRPF mutations are associated with generalized defects in spliceosome formation and pre-mRNA splicing in patients with retinitis pigmentosa. Hum Mol Genet. 2011;20:2116–30. https://doi.org/10.1093/hmg/ddr094.
148. den Hollander AI, McGee TL, Ziviello C, Banfi S, Dryja TP, Gonzalez-Fernandez F, et al. A homozygous missense mutation in the IRBP gene (RBP3) associated with autosomal recessive retinitis pigmentosa. Invest Ophthalmol Vis Sci. 2009;50:1864–72. https://doi.org/10.1167/iovs.08-2497.
149. Sarkar H, Moosajee M. Retinol dehydrogenase 12 (RDH12): role in vision, retinal disease and future perspectives. Exp Eye Res. 2019;188:107793.
150. Agrawal SA, Burgoyne T, Eblimit A, Bellingham J, Parfitt DA, Lane A, et al. REEP6 deficiency leads to retinal degeneration through disruption of ER homeostasis and protein trafficking. Hum Mol Genet. 2017;26:2667–77. https://doi.org/10.1093/hmg/ddx149.
151. Ba-Abbad R, Leys M, Wang X, Chakarova C, Waseem N, Carss KJ, et al. Clinical features of a retinopathy associated with a dominant allele of the RGR gene. Invest Ophthalmol Vis Sci. 2018;59:4812–20. https://doi.org/10.1167/iovs.18-25061.
152. Hargrave PA. Rhodopsin structure, function, and topography the Friedenwald lecture. Invest Ophthalmol Vis Sci. 2001;42:3–9. Available: http://www.ncbi.nlm.nih.gov/pubmed/11133841
153. Lima de Carvalho JR, Kim HJ, Ueda K, Zhao J, Owji AP, Yang T, et al. Effects of deficiency in the RLBP1-encoded visual cycle protein CRALBP on visual dysfunction in humans and mice. J Biol Chem. 2020;295:6767–80. https://doi.org/10.1074/jbc.RA120.012695.
154. Loewen CJR, Molday RS. Disulfide-mediated oligomerization of peripherin/Rds and Rom-1 in photoreceptor disk membranes: implications for photoreceptor outer segment morphogenesis and degeneration. J Biol Chem. 2000;275:5370–8.
155. Liu Q, Lyubarsky A, Skalet JH, Pugh EN, Pierce EA. RP1 is required for the correct stacking of outer segment discs. Invest Ophthalmol Vis Sci. 2003;44:4171–83.
156. Yamashita T, Liu J, Gao J, LeNoue S, Wang C, Kaminoh J, et al. Essential and synergistic roles of RP1 and RP1L1 in rod photoreceptor axoneme and retinitis pigmentosa. J Neurosci. 2009;29:9748–60. https://doi.org/10.1523/JNEUROSCI.5854-08.2009.
157. Schwarz N, Lane A, Jovanovic K, Parfitt DA, Aguila M, Thompson CL, et al. Arl3 and RP2 regulate the trafficking of ciliary tip kinesins. Hum Mol Genet. 2017;26:2480–92. https://doi.org/10.1093/hmg/ddx143.
158. Moiseyev GCY, Takahashi Y, Wu BX, Ma J. RPE65 is the isomerohydrolase in the retinoid visual cycle. Proc Natl Acad Sci U S A. 2005;102:12413–8.

159. Megaw RD, Soares DC, Wright AF. RPGR: its role in photoreceptor physiology, human disease, and future therapies. Exp Eye Res. 2015;138:32–41.
160. Gurevich VV, Gurevich EV, Cleghorn WM. Arrestins as multi-functional Signaling adaptors. Handbook of experimental pharmacology. Handb Exp Pharmacol. 2008;186:15–37. https://doi.org/10.1007/978-3-540-72843-6_2.
161. Corton M, Avila-Fernández A, Campello L, Sánchez M, Benavides B, López-Molina MI, et al. Identification of the photoreceptor transcriptional co-repressor SAMD11 as novel cause of autosomal recessive retinitis pigmentosa. Sci Rep. 2016;6:1–13. https://doi.org/10.1038/srep35370.
162. Jin ZB, Huang XF, Lv JN, Xiang L, Li DQ, Chen J, et al. SLC7A14 linked to autosomal recessive retinitis pigmentosa. Nat Commun. 2014;5:3517. https://doi.org/10.1038/ncomms4517.
163. MacLaren RE, Yusuf IH, Birtel J, Shanks ME, Clouston P, Downes SM, et al. Clinical characterization of retinitis pigmentosa associated with variants in SNRNP200. JAMA Ophthalmol. 2019;137:1295–300. https://doi.org/10.1001/jamaophthalmol.2019.3298.
164. Dharmat R, Eblimit A, Robichaux MA, Zhang Z, Nguyen TMT, Jung SY, et al. SPATA7 maintains a novel photoreceptor-specific zone in the distal connecting cilium. J Cell Biol. 2018;217:2851–65. https://doi.org/10.1083/jcb.201712117.
165. Liu Y, Chen X, Xu Q, Gao X, Tam POS, Zhao K, et al. SPP2 mutations cause autosomal dominant retinitis pigmentosa. Sci Rep. 2015;5:1–10. https://doi.org/10.1038/srep14867.
166. Chakarova CF, Khanna H, Shah AZ, Patil SB, Sedmak T, Murga-Zamalloa CA, et al. TOPORS, implicated in retinal degeneration, is a cilia-centrosomal protein. Hum Mol Genet. 2011;20:975–87. https://doi.org/10.1093/hmg/ddq543.
167. Sharma TP, Wiley LA, Whitmore SS, Anfinson KR, Cranston CM, Oppedal DJ, et al. Patient-specific induced pluripotent stem cells to evaluate the pathophysiology of TRNT1-associated retinitis pigmentosa. Stem Cell Res. 2017;21:58–70. https://doi.org/10.1016/j.scr.2017.03.005.
168. Goyal S, Jäger M, Robinson PN, Vanita V. Confirmation of TTC8 as a disease gene for nonsyndromic autosomal recessive retinitis pigmentosa (RP51). Clin Genet. 2016;89:454–60. https://doi.org/10.1111/cge.12644.
169. Lobo GP, Au A, Kiser PD, Hagstrom SA. Involvement of endoplasmic reticulum stress in TULP1 induced retinal degeneration. PLoS One. 2016;11:e0151806. https://doi.org/10.1371/journal.pone.0151806.
170. French LS, Mellough CB, Chen FK, Carvalho LS. A review of gene, drug and cell-based therapies for usher syndrome. Front Cell Neurosci. 2020;14:183. https://doi.org/10.3389/fncel.2020.00183.
171. Avila-Fernandez A, Perez-Carro R, Corton M, Lopez-Molina MI, Campello L, Garanto A, et al. Whole-exome sequencing reveals ZNF408 as a new gene associated with autosomal recessive retinitis pigmentosa with vitreal alterations. Hum Mol Genet. 2015;24:4037–48. https://doi.org/10.1093/hmg/ddv140.
172. Li L, Nakaya N, Chavali VRM, Ma Z, Jiao X, Sieving PA, et al. A mutation in ZNF513, a putative regulator of photoreceptor development, causes autosomal-recessive retinitis pigmentosa. Am J Hum Genet. 2010;87:400–9. https://doi.org/10.1016/j.ajhg.2010.08.003.
173. Wald G. The molecular basis of visual excitation. Nature. 1968;219:800–7.
174. Gurevich VV, Gurevich EV, Cleghorn WM. Arrestins as multi-functional signaling adaptors. In: Handbook of experimental pharmacology. 2008. p. 15–37.
175. Krispel CM, Chen D, Melling N, Chen YJ, Martemyanov KA, Quillinan N, Arshavsky VY, Wensel TG, Chen CK, Burns ME. RGS expression rate-limits recovery of rod photoresponses. Neuron. 2006;51:409–16.
176. Koch KW, Stryer L. Highly cooperative feedback control of retinal rod guanylate cyclase by calcium ions. Nature. 1988;334:64–6.
177. Haeseleer F, Sokal I, Li N, Pettenati M, Rao N, Bronson D, Wechter R, Baehr W, Palczewski K. Molecular characterization of a third member of the guanylyl cyclase-activating protein subfamily. J Biol Chem. 1999;274:6526–35.
178. Tachibanaki S, Arinobu D, Shimauchi-Matsukawa Y, Tsushima S, Kawamura S. Highly effective phosphorylation by G protein-coupled receptor kinase 7 of light-activated visual pigment in cones. Proc Natl Acad Sci U S A. 2005;102:9329–34.
179. Tachibanaki S, Tsushima S, Kawamura S. Low amplification and fast visual pigment phosphorylation as mechanisms characterizing cone photoresponses. Proc Natl Acad Sci U S A. 2001;98:14044–9.
180. Trehan A, Cañada FJ, Rando RR. Inhibitors of retinyl ester formation also prevent the biosynthesis of 11-cis-retinol. Biochemistry. 1990;29:309–12.
181. Saari JC, Nawrot M, Kennedy BN, Garwin GG, Hurley JB, Huang J, Possin DE, Crabb JW. Visual cycle impairment in cellular retinaldehyde binding protein (CRALBP) knockout mice results in delayed dark adaptation. Neuron. 2001;29:739–48.
182. Moiseyev G, Chen Y, Takahashi Y, Wu BX, Ma J. RPE65 is the isomerohydrolase in the retinoid visual cycle. Proc Natl Acad Sci U S A. 2005;102:12413–8.
183. Lee L. Mechanisms of mammalian ciliary motility: insights from primary ciliary dyskinesia genetics. Gene. 2011;473:57–66.
184. Goetz SC, Anderson KV. The primary cilium: a signalling centre during vertebrate development. Nat Rev Genet. 2010;11:331–44.
185. Chen HY, Kelley RA, Li T, Swaroop A. Primary cilia biogenesis and associated retinal ciliopathies. SCDB. 2020; https://doi.org/10.1016/j.semcdb.2020.07.013.

186. Prevo B, Scholey JM, Peterman EJG. Intraflagellar transport: mechanisms of motor action, cooperation, and cargo delivery. FEBS J. 2017;284:2905–31.
187. Blacque OE, Reardon MJ, Li C, et al. Loss of C. elegans BBS-7 and BBS-8 protein function results in cilia defects and compromised intraflagellar transport. Genes Dev. 2004;18:1630–42.
188. Schwarz N, Lane A, Jovanovic K, et al. Arl3 and RP2 regulate the trafficking of ciliary tip kinesins. Hum Mol Genet. 2017;26:2480–92.
189. Nakayama K, Katoh Y. Architecture of the IFT ciliary trafficking machinery and interplay between its components. Crit Rev Biochem Mol Biol. 2020; https://doi.org/10.1080/10409238.2020.1768206.
190. Zaghloul NA, Katsanis N. Mechanistic insights into Bardet-Biedl syndrome, a model ciliopathy. J Clin Invest. 2009;119:428–37. https://doi.org/10.1172/JCI37041.
191. Weihbrecht K, Goar WA, Pak T, Garrison JE, DeLuca AP, Stone EM, Scheetz TE, Sheffield VC. Keeping an Eye on Bardet-Biedl Syndrome: A Comprehensive Review of the Role of Bardet-Biedl Syndrome Genes in the Eye. Med Res Arch. 2017;5 https://doi.org/10.18103/mra.v5i9.1526.
192. Gonçalves J, Pelletier L. The ciliary transition zone: finding the pieces and assembling the gate. Mol Cells. 2017;40:243–53.
193. Inoue T, Lin YC, Niewiadomski P, Lin B, Nakamura H, Phua SC, Jiao J, Levchenko A, Inoue T, Rohatgi R. Chemically inducible diffusion trap at cilia reveals molecular sieve-like barrier. Nat Chem Biol. 2013;9:437–43.
194. Sang L, Miller JJ, Corbit KC, et al. Mapping the NPHP-JBTS-MKS protein network reveals ciliopathy disease genes and pathways. Cell. 2011;145:513–28.
195. Dharmat R, Eblimit A, Robichaux MA, et al. SPATA7 maintains a novel photoreceptor-specific zone in the distal connecting cilium. J Cell Biol. 2018;217:2851–65.
196. Eblimit A, Nguyen TMT, Chen Y, et al. Spata7 is a retinal ciliopathy gene critical for correct RPGRIP1 localization and protein trafficking in the retina. Hum Mol Genet. 2015;24:1584–601.
197. Steinberg RH, Fisher SK, Anderson DH. Disc morphogenesis in vertebrate photoreceptors. J Comp Neurol. 1980;190:501–18.
198. Salinas RY, Pearring JN, Ding JD, Spencer WJ, Hao Y, Arshavsky VY. Photoreceptor discs form through peripherin dependent suppression of ciliary ectosome release. J Cell Biol. 2017;216:1489–99.
199. Strayve D, Makia MM, Kakakhel M, Sakthivel H, Conley SM, Al-Ubaidi MR, Naash MI. ROM1 contributes to phenotypic heterogeneity in PRPH2-associated retinal disease. Hum Mol Genet. 2020; https://doi.org/10.1093/hmg/ddaa160.
200. Yang Z, Chen Y, Lillo C, et al. Mutant prominin 1 found in patients with macular degeneration disrupts photoreceptor disk morphogenesis in mice. J Clin Invest. 2008;118:2908–16.
201. Yamashita T, Liu J, Gao J, et al. Essential and synergistic roles of RP1 and RP1L1 in rod photoreceptor axoneme and retinitis pigmentosa. J Neurosci. 2009;29:9748–60.
202. Ishikawa M, Sawada Y, Yoshitomi T. Structure and function of the interphotoreceptor matrix surrounding retinal photoreceptor cells. Exp Eye Res. 2015;133:3–18.
203. Al-Ubaidi MR, Naash MI, Conley SM. A perspective on the role of the extracellular matrix in progressive retinal degenerative disorders. Invest Ophthalmol Vis Sci. 2013;54:8119–24.
204. Hollyfield JG. Hyaluronan and the functional organization of the interphotoreceptor matrix. Invest Ophthalmol Vis Sci. 1999;40:2767–9.
205. van Huet RA, Collin RW, Siemiatkowska AM, et al. IMPG2-associated retinitis pigmentosa displays relatively early macular involvement. Invest Ophthalmol Vis Sci. 2014;55:3939–53.
206. Zhang Q, Xu M, Verriotto JD, Li Y, Wang H, Gan L, Lam BL, Chen R. Next-generation sequencing-based molecular diagnosis of 35 Hispanic retinitis pigmentosa probands. Sci Rep. 2016;6:1–8.
207. den Hollander AI, McGee TL, Ziviello C, Banfi S, Dryja TP, Gonzalez-Fernandez F, Ghosh D, Berson EL. A homozygous missense mutation in the IRBP gene (RBP3) associated with autosomal recessive retinitis pigmentosa. Invest Ophthalmol Vis Sci. 2009;50:1864–72.
208. Littink KW, van den Born LI, Koenekoop RK, et al. Mutations in the EYS gene account for approximately 5% of autosomal recessive retinitis pigmentosa and cause a fairly homogeneous phenotype. Ophthalmology. 2010;117:2026–33, 2033.e1–7.
209. Inoue Y, Yoneda M, Miyaishi O, Iwaki M, Zako M. Hyaluronan dynamics during retinal development. Brain Res. 2009;1256:55–60.
210. Alfano G, Kruczek PM, Shah AZ, Kramarz B, Jeffery G, Zelhof AC, Bhattacharya SS. EYS is a protein associated with the ciliary axoneme in rods and cones. PLoS One. 2016; https://doi.org/10.1371/journal.pone.0166397.
211. Lu Z, Hu X, Liu F, et al. Ablation of EYS in zebrafish causes mislocalisation of outer segment proteins. F-actin disruption and cone-rod dystrophy. Sci Rep. 2017; https://doi.org/10.1038/srep46098.
212. Messchaert M, Dona M, Broekman S, Peters TA, Corral-Serrano JC, Slijkerman RWN, van Wijk E, Collin RWJ. Eyes shut homolog is important for the maintenance of photoreceptor morphology and visual function in zebrafish. PLoS One. 2018;13:1–16.
213. Pruett RC. Retinitis pigmentosa: clinical observations and correlations. Trans Am Ophthalmol Soc. 1983;81:693–735.
214. Fishman GA, Anderson RJ, Lourenco P, Lourenq P, Lourenco P. Prevalence of posterior subcapsular lens opacities in patients with retinitis pigmentosa. Br J Ophthalmol. 1985;69:263–6.

215. Berson EL, Rosner B, Simonoff E. Risk factors for genetic typing and detection in retinitis pigmentosa. Am J Ophthalmol. 1980;89:763–75.
216. Yoshida N, Ikeda Y, Murakami Y, Nakatake S, Fujiwara K, Notomi S, Hisatomi T, Ishibashi T. Factors affecting visual acuity after cataract surgery in patients with retinitis pigmentosa. Ophthalmology. 2015;122:903–8.
217. Bakthavatchalam M, Lai FHP, Rong SS, Ng DS, Brelen ME. Treatment of cystoid macular edema secondary to retinitis pigmentosa: a systematic review. Surv Ophthalmol. 2018;63:329–39.
218. Huang Q, Chen R, Lin X, Xiang Z. Efficacy of carbonic anhydrase inhibitors in management of cystoid macular edema in retinitis pigmentosa: a meta-analysis. PLoS One. 2017;12:e0186180.
219. Thobani A, Fishman GA. The use of carbonic anhydrase inhibitors in the retreatment of cystic macular lesions in retinitis pigmentosa and X-linked retinoschisis. Retina. 2011;31:312–5.
220. Veritti D, Sarao V, De Nadai K, Chizzolini M, Parmeggiani F, Perissin L, Lanzetta P. Dexamethasone implant produces better outcomes than oral acetazolamide in patients with cystoid macular edema secondary to retinitis pigmentosa. J Ocul Pharmacol Ther. 2020;36:190–7.
221. Strong S, Liew G, Michaelides M. Retinitis pigmentosa-associated cystoid macular oedema: pathogenesis and avenues of intervention. Br J Ophthalmol. 2017;101:31–7.
222. Ikeda Y, Yoshida N, Murakami Y, Nakatake S, Notomi S, Hisatomi T, Enaida H, Ishibashi T. Long-term surgical outcomes of epiretinal membrane in patients with retinitis pigmentosa. Sci Rep. 2015; https://doi.org/10.1038/srep13078.
223. Suzuki K, Tsunekawa Y, Hernandez-Benitez R, et al. In vivo genome editing via CRISPR/Cas9 mediated homology-independent targeted integration. Nature. 2016;540:144–9.
224. Collin RWJ, Garanto A. Applications of antisense oligonucleotides for the treatment of inherited retinal diseases. Curr Opin Ophthalmol. 2017;28:260–6.
225. Brito-García N, Del Pino-Sedeño T, Trujillo-Martín M, Coco RM, Rodríguez De La Rúa E, Del Cura-González I, Serrano-Aguilar P. Effectiveness and safety of nutritional supplements in the treatment of hereditary retinal dystrophies: a systematic review. Eye. 2017;31:273–85.
226. Schwartz SG, Wang X, Chavis P, Kuriyan AE, Abariga SA. Vitamin A and fish oils for preventing the progression of retinitis pigmentosa. Cochrane database Syst Rev. 2020;6:CD008428.
227. Chakradhar S. An eye to the future: researchers debate best path for stem cell-derived therapies. Nat Med. 2016;22:116–9.

5 Syndromic Retinitis Pigmentosa

Chang Ki Yoon

5.1 Syndromic Retinitis Pigmentosa

Typical retinitis pigmentosa (RP) is defined as disease confined to eyeball. In some cases, mutations in known causal genes of RP result in the phenotype of RP and extraocular manifestations simultaneously. These genes are listed in Table 5.1. Moreover, there are systemic multi-organ disorders that show pigmentary retinopathy. Etiologies are variable including drug toxicity, infection, monogenic mutation. Some of these diseases have curable etiology or strategies to relieve or retard some conditions. Therefore, differential diagnosis is required to discriminate the cause of pigmentary retinopathy. A multidisciplinary approach is needed because systemic manifestations are quite heterogenous. In this chapter, inherited syndromic disorders showing typical pigmentary retinopathy will be described. Syndromic RP in this chapter includes Usher syndrome, ciliopathy, inborn errors of metabolism, and mitochondrial disorders (Table 5.2).

C. K. Yoon (✉)
Department of Ophthalmology, Seoul National University Hospital and Seoul National University College of Medicine, Seoul, Republic of Korea

5.2 Usher Syndrome

Usher syndrome is autosomal recessive disorder having retinopathy and sensorineural hearing loss (SNHL). Usher syndrome is most common syndromic RP, which accounts for 18% of RP [1]. Prevalence of Usher syndrome is reported to be 3.2–6.2 cases per 100,000 [2]. It comprises about 50% of total patients who have both blindness and deafness in the USA.

Usher syndrome is clinically classified into three types. Type 1 shows congenital SNHL, speech impairment, vestibular dysfunction, and retinopathy of childhood onset. Type 2 shows moderate, nonprogressive hearing deficit without vestibular dysfunction and milder, later-onset retinopathy [3]. In type 3, most rare form, hearing loss is found lately between the second and fourth decades of life and progresses slowly. Retinopathy may start in adulthood. Type 1 and type 2 comprise 33% and 67% of usher syndrome. And the rarest type 3 is 2–4% [4]. Type 3 is reported to be 40% in Finland or Ashkenazi Jewish populations [5].

In type 1 Usher, one of the earliest signs is vestibular dysfunction. It can manifest as motor development delay in childhood or nonprogressive ataxia in adulthood. Although affected patients overcome areflexia through vision before visual loss, they are prone to fall down and feel difficulty in activity requiring balancing. This is

H.-G. Yu (ed.), *Inherited Retinal Disease*, https://doi.org/10.1007/978-981-16-7337-5_5

Table 5.1 Genes underlying both syndromic and non-syndromic IRDs(RPs)

Genes	Syndromic IRD	Non-syndromic IRD
ABDH12	PHARC	arRP
AHI1	JBTS3	arRP
ARLBP2	RP with situs inversus	arRP
ARL3	JBTS35	adRP
ARL6	BBS3	arRP
BBS2	BBS2	arRP
C8ORF37	BBS2	arRP
CC2D2A	JBTS9, NKS6	arRP
CEP290	BBS14, JBTS5, MKS4, SLSN6	arLCA
CLN3	CLN3	arRP
CLRN1	USH3A	arRP
CWC27	RPSKA	arRP
DHDDS	CDG1BB	arRP
FLVCR1	PCARP	arRP
HGSNAT	MPS3C	arRP
IFT40	SRTD9 with/without polydactyly	arRP
IQCB1	SLSN5	arLCA
MVK	HIDS, MEVA	arRP
OFD1	JBTS10	XLRP
RPGR	RP, sinorespiratory infections and deafness	XLRP
TTC8	BBS8	arRP
USH2A	USH2A	arRP

arRP, autosomal recessive retinitis pigmentosa; arLCA, autosomal recessive Leber's congenital amaurosis; JBTS, Joubert syndrome

usually found at neonatal screening and suspected in infants where screening is not available. Hearing defect in type 2 is mild in low frequency and severe in high frequency. Hearing deficits do not usually progress. Vestibular function is usually normal. Some patients with type 2 have ataxia, which is supposed to be due to cerebellar atrophy. Night blindness develops around 15 years in type 1 while it presents variably until the thirties and after adolescent mostly in type 2 and 3 [3]. Visual prognosis is better in type 2 than type 1. While most patients lost vision around 15 years in type 1, those of type 2 preserve their vision longer. Proportion of patients who preserve at least 20/40 vision is 69% in type 1 and 94% in type 2. vision better than 20/80 was 89% in type 1 and 98% in type 2. In forties, 77% of type 1 and 95% of type 2 preserve better than 20/200 vision [4]. Macular lesion is well visualized in fluorescein angiogram. Foveal lesions were seen on fluorescein angiogram more frequently and at an earlier age in type 1 as compared with type 2. And foveal lesion is also more frequently found in type 1 than type 2. Posterior subcapsular cataract is observed in about 50% of both type 1 and 2. Electroretinogram is always profoundly abnormal. Retinal pigmentation is barely observed in early childhood. Numerous subtle retinal pigmentations can be mistaken as rubella retinopathy or some other retinal disease.

Simultaneous visual and auditory dysfunction requires sophisticated educational and social support for children having Usher. Although, visual rehabilitation is not available now, cochlear implant helps hearing recovery and language development for affected children.

Until now, 16 genes are reported to be associated with Usher syndrome. Genes related to type 1 include *MYO7A, USH1C, CDH23, PCDH15, USH1G, ESPN,* type 2 include *USH2A, ADGRV1, DFNB31*. Type 3 genes are *CLRN1* and *HARS*, and atypical Usher syndrome genes are *ABHD12, ARSG, CEP250, CEP78, and CIB2*. Genes associated with Usher syndrome mostly express proteins in hair bundle and ribbon synapse, which play an essential role in mechanoelectrical trans-

Table 5.2 Syndromic retinitis pigmentosa and associated causal genes

Disease	Genes
Usher syndrome	ABHD12, ADGRV1, ARSG, CDH23, CEP250, CEP78, CIB2, CLRN1, DFNB31, ESPN, HARS, MYO7A, PCDH15, USH1C, USH1G, USH2A
Ciliopathies	
Bardet-Biedl syndrome	ADIPOR1, ARL6, BBIP1, BBS1, BBS2, BBS4, BBS5, BBS7, BBS9, BBS10, BBS12, C8orf37, CEP19, CEP290, IFT172, IFT27, INPP5E, KCNJ13, LZTFL1, MKKS, MKS1, NPHP1, SDCCAG8, TRIM32, TTC8
Cohen syndrome	VPS13B (COH1)
Joubert syndrome	CEP120, OFD1, CC2D2A, TCTN1, TCTN2, MKS1, B9D1, TMEM67, TMEM216, TMEM231, CEP290, AIH1, NPHP1, INPP5E, RPGRIP1L, PDE6D, CPLANE1, CSPP1, INPP5E, KIAA0586
Senior-Løken syndrome	NPHP1, INVS/NPHP2, NPHP3, NPHP4, IQCB1/NPHP5, CEP290/NPHP6, SDCCAG8/NPHP10, WDR19/NPHP13, CEP164, TRAF3IP1
Sensenbrenner syndrome (cranioectodermal dysplasia)	IFT122, WDR35, IFT140, IFT43, IFT52, WDR19
Short-rib thoracic dysplasia with or without polydactyly (includes Jeune, Mainzer-Saldino, Ellis-van Creveld, and short-rib polydactyly syndrome)	IFT80, DYNC2H1, TTC21B, WDR19, NEK1, WDR35, WDR60, IFT140, IFT172, WDR34, CEP120, KIAA0586, DYNC2LI1, IFT52, TCTEX1D2, IFT43, IFT81, INTU
Inborn errors of metabolism	
Alfa-tocopherol transfer protein deficiency (familial isolated vitamin E deficiency)	TTPA
Bassen-Kornzweig syndrome (abetalipoproteinemia)	MTTP
Mucopolysaccharidoses	IDUA, IDS, HSS, NAGLU, HGSNAT, GNS, GALNS, GLB1, ARSB, GUSB, HYAL1
Neuronal ceroid-lipofuscinoses	PPT1, TPP1, CLN3, DNAJC5, CLN5, CLN6, MFSD8, CLN8, CTSD, GRN, ATP13A2, CTSF, KCTD7
Refsum disease (phytanic acid oxidase deficiency)	PHYH, PEX7, PEX1, PEX2, PEX26
Mevalonate kinase deficiency	MVK
HARP syndrome (hypoprebetalipoproteinemia, acanthocytosis, RP, and pallidal degeneration)	PANK2
PHARC syndrome (polyneuropathy, hearing loss, ataxia, RP, and cataract)	ABHD12
Mitochondrial disorders	
Kearns-Sayre syndrome	
MELAS	
NARP syndrome (neuropathy, ataxia, and RP)	

duction (MET) and neurotransmission, respectively. Usher syndrome proteins interactively form a molecular complex to develop and maintain hair bundle function [6]. USH1 proteins form heteromeric structure to apical interstereocilia development, which is necessary to cohesive stereocilia formation and hair bundle development. In adult, USH1 Protein plays a crucial role in MET complex. USH1 protein forms tip-link with cadherin-23 and postcadherin-15 that function as gatekeeper of MET channel complex. USH2 proteins are not participating stereocilia complex but forms ankle link complex of base of stereocilia and play an essential role in hair bundle morphogenesis. This structure act in hair bundle development that forms the typical U or V shape of inner hair cell and outer hair cell [7, 8]. USH3 protein, clarin-1, is likely to be necessary for synaptic active zone between MET and inner hair cells. Hair bundle defect from *USH* gene mutation prohibit MET process and result in hearing loss and vestibular areflexia [9]. Most of

Usher syndrome is primarily associated with primary cilia abnormality that Usher syndrome can be included in ciliopathy.

Usher proteins are observed at connecting cilium, periciliary membrane complex, inner and outer segments of photoreceptors. Ethnic difference is not found between Asian and European ancestry. USH1 proteins have been proposed to form a protein network mediating membrane–membrane coupling between photoreceptor outer segment and the surrounding calyceal processes [7]. MYO7A protein transport melanosome from retinal pigment epithelium (RPE) to apical process, induce phagocytosis and intracellular movement, and helps translocation of RPE65 for visual pigment recycle. *MYO7A* interact with rhodopsin adaptor protein complex, including Spectrin-βV, Kinesin II and dynein, and helps rhodopsin transportation. *MYO7A* is presumed to play a significant role in the transportation of proteins and organelle in RPE and photoreceptors. Retinal abnormalities observed in *MYO7A* mutant animal model are recovered after inserting *MYO7A* cDNA using adeno-associated virus (AAV) and lentivirus. This supports the MYO7A causal relation in Usher syndrome [8].

USH2 protein complex is known to be associated with protein transportation through connecting cilium in periciliary membrane complex. The USH2 proteins (usherin, Adgrvr1, and whirlin) have been detected in a spatially restricted inner segment membrane region that surrounds the photoreceptor connecting cilium, the periciliary membrane complex region [6].

5.3 Ciliopathy

Ciliopathy is a major part of syndromic RP. Cilium is an evolutionary conserved, ubiquitous microtubule-based organelle, which is essential for the development and maintenance of cells. Cilium contains motile and immotile cilium. Motile cilium presents in specific cells like spermatozoa, respiratory tract epithelium. Non-motile cilia, also called primary cilia, have a structure of 9-0 microtubule doublet. Primary cilia sense mechanical stimulation and chemicals, mediate signal transduction that also called "antenna" of the cell [10]. Dysfunction of primary cilia results in ciliopathy. This entity of disease involves multiple organs including retinopathy, cystic kidney disease, obesity, liver dysfunction, skeletal anomaly, congenital heart disease, and central nervous system developmental disease [11]. Retinopathy is most highly penetrant up to 50% of affected patients.

5.3.1 Bardet-Biedle Syndrome

Bardet reported the patient having retinopathy, polydactyly, and congenital obesity in 1920. Biedle added mental retardation and hypogenitalism in 1922. This disease is now called Bardet-Biedle syndrome (BBS). Additionally, paraplegia and renal abnormality are included. Prevalence is reported to be 1:160,000. Bedouin of Arab, who have more consanguineous marriage than other ethnicities, shows 1:13,500 prevalence [12]. Founder effect may predispose the prevalence of 1:17,500 in New Foundland, Canada [13].

Retinopathy of BBS involves central vision early and shows less pigmentation than typical RP. Macular abnormality and RPE/choriocapillary atrophy are observed in early life [14]. Macular abnormality includes macular epiretinal membrane and leakage in fluorescein angiogram. Electroretinogram usually shows cone-rod type pattern. Retina sometimes shows less pigmentary deposit or multiple white patches. Nyctalopia presents at average 8.5 years old and legal blindness developed at average 15.5 [1]. Another study reported that 73% were blind at 20 and 86% at 30 [14].

Five cardinal features are incompletely manifested in most of the cases. Schachat and Maumenee suggested that diagnosis of BBS can be confirmed only when at least four of five cardinal features are presented and one of them is retinopathy [15]. Pigmentary retinopathy is found in 90–100% of cases with electroretinogram abnormality in almost all of the cases [13]. Mental retardation is reported to exist in 40–85% of cases, and mild in half of cases. Mental retardation is generally regarded as not an essential feature of BBS. Although obesity is observed in most cases, sometimes patients maintain normal weight from diet and exercise. Polydactyly is present in 75% of cases, is postaxial, and may involve any or all extremities. Syndactyly or brachydactyly is present in 14.4% of patients [14]. Both are considered equivalent as polydactyly when confirming diagnosis [13]. Hypogenitalism is present in about half of patients after puberty. Infertility is particularly prominent in male Bardet–Biedl patients although rare patients remain fertile and become father. Vaginal atresia, urogenital sinuses, uterine and ovarian hypoplasia and congenital hydrometrocolpos have been described in female BBS. Clinical features of these patients overlap with diagnostic criteria of McKusick–Kaufman syndrome.

Renal abnormality is most common in noncardinal features around 46–96% [16]. Renal abnormality, including cysts, agenesis, and scarring, is asserted as sixth cardinal feature because uremia is fatal. Coincidence of renal abnormality and hepatic fibrosis is reported. Cardiac anomaly is present in half of Bedouin familial cases [17]. CNS-related ataxia, abnormal gait, facial hypotony, and high palate are also reported to present in BBS cases.

Until now, 25 genes have been identified to cause BBS phenotype [18]. Their proteins are involved in lipid homeostasis, intraflagellar transport, establishing planar cell polarity, and regulation of intracellular trafficking and centrosomal functions [19]. The core BBS machinery consists of the octameric BBSome and the small GTPase. Eight proteins (encoded by *BBS1, BBS2, BBS4, BBS5, BBS7, BBS8, BBS9*, and *BBIP1*) comprise BBSome complex, which is protein complex plays an adaptor role in transportation and recycle of ciliary membrane proteins. *BBS3 (ARL6) MKKS, BBS10*, and *BBS12* take part in making chaperone complex. *IFT172* and *IFT27* form proteins of intraflagellar transport. MKS1 is a component of flagella basal body. Proteins of *ARL6, CEP290*, and *TTC8* are observed around connecting cilium. Defects in connecting cilium, vesicular and intraflagellar transport system are suggested as disease causing mechanism of BBS [20, 21]. One meta-analysis revealed that BBS2, BBS7, and BBS9 are more essential for renal development and function than peripheral compartment including BBS1, BBS4, and BBS8 (TTC8). And a mutation in ARL6 causes less severe disease [22].

5.3.2 Senior Loken Syndrome

Senior Loken Syndrome (SLS) is characterized by pigmentary retinopathy and medullary cystic kidney disease called nephronophthisis (NPHP) [23]. NPHP is characterized by the development of fluid-filled cysts known as cystic dilation within the kidney leading to polyuria, polydipsia, weakness, fatigue, and eventually end-stage renal disease. NPHP is the most frequent genetic cause of renal failure in children and adolescents. Typical pathologic triad consists of corticomedullary cysts, tubular basement membrane, and interstitial fibrosis. Retinopathy is presented as RP, Leber congenital amaurosis (LCA), or sector RP. Visual symptom such as photophobia and nystagmus can occur in the few years of later in childhood [24].

Nine genes of 25 known NPHP genes are identified to cause SLS (*NPHP1, SLSN3, NPHP4, IQCB1/NPHP5, CEP290/NPHP6, SDCCAG8, WDR19/NPHP13, TRAF3IP1, and CEP164*). NPHP genes are expressed in primary cilia, basal bodies, or centrosomes in kidney epithelial cells [25]. SLS genes are likely to be involved in ciliogenesis and regulation of ciliary protein trafficking. They localize to cilia at the ciliary transition zone, inversin compartment, or subunits of the IFT complexes. *IQCB1* (encode a protein NPHP5) plays cilia functioning through protein complex with RPGR, calmodulin, and NPHP6. Moreover, *IQCB1* is suggested to play role in the transport of proteins to the OS [26].

5.3.3 Joubert Syndrome

Common symptoms of Joubert syndrome include hypoplasia of cerebellar vermis, dysregulation of breath, general developmental delay, loss of voluntary muscle coordination, and eye disease. Additionally polydactyly, hepatic fibrosis, renal disease, and retinal dystrophy are manifested that such case is referred to as cerebello-oculo-renal syndrome. Ocular motor apraxia is most common ocular symptom. Strabismus and nystagmus follow. Ptosis, chorioretinal coloboma, and optic atrophy are also reported. Retinopathy is observed in 38%. Twenty-eight genes are known to be involved in the pathogenesis of Joubert syndrome [27]. Except for *OFD1*, Joubert syndrome is inherited in an autosomal recessive pattern. *AHI1, INPPtE, ARL13B*, and *CC2D2A* are most common causal genes. *AHI1* (Abelson's helper integration 1) has been found to play a crucial role in vesicular trafficking, which is necessary for normal function of photoreceptor outer segment [28].

5.3.4 Alagille Syndrome

Alagille Syndrome (ALGS) is an autosomal dominant, multisystem disorder with variable phenotypic penetrance. Variable clinical features include hepatic dysfunction caused by bile duct paucity, cardiac disease, ocular abnormalities, skeletal anomalies, and characteristic facial features. ALGS is caused mostly (about 90%) by mutations in JAGGED1 (*JAG1*), which encodes the ligand JAGGED1 in the notch signaling pathway. Rarely, *NOTCH2* mutation results in ALGS [29]. Optic disc drusen, angulated retinal vessels, pigmentary retinopathy, and a posterior embryotoxon are reported as ocular manifestations.

5.4 Retinopathy Associated with Inborn Errors of Metabolism

5.4.1 Neuronal Ceroid Lipofuscinoses

Neuronal ceroid lipofuscinoses (NCL) are neurodegenerative lysosomal storage diseases. They are characterized by the accumulation of lysosomal storage material and progressive neurological deterioration with dementia, epilepsy, retinopathy, motor disturbances, and early death. The disease is classified into groups according to the age at which symptoms usually appear. The main alerting symptoms are a newly observed psychomotor abnormality followed by evident dementia [30].

1. Infantile onset NCL (INCL)

   This is associated with dysfunction of the lysosomal enzyme cathepsin D (encoded by *CTSD*) and palmitoyl protein thioesterase 1 (encoded by *CLN1*). Patients having former mutations are born with microcephaly and seizures. The latter, develops in second half of the first year of life, is more frequent. This is characterized by a decreased muscle tone and decreased social interactions, followed by a dramatic loss of psychomotor functions, myoclonus, seizures, and visual failure. Ultimately patients develop spasticity and a vegetative state.
2. Late infantile onset NCL (LINCL)

   The most prevalent and typical form in this group is caused by *CLN2*, encoding lysosomal enzyme tripeptidyl peptidase 1 (TPP1). Acquisition of speech may be delayed in some patients. Motor decline with clumsiness and ataxia, deterioration of speech, and epilepsy are occurred between 2 and 4 years of age. After third year of life, loss of motor function, language, vision, and swallowing ability progresses rapidly, leading to death around the middle teenage years. Mutations in the *CLN1, CLN5, CLN6, CLN7, CLN8*, and *CLN14* genes are rare. They manifest later and progress slower than *CLN2* mutation.
3. Juvenile onset NCL (JNCL)

   This is a most prevalent form of NCL. It is caused by dysfunction of lysosomal membrane protein (encoded by *CLN3*). Onset is between 4 and 7 years of age with insidious visual failure due to a pigmentary retinopathy. Cognitive decline and abnormal became apparent. Seizure develops at around 10 years of age followed by a movement disorder, speech and swallowing difficulties. Patients usually deceased in the third decade. Rarely, this form of NCL is caused by mutations in the *CLN1, CLN2, CLN5, CLN7, CLN8, CLN10, or CLN12* genes.

4. Adult onset NCL (ANCL)

   Although this is inherited as autosomal recessive pattern, autosomal dominant type has been reported. This extremely rare form of NCL starts with cognitive impairment and depression in mid-thirties. Ataxia, parkinsonism, and epilepsy followed with or without visual failure.

Other atypical forms of NCL are also reported. One of the variant forms is found only in the Finnish population. INCL has an incidence of 1:50,000 in Scandinavia and 1:100,000 worldwide. In Germany, incidence of LINCL is 0.46 per 100,000 and that of JNCL is 0.71 per 100,000 [31].

Retinopathy involves central vision first and eventually result in a severe visual loss in childhood forms (1–3 of above forms). The ERG becomes abnormal early in the course of childhood forms and is usually abolished within a few years. The ERG becomes undetectable for LINCL between 3 and 4 years and for JNCL between 5 and 7 years of age [32]. However, visual symptoms and electrophysiologic abnormality are rare on ANCL. The abnormal ERG pattern varies between disease subtypes.

Accumulation of storage material that is autofluorescent, sudanophilic, and periodic acid-Schiff-positive within lysosomes in neurons and other cells. The storage material is a complex mixture of lipoproteins and hydrophobic peptides. Deposit patterns observed on electron microscopy can be used for diagnosis and classification. Granular inclusions are seen in INCL, curvilinear inclusions predominate in LINCL and fingerprint inclusions are seen in JNCL [33].

An NCL must be suspected in children and young adults who initially developed normally but then present with an unexplained progressive neurological disorder. The diagnostic approaches to specific NCL form strongly depend on the age at manifestation and the definitive diagnosis is increasingly based on molecular genetic testing. In special cases, electron microscopic analysis may be helpful to confirm the diagnosis.

5.4.2 Refsum Disease

Refsum disease is characterized by progressive neurologic deficit, sensorineural hearing loss, liver disease, skeletal abnormality, and pigmentary retinopathy. This disease includes two types of peroxisomal disorder. One is infantile Refsum disease (IRD), which is caused by deficit of peroxisome production, and the other is adult Refsum disease (ARD) caused by dysfunction of peroxisomal enzyme. Peroxism is a single membrane bound organelle which exists in most of eukaryotic cells. Peroxisome contains enzymes such as catalase, hydroxylase and oxidase, participate in oxidative processes. Blood phytanic acid levels increase moderately in IRD and highly in ARD.

IRD presents with craniofacial anomaly, severe hypotony, psychomotor retardation, and hepatic dysfunction within 6 months, severe hearing loss in 1 year of age [34]. Ocular manifestation includes nystagmus, visual decline, retinitis punctata albescence at midperiphery, optic atrophy, and cataract. Electroretinogram is impaired early and sometimes shows electronegative pattern. Affected individuals lose their life in second and third decades in most cases. Mutations in at least 12 different genetic loci have been implicated in IRD, such as *PEX1, PEX2*, and *PEX26*, and most commonly affect peroxisomal matrix protein import and targeting [35].

ARD is an autosomal recessive disease, also called heredopathia atactica polyneuritiformis. Survival for ARD is until the 4th–5th decade. Ataxia, weakness in the extremities, and nyctalopia are early symptoms. Progressive peripheral neuropathy and peripheral muscle wasting usually follow. Cardiac conduction defects occur in early adulthood. Other common findings include paresthesia, anosmia, deafness, dry skin, epiphyseal dysplasia, and spondylitis. Pigmentary retinopathy is not evident until the third decade. ERG responses are severely impaired or nonrecordable at all ages. Phytanic acid levels in blood and urine are always highly elevated. Protein levels in cerebrospinal fluid (CSF) are elevated in typical cases. Phytanoyl-coenzyme A hydroxylase (PAHX encoded by *PHYH*) is deficient in 90% of cases or type 2 peroxisomal targeting signal receptor (PTS2 encoded by *PEX7*) is deficient in less than 10% of cases [36, 37]. PAHX is a peroxisomal protein that catalyzes the first step in the alpha-oxidation of phytanic acid. Defect of *PHYH* leads to enzymatically inactive protein and dysregulates the downward pathways resulting in phytanic acid accumulation.

Dietary restriction of phytanic acid can limit progression of disease and often improve ichthyosis, neurologic deficits, and cardiac disease. Very high blood plasma levels of phytanic acid can be life threatening. Blood plasma filtration can be applied in such conditions [38].

5.5 Retinopathy Associated with Mitochondrial Disorders

5.5.1 Kearn-Sayre Syndrome

Kearn-Sayre Syndrome (KSS) is a chronic progressive external ophthalmoplegia (CPEO) plus syndrome. Characteristic clinical features include CPEO symptoms, progressive bilateral ophthalmoparesis, and ptosis plus pigmentary retinopathy under the age of 20 years and cardiac conduction block. CSF protein concentration elevation or cerebral ataxia, deafness, small statures are also manifested [39]. The prevalence of KSS is estimated to be 1–3 per 100,000 based on population study [40].

KSS is sporadic in 90% of cases and associated with large-scale mitochondrial DNA. KSS clinical feature is much broader and requires a multidisciplinary approach to diagnose appropriately. The salt-and-pepper retinopathy is most prominent in the posterior pole or peripapillary rather than mid-peripheral retina. Pigmentary change shows mottled appearance more frequently than bony spicule [40]. RPE atrophy, revealing underlying choroidal vessel, is called "choroidal sclerosis." Histopathologic studies suggest that RPE dysfunction is the causative mechanism for retinal degeneration. Electroretinography abnormality is usually mild compared to RP. Visual symptom presents in about 50% of patients and this is also rather mild.

5.5.2 Mitochondrial Encephalomyopathy, Lactic Acidosis, and Stroke-Like Episodes

Mitochondrial Encephalomyopathy, Lactic Acidosis, and Stroke-Like Episodes (MELAS) is a multisystem disorder with protean manifestations. Majority of affected individuals (65–76%) present at or before age of 20 years. MELAS is suggested to be the most common maternally inherited mitochondrial disorder with a minimum prevalence of 0.18/100,000 in Japan [41]. Common clinical manifestations include stroke-like episodes, encephalopathy with seizures and/or dementia, muscle weakness and exercise intolerance, normal early psychomotor development, recurrent headaches, recurrent vomiting, hearing impairment, peripheral neuropathy, learning disability, and short stature. Pigmentary retinopathy is observed in about 25% of affected patients [39]. Lactic acidosis both in blood and CSF is very common. Muscle biopsy and modified Gomori stain shows "ragged red fibers." This presents mitochondrial proliferation below the plasma membrane.

The diagnosis is established when it fulfills certain clinical diagnosis criteria and finds pathogenic variants in mitochondrial gene testing. m.3243A>G pathogenic variant in *MT-TL1* is present in about 80% of patients. m.3271T>C and m.3252A>G in MT-TL1 and m.13513G>A in *MT-ND5* follows in less than 10% proportions. And other genes are reported rarely. Heteroplasmy in mitochondrial disorders results in varying tissue distribution that pathogenic variant is possibly not detected in leukocytes. In such a case genetic testing should be performed in other tissues [42].

References

1. Koenig R. Bardet-Biedl syndrome and Usher syndrome. Dev Ophthalmol. 2003;37:126–40. Available at: https://pubmed.ncbi.nlm.nih.gov/12876834/. Accessed 21 Dec 2020
2. Blanco-Kelly F, Jaijo T, Aller E, et al. Clinical aspects of usher syndrome and the USH2A gene in a cohort of 433 patients. JAMA Ophthalmol. 2015;133:157–64.

3. Fishman GA, Kumar A, Joseph ME, et al. Usher's syndrome: ophthalmic and neuro-otologic findings suggesting genetic heterogeneity. Arch Ophthalmol. 1983;101:1367–74. Available at: http://lps3.pubmed.ncbi.nlm.nih.gov.libproxy.snu.ac.kr/6604514/. Accessed 21 Dec 2020
4. Piazza L, Fishman GA, Farber M, et al. Visual acuity loss in patients with Usher's syndrome. Arch Ophthalmol. 1986;104:1336–9. Available at: https://pubmed.ncbi.nlm.nih.gov/3753284/. Accessed 21 Dec 2020
5. Ness SL, Ben-Yosef T, Bar-Lev A, et al. Genetic homogeneity and phenotypic variability among Ashkenazi Jews with Usher syndrome type III. J Med Genet. 2003;40:767–72. Available at: http://lps3.pubmed.ncbi.nlm.nih.gov.libproxy.snu.ac.kr/14569126/ Accessed 21 Dec 2020
6. Géléoc GGS, El-Amraoui A. Disease mechanisms and gene therapy for Usher syndrome. Hear Res. 2020;394
7. El-Amraoui A, Petit C. The retinal phenotype of Usher syndrome: pathophysiological insights from animal models. Comptes Rendus Biol. 2014;337:167–77. Available at: http://lps3.pubmed.ncbi.nlm.nih.gov.libproxy.snu.ac.kr/24702843/. Accessed 1 Mar 2021
8. Mathur P, Yang J. Usher syndrome: hearing loss, retinal degeneration and associated abnormalities. Biochim Biophys Acta Mol Basis Dis. 2015;1852:406–20. Available at: https://doi.org/10.1016/j.bbadis.2014.11.020.
9. Geng R, Melki S, Chen DHC, et al. The mechanosensory structure of the hair cell requires clarin-1, a protein encoded by Usher syndrome III causative gene. J Neurosci. 2012;32:9485–98. Available at: http://lps3.pubmed.ncbi.nlm.nih.gov.libproxy.snu.ac.kr/22787034/. Accessed 1 Mar 2021
10. Chen HY, Kelley RA, Li T, Swaroop A. Primary cilia biogenesis and associated retinal ciliopathies. Scdb. 2020. Available at: https://doi.org/10.1016/j.semcdb.2020.07.013.
11. Reiter JF, Leroux MR. Genes and molecular pathways underpinning ciliopathies. Nat Rev Mol Cell Biol. 2017;18:533–47. Available at: https://www.ncbi.nlm.nih.gov/pmc/articles/PMC5851292/?report=abstract. Accessed 26 Dec 2020.
12. Farag TI, Teebi AS. High incidence of Bardet Biedl syndrome among the Bedouin. Clin Genet. 1989;36:463–4. Available at: https://pubmed.ncbi.nlm.nih.gov/2591073/. Accessed 27 Dec 2020
13. Green JS, Parfrey PS, Harnett JD, et al. The cardinal manifestations of Bardet–Biedl syndrome, a form of Laurence–Moon–Biedl syndrome. N Engl J Med. 1989;321:1002–9. Available at: https://pubmed.ncbi.nlm.nih.gov/2779627/. Accessed 27 Dec 2020
14. Klein D, Ammann F. The syndrome of Laurence-Moon-Bardet-Biedl and allied diseases in Switzerland. Clinical, genetic and epidemiological studies. J Neurol Sci. 1969;9:479–513. Available at: https://pubmed.ncbi.nlm.nih.gov/5367041/. Accessed 7 Feb 2021
15. Schachat AP, Maumenee IH. Bardet-Biedl syndrome and related disorders. Arch Ophthalmol. 1982;100:285–8. Available at: http://lps3.pubmed.ncbi.nlm.nih.gov.libproxy.snu.ac.kr/7065946/. Accessed 28 Dec 2020
16. Zacchia M, Di Iorio V, Trepiccione F, et al. The kidney in Bardet-Biedl syndrome: possible pathogenesis of urine concentrating defect. Kidney Dis. 2017;3:57–65. Available at: http://lps3.pubmed.ncbi.nlm.nih.gov.libproxy.snu.ac.kr/28868293/. Accessed 1 Mar 2021
17. Elbedour K, Zucker N, Zalzstein E, et al. Cardiac abnormalities in the Bardet-Biedl syndrome: echocardiographic studies of 22 patients. Am J Med Genet. 1994;52:164–9. Available at: http://lps3.pubmed.ncbi.nlm.nih.gov.libproxy.snu.ac.kr/7802002/. Accessed 28 Dec 2020
18. Anon. RetNet—Retinal Information Network. Available at: https://sph.uth.edu/retnet/. Accessed 9 Feb 2016.
19. Tsang SH, Aycinena ARP, Sharma T. Ciliopathy: Bardet-Biedl syndrome. In: Advances in experimental medicine and biology. Vol 1085. New York: Springer; 2018. p. 171–4.
20. Satta M, Castro-Sánchez S, Valverde D. Bardet-Biedl syndrome as a chaperonopathy: dissecting the major role of chaperonin-like BBS proteins (BBS6-BBS10-BBS12). Front Mol Biosci. 2017;4:55. Available at: www.frontiersin.org.
21. Zaghloul NA, Katsanis N. Mechanistic insights into Bardet-Biedl syndrome, a model ciliopathy. J Clin Invest. 2009;119:428–37.
22. Niederlova V, Modrak M, Tsyklauri O, et al. Meta-analysis of genotype-phenotype associations in Bardet-Biedl syndrome uncovers differences among causative genes. Hum Mutat. 2019;40:2068–87.
23. Senior B, Friedmann AI, Braudo JL. Juvenile familial nephropathy with tapetoretinal degeneration. A new oculorenal dystrophy. Am J Ophthalmol. 1961;52:625–33. Available at: http://lps3.pubmed.ncbi.nlm.nih.gov.libproxy.snu.ac.kr/13910672/. Accessed 25 Feb 2021
24. Tsang SH, Aycinena ARP, Sharma T. Ciliopathy: Senior-Løken syndrome. In: Advances in experimental medicine and biology. Vol 1085. New York: Springer; 2018. p. 175–8.
25. Luo F, Tao YH. Nephronophthisis: a review of genotype–phenotype correlation. Nephrology. 2018;23:904–11. Available at: https://pubmed.ncbi.nlm.nih.gov/29717526/. Accessed 1 Mar 2021
26. Ronquillo CC, Bernstein PS, Baehr W. Senior-Løken syndrome: a syndromic form of retinal dystrophy associated with nephronophthisis. Vis Res. 2012;75:88–97.
27. Wang SF, Kowal TJ, Ning K, et al. Review of ocular manifestations of Joubert syndrome. Genes (Basel). 2018;9. Available at: http://lps3.pubmed.ncbi.nlm.nih.gov.libproxy.snu.ac.kr/30518138/. Accessed 23 Dec 2020
28. Westfall JE, Hoyt C, Liu Q, et al. Retinal degeneration and failure of photoreceptor outer segment formation

in mice with targeted deletion of the Joubert syndrome gene, Ahi1. J Neurosci. 2010;30:8759–68. Available at: https://pubmed.ncbi.nlm.nih.gov/20592197/. Accessed 26 Feb 2021
29. Mitchell E, Gilbert M, Loomes KM. Alagille syndrome. Clin Liver Dis. 2018;22:625–41. Available at: http://lps3.pubmed.ncbi.nlm.nih.gov.libproxy.snu.ac.kr/30266153/. Accessed 1 Mar 2021
30. Kohlschütter A, Schulz A, Bartsch U, Storch S. Current and emerging treatment strategies for neuronal ceroid lipofuscinoses. CNS Drugs. 2019;33:315–25. Available at: https://doi.org/10.1007/s40263-019-00620-8. Accessed 28 Dec 2020.
31. Claussen M, Heim P, Knispel J, et al. Incidence of neuronal ceroid-lipofuscinoses in West Germany: variation of a method for studying autosomal recessive disorders. Am J Med Genet. 1992;42:536–8. Available at: http://lps3.pubmed.ncbi.nlm.nih.gov.libproxy.snu.ac.kr/1609834/. Accessed 28 Dec 2020
32. Goebel HH. The neuronal ceroid-lipofuscinoses. Semin Pediatr Neurol. 1996;3:270–8.
33. Arsenio-Nunes ML, Goutières F, Aicardi J. An ultramicroscopic study of skin and conjunctival biopsies in chronic neurological disorders of childhood. Ann Neurol. 1981;9:163–73. Available at: http://lps3.pubmed.ncbi.nlm.nih.gov.libproxy.snu.ac.kr/7235631/. Accessed 1 Mar 2021
34. Poll-The BT, Saudubray JM, Ogier H, et al. Infantile Refsum's disease: biochemical findings suggesting multiple peroxisomal dysfunction. J Inherit Metab Dis. 1986;9:169–74. Available at: http://lps3.pubmed.ncbi.nlm.nih.gov.libproxy.snu.ac.kr/2427795/. Accessed 28 Feb 2021
35. Kumar R, De Jesus O. Refsum disease. StatPearls; 2021. Available at: http://www.ncbi.nlm.nih.gov/pubmed/32809453. Accessed 28 Feb 2021.
36. Jansen GA, Ofman R, Ferdinandusse S, et al. Refsum disease is caused by mutations in the phytanoyl-coa hydroxylase gene. Nat Genet. 1997;17:193. Available at: https://pubmed.ncbi.nlm.nih.gov/9326940/. Accessed 29 Dec 2020
37. Jansen GA, Waterham HR, Wanders RJA. Molecular basis of refsum disease: sequence variations in phytanoyl-CoA hydroxylase (PHYH) and the PTS2 receptor (PEX7). Hum Mutat. 2004;23:209–18. Available at: https://pubmed.ncbi.nlm.nih.gov/14974078/. Accessed 29 Dec 2020
38. Rüether K, Baldwin E, Casteels M, et al. Adult refsum disease: a form of tapetoretinal dystrophy accessible to therapy. Surv Ophthalmol. 2010;55:531–8. Available at: http://lps3.pubmed.ncbi.nlm.nih.gov.libproxy.snu.ac.kr/20850855/. Accessed 28 Feb 2021
39. Kisilevsky E, Freund P, Margolin E. Mitochondrial disorders and the eye. Surv Ophthalmol. 2020;65:294–311. Available at: https://doi.org/10.1016/j.survophthal.2019.11.001.
40. Schaefer AM, McFarland R, Blakely EL, et al. Prevalence of mitochondrial DNA disease in adults. Ann Neurol. 2008;63:35–9. Available at: http://lps3.pubmed.ncbi.nlm.nih.gov.libproxy.snu.ac.kr/17886296/. Accessed 28 Feb 2021
41. Yatsuga S, Povalko N, Nishioka J, et al. MELAS: a nationwide prospective cohort study of 96 patients in Japan. Biochim Biophys Acta Gen Subj. 1820;2012:619–24. Available at: http://lps3.pubmed.ncbi.nlm.nih.gov.libproxy.snu.ac.kr/21443929/. Accessed 1 Mar 2021
42. Agier V, Auré K, Lombès A. MELAS syndrome. Drugs Future. 2009;34:237–41. Available at: http://lps3.www.ncbi.nlm.nih.gov.libproxy.snu.ac.kr/books/NBK532959/. Accessed 1 Mar 2021

Leber Congenital Amaurosis/ Early-Onset Severe Retinal Dystrophy

6

Michalis Georgiou and Michel Michaelides

Abstract

Leber congenital amaurosis/early-onset severe retinal dystrophy (LCA/EOSRD) is a genetically and phenotypically heterogeneous group of inherited retinal diseases with widely overlapping features. Herein we present in a comprehensive and concise manner the clinical features, molecular genetics, treatment principles, novel treatment methods, and retinal imaging findings of LCA/EOSRD, emphasizing in some of the most common genotypes: *GUCY2D*, *CEP290*, *CRB1*, *RDH12*, *RPE65*, *TULP1*, *AIPL1*, and *NMNAT1*.

Keywords

Leber congenital amaurosis · LCA · Early-onset severe retinal dystrophy · EOSRD · *GUCY2D* · *CEP290* · *CRB1* · *RDH12* · *RPE65* · *TULP1* · *AIPL1* · *NMNAT1* · Clinical features · Retinal imaging · OCT · FAF

M. Georgiou · M. Michaelides (✉)
UCL Institute of Ophthalmology, University College London, London, UK

Moorfields Eye Hospital NHS Foundation Trust, London, UK
e-mail: michel.michaelides@ucl.ac.uk

6.1 Introduction

Leber congenital amaurosis (LCA) and early-onset severe retinal dystrophy (EOSRD) are a group of both phenotypically and genetically heterogeneous inherited retinal diseases, characterized by severe congenital/early-onset visual loss, nystagmus, and amaurotic pupils, leading into blindness and lifelong morbidity for the patients. Below we present the clinical features, molecular genetics, treatment principles, novel treatment methods, and retinal imaging findings of LCA/EOSRD, and we further emphasize in selected genotypes: *GUCY2D*, *CEP290*, *CRB1*, *RDH12*, *RPE65*, *TULP1*, *AIPL1*, and *NMNAT1*.

6.2 Clinical Features

6.2.1 Signs and Symptoms

Clinical presentation of LCA/EOSRD includes severe congenital/early infancy visual loss, amaurotic pupils, nystagmus and a markedly abnormal or undetectable full-field electroretinogram (ERG) [1]. LCA is characterized by roving eye movements or nystagmus, poor pupillary light responses, oculodigital sign (poking, rubbing, and/or pressing of the eyes), undetectable or severely abnormal full-field electroretinogram (ERG), and severe visual impairment from birth

H.-G. Yu (ed.), *Inherited Retinal Disease*, https://doi.org/10.1007/978-981-16-7337-5_6

or the first few months of life. EOSRD is characterized by the onset of visual impairment typically after infancy but before 5 years old, with minimal full-field ERG preservation and variably preserved visual acuity.

Patients with LCA/EOSRD usually present with the non-syndromic disease, with confined ocular manifestations, signs, and symptoms. However, some affected infants may at an older age, develop manifestations from other systems, particularly renal disease, including *IQCB1*-, *IFT140*-, and *CEP290*-associated LCA, which can lead to syndromic disease, including Joubert syndrome and Senior-Loken syndrome, with nephronophthisis and the subsequent development of end-stage renal disease.

6.2.2 Fundus Findings

The fundus in LCA/EOSRD can appear normal at presentation [2] or show a variety of retinal abnormalities, including pigmentary retinopathy, white deposits at the level of the retinal pigment epithelium [3], vascular attenuation, or pseudo papilledema and macular atrophy. Those with a normal fundus appearance at birth usually develop pigmentary retinopathy, optic disc pallor, and vascular attenuation with time. Other late changes include optic disc drusen, keratoconus, and lens opacities.

6.3 Retinal Imaging

Multimodal retinal imaging can facilitate diagnosis and monitor disease progression, as well as being a useful tool for the identification of endpoints in the ongoing and anticipated therapeutic trials.

Optical coherence tomography (OCT) can be used to investigate the retinal structure in LCA/EOSRD and monitor disease progression. Depending on the genotype, patients can have relatively preserved outer retinal structure on OCT (even into late adulthood), although foveal cone outer segment abnormalities and foveal cone loss can be common early in life. Fundus autofluorescence (FAF) findings are variable; normal, reduced AF, central foveal hyperautofluorescence, and/or a perimacular ring of increased AF has been reported. Specific imaging findings for selected genotypes are presented later in the chapter.

6.4 Molecular Genetics

LCA/EOSRD is typically inherited in an autosomal recessive manner. Rarely heterozygous pathogenic variants in *CRX*, *OTX2*, or *IMPDH1*, can lead to autosomal dominant LCA/EOSRD. In total, the reported LCA/EOSRD-associated genes ($n = 25$) account for approximately 70–80% of cases [4, 5], with more genes yet to be identified. These genes encode proteins with a diverse range of retinal functions, including photoreceptor development/integrity, the visual cycle and phototransduction [1]. The most common causative genes *are CEP290* [6], *GUCY2D* [2], *CRB1* [7], and *RPE65* [4, 5, 8].

Molecular genetic testing is crucial for accurate diagnosis and for access to current or anticipated treatments or participation in clinical trials. Gene-targeted testing, typically done using multigene panel tests, requires prior characterization of the causative gene as a "retinal dystrophy gene." Genomic testing (whole genome sequencing) enables the clinician to explore genes not previously known to be associated with retinal dystrophy and/or identification of complex genetic alterations [9].

6.5 Treatment Principles

6.5.1 Symptomatic Management

Management of most forms of LCA/EOSRD is symptomatic. The rate of visual loss varies, with some genes associated with faster progression. Affected children benefit from correction of refractive error, use of low vision aids when possible, and optimal access to educational and work-related opportunities. Infants with severe visual impairment may also have delays or difficulties with speech, social skills, and behaviour, highlighting the importance of a multi-specialist approach.

6.5.2 Novel Treatment Methods

It is of paramount importance to molecularly characterize LCA/EOSRD patients in order to facilitate access to, and potential benefit from, the ongoing advances in the field. The first FDA- and EMA-approved gene therapy is available for LCA/EOSRD-associated with *RPE65* [10, 11], and there are multiple other trials underway for LCA/EOSRD and other inherited retinal diseases. Following successful gene supplementation therapy in experimental models of *AIPL1*-, *RDH12*-, *GUCY2D*-, and *RPGRIP*-associated LCA, clinical trials in these subsets of LCA are either ongoing or likely in the future. A different gene therapy technique utilizing antisense oligonucleotide-mediated exon skipping to abrogate the disease-causing variant is also showing promise [12]. A phase 3 clinical trial investigating the safety and efficacy of intravitreal injections of this type of therapy for *CEP290*-associated LCA is ongoing.

6.6 Specific Causes of LCA/EOSRD

GUCY2D, *CEP290*, *CRB1*, *RDH12*, and *RPE65* are the most common causes of LCA/EOSRD, and they are presented below, together with *TULP1*, *AIPL1*, and *NMNAT1 due to distinctive findings, in greater detail.*

6.6.1 *GUCY2D*-LCA/EOSRD

Patients with GUCY2D-LCA/EOSRD (OMIM 600179) often have relatively normal fundi, in contrast to most other LCA/EOSRD genotypes [2]. *GUCY2D* encodes retinal guanylate cyclase-1 (RetGC1), which plays an important role in photoreceptor recovery following phototransduction, thereby disease-causing variants in *GUCY2D* and subsequent RetGC1 deficiency result in the biochemical equivalent of chronic light exposure [1]. There can be relatively preserved outer retinal structure on OCT in many patients (even into late adulthood, Fig. 6.1a), although foveal cone outer segment abnormalities and foveal cone loss have been observed [2, 13]. FAF findings are variable; normal, central foveal hyperautofluorescence, and/or a perimacular ring of increased AF have been reported (Fig. 6.1a) [2]. A phase 1/2 gene therapy trial (NCT03920007) is ongoing for subretinal administration of SAR439483.

6.6.2 *CEP290*-LCA/EOSRD

CEP290 is localized to the connecting cilia of photoreceptors and the centromeres. OCT studies of *CEP290*-LCA/EOSRD (OMIM 610142) have shown that despite profound cone dysfunction, the foveal architecture is structurally preserved until the fourth decade of life in some patients; although with abnormal inner and outer segments, in contrast to the early loss of rod photoreceptors [6, 13]. FAF imaging reveals a perifoveal hyperautofluorescent ring in most patients (Fig. 6.1b), and areas of decreased signal in older patients (pigmentary retinopathy) [6]. Phase 1/2 (AGN-151587 (EDIT-101), NCT03872479) and Phase 2/3 (sepofarsen (QR-110), NCT03913143) antisense oligonucleotide-mediated exon skipping, gene therapy trials are ongoing for patients with compound heterozygous or homozygous intron 26 c.2991+1655A>G *CEP290* variant. That specific intronic variant is the most common disease-causing variant, having been identified in at least one allele in 58–77% of *CEP290*-LCA patients [6, 14].

6.6.3 *CRB1*-LCA/EOSRD

CRB1 is a major component of the outer limiting membrane and co-localizes with the zonula adherens, and likely has a role in retinal development [1]. *CRB1*-associated disease (OMIM 604210) has nummular pigmentation, maculopathy, relative preservation of para-arteriolar RPE, intraretinal

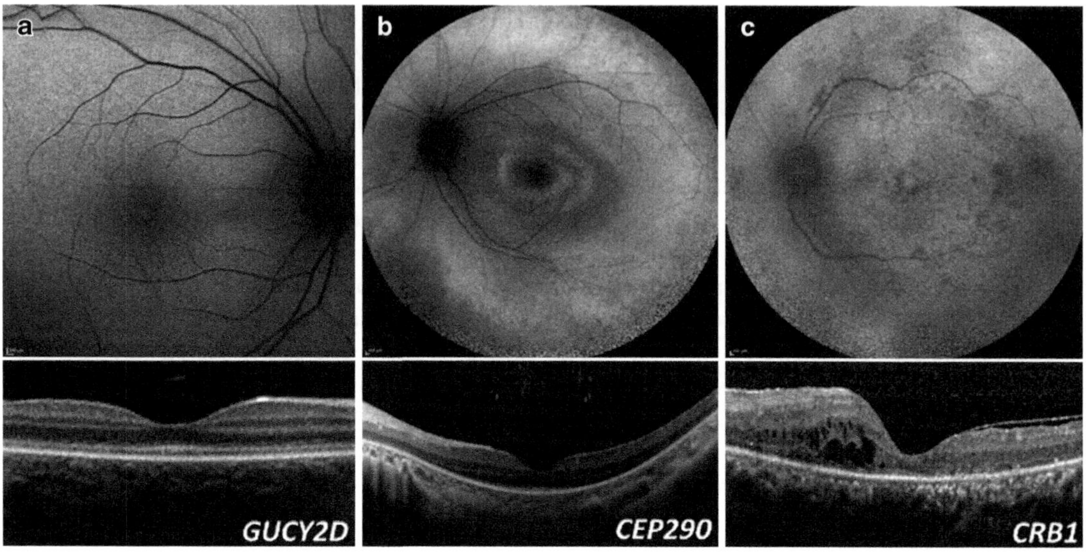

Fig. 6.1 Retinal imaging of *GUCY2D*, *CEP290*, and *CRB1*—Leber congenital amaurosis/early-onset severe retinal dystrophy (LCA/EOSRD). (**a**–**c**) Fundus autofluorescence (FAF) imaging with corresponding horizontal trans-foveal optical coherence tomography (OCT). (**a**) *GUCY2D*-LCA/EOSRD; relatively preserved outer retinal structure on OCT and normal-appearing FAF. (**b**) *CEP290*-LCA/EOSRD; preserved foveal architecture on OCT, despite the profound functional loss, and FAF imaging with a perifoveal hyperautofluorescent ring. (**c**) *CRB1*-LCA/EOSRD; nummular pigmentation, maculopathy, relative preservation of para-arteriolar RPE on FAF, and intraretinal cystoid spaces on OCT

nal cystoid spaces, with retinal thickening and loss of lamination on OCT (Fig. 6.1c) [15]. Not all findings are present in all patients. Altered retinal lamination with increased RNFL thickness; is a rather unique finding for *CRB1* compared to other LCA/EOSRD genotypes [16]. *CRB1* variants can be associated with a range of phenotypes and corresponding retinal imaging findings, including retinitis pigmentosa [17], Coats-like vasculopathy, and maculopathy [18].

6.6.4 *RDH12*-LCA/EOSRD

RDH12 is a photoreceptor retinoid metabolism protein. *RDH12*-associated disease (OMIM 608830), which gives rise to an EOSRD phenotype, is characterized by early-dense intraretinal pigment migration and maculopathy [19]. OCT reveals severe loss of structure, often from 10 years of age [20]. Macular atrophy is a universal finding on FAF (centrally decreased signal), and with disease progression, the area of atrophy extends peripherally in a variegated watercolour-like pattern (Fig. 6.2a), which usually corresponds to the retinal vasculature [20]. Recently the phenotypic spectrum of *RDH12 has been extended to include* later onset and milder phenotypes [21, 22]. Similar to the successful treatment of *RPE65*-LCA/EOSRD, another retinoid metabolism protein, *RDH12*-associated disease, is a potential target for gene therapy which is being actively investigated [23].

6.6.5 *RPE65*-LCA/EOSRD

As mentioned above RPE65 is a retinoid cycle protein. *RPE65*-deficiency (OMIM 180069) is associated with reduced or absent AF on FAF imaging, suggesting low or absent levels of lipofuscin in the RPE (Fig. 6.2b) [3, 24]. OCT studies have demonstrated relatively normal retinal thickness in some patients, with more commonly a central macular area of the relatively preserved retina with a surrounding ring of thinning or more widespread retinal loss (Fig. 6.2b) [3, 25]. There is an FDA- and EMA-approved gene ther-

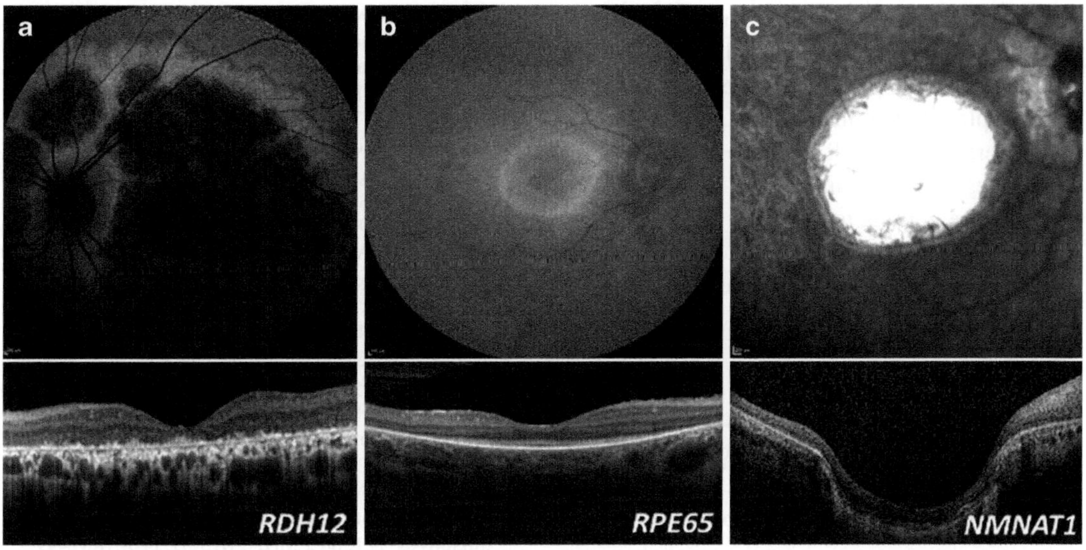

Fig. 6.2 Retinal imaging of *RDH12*, *RPE65* and *NMNAT1*—Leber congenital amaurosis/early-onset severe retinal dystrophy (LCA/EOSRD). (**a**) *RDH12*-LCA/EOSRD; FAF shows a centrally decreased signal with atrophy extending peripherally in a variegated watercolour-like fashion. OCT shows severe loss of structure and macular atrophy. (**b**) *RPE65*-EOSRD; the reduced signal on FAF imaging and OCT showing the preserved structure at the central macula. (**c**) *NMNAT1*-LCA; near-infrared imaging and corresponding OCT scan, of a patient with severe and extensive maculopathy

apy for *RPE65*-EOSRD (Luxturna (Voretigene neparvovec-rzyl), Spark Therapeutics), and ongoing Phase1/2 trials for other vectors (NCT02946879, AAV2/5 - OPTIRPE65).

6.6.6 *TULP1, AIPL1,* and *NMNAT1*-LCA

TULP1 (OMIM 602280), *AIPL1* (OMIM 604323) and *NMNAT1* (OMIM 608700) are uncommon genetic causes of LCA and are clinically characterized by early maculopathy.

TULP1 is expressed exclusively in the retina and is involved in protein trafficking, including the transport of rhodopsin [26]. A perifoveal ring of increased signal on FAF, and a thinned retina, with photoreceptor loss on OCT are common findings. A salt-and-pepper retinopathy with midperipheral RPE atrophy can develop with age [27].

NMNAT1 encodes nicotinamide mononucleotide adenylyltransferase 1, and participates in coenzyme NAD biosynthesis, which is neuroprotective [28]. *NMNAT1* maculopathy typically is severe, early-onset and extensive (Fig. 6.2c), with pigment clumping (including nummular pigmentation), both visible on FAF and OCT [29]. Similar to *RDH12*, the phenotypic spectrum of *NMNAT1 has been extended to the later* onset and a milder phenotype [28].

In *AIPL1*-LCA no patient is identified in the literature with residual outer retinal structure beyond the age of 4 years [13, 30]. *AIPL1* encodes Aryl-hydrocarbon-interacting-protein-like 1—a photoreceptor-specific co-chaperone that interacts specifically with the molecular chaperone HSP90 and modulates the stability of and assembly of the HSP90 with retinal cGMP phosphodiesterase [31]. A compassionate use gene therapy study is ongoing for *AIPL1*-LCA.

6.7 Concluding Remarks and Future Prospects

Advances in molecular genetic techniques have greatly simplified molecular diagnosis. Similarly, advances in retinal imaging and retinal function testing have improved knowledge of disease natural history, which is key to identifying treatment effects in clinical trials of novel therapies. The ongoing challenge, which is becoming increasingly explored in clinical trials, is to develop novel therapies that will improve function and/or slow degeneration.Financial DisclosuresThe authors have nothing to disclose.

Conflicting Interests The authors declare that there is no conflict of interest.

Contributors MG reviewed the literature, drafted the chapter and provided critical revision. MM conceived, supervised, and revised the chapter. Manuscript writing: All authors. Final approval of manuscript: All authors

Ethical Statement The authors are accountable for all aspects of the work in ensuring that questions related to the accuracy or integrity of any part of the work are appropriately investigated and resolved.

References

1. Kumaran N, Moore AT, Weleber RG, et al. Leber congenital amaurosis/early-onset severe retinal dystrophy: clinical features, molecular genetics and therapeutic interventions. Br J Ophthalmol. 2017;101(9):1147–54.
2. Bouzia Z, Georgiou M, Hull S, et al. GUCY2D-associated leber congenital amaurosis: a retrospective natural history study in preparation for trials of novel therapies. Am J Ophthalmol. 2020;210:59–70.
3. Kumaran N, Georgiou M, Bainbridge JWB, et al. Retinal structure in RPE65-associated retinal dystrophy. Invest Ophthalmol Vis Sci. 2020;61(4):47.
4. den Hollander AI, Roepman R, Koenekoop RK, et al. Leber congenital amaurosis: genes, proteins and disease mechanisms. Prog Retin Eye Res. 2008;27(4):391–419.
5. Xu K, Xie Y, Sun T, et al. Genetic and clinical findings in a Chinese cohort with Leber congenital amaurosis and early onset severe retinal dystrophy. Br J Ophthalmol. 2019; https://doi.org/10.1136/bjophthalmol-2019-314281.
6. Sheck L, Davies WIL, Moradi P, et al. Leber congenital amaurosis associated with mutations in CEP290, clinical phenotype, and natural history in preparation for trials of novel therapies. Ophthalmology. 2018;125(6):894–903.
7. van den Hurk JA, Rashbass P, Roepman R, et al. Characterization of the Crumbs homolog 2 (CRB2) gene and analysis of its role in retinitis pigmentosa and Leber congenital amaurosis. Mol Vis. 2005;11:263–73.
8. Gu SM, Thompson DA, Srikumari CR, et al. Mutations in RPE65 cause autosomal recessive childhood-onset severe retinal dystrophy. Nat Genet. 1997;17(2):194–7.
9. Pontikos N, Arno G, Jurkute N, et al. Genetic basis of inherited retinal disease in a molecularly characterised cohort of over 3000 families from the United Kingdom. Ophthalmology. 2020;127(10):1384–94.
10. Jacobson SG, Cideciyan AV, Ratnakaram R, et al. Gene therapy for Leber congenital amaurosis caused by RPE65 mutations: safety and efficacy in 15 children and adults followed up to 3 years. Arch Ophthalmol. 2012;130(1):9–24.
11. Bainbridge JW, Mehat MS, Sundaram V, et al. Long-term effect of gene therapy on Leber's congenital amaurosis. N Engl J Med. 2015;372(20):1887–97.
12. Cideciyan AV, Jacobson SG, Drack AV, et al. Effect of an intravitreal antisense oligonucleotide on vision in Leber congenital amaurosis due to a photoreceptor cilium defect. Nat Med. 2019;25(2):225–8.
13. Pasadhika S, Fishman GA, Stone EM, et al. Differential macular morphology in patients with RPE65-, CEP290-, GUCY2D-, and AIPL1-related Leber congenital amaurosis. Invest Ophthalmol Vis Sci. 2010;51(5):2608–14.
14. McAnany JJ, Genead MA, Walia S, et al. Visual acuity changes in patients with Leber congenital amaurosis and mutations in CEP290. JAMA Ophthalmol. 2013;131(2):178–82.
15. Kousal B, Dudakova L, Gaillyova R, et al. Phenotypic features of CRB1-associated early-onset severe retinal dystrophy and the different molecular approaches to identifying the disease-causing variants. Graefes Arch Clin Exp Ophthalmol. 2016;254(9):1833–9.
16. Jacobson SG, Cideciyan AV, Aleman TS, et al. Crumbs homolog 1 (CRB1) mutations result in a thick human retina with abnormal lamination. Hum Mol Genet. 2003;12(9):1073–8.
17. Talib M, van Schooneveld MJ, van Genderen MM, et al. Genotypic and phenotypic characteristics of CRB1-associated retinal dystrophies: a long-term follow-up study. Ophthalmology. 2017;124(6):884–95.
18. Khan KN, Robson A, Mahroo OAR, et al. A clinical and molecular characterisation of CRB1-associated maculopathy. Eur J Hum Genet. 2018;26(5):687–94.
19. Schuster A, Janecke AR, Wilke R, et al. The phenotype of early-onset retinal degeneration in persons with RDH12 mutations. Invest Ophthalmol Vis Sci. 2007;48(4):1824–31.
20. Fahim AT, Bouzia Z, Branham KH, et al. Detailed clinical characterisation, unique features and natural history of autosomal recessive RDH12-associated retinal degeneration. Br J Ophthalmol. 2019;103(12):1789–96.

21. Scott HA, Place EM, Ferenchak K, et al. Expanding the phenotypic spectrum in RDH12-associated retinal disease. Cold Spring Harb Mol Case Stud. 2020;6(1).
22. Ba-Abbad R, Arno G, Robson AG, et al. Macula-predominant retinopathy associated with biallelic variants in RDH12. Ophthalmic Genet. 2020;1–4.
23. Fahim AT, Thompson DA. Natural history and genotype-phenotype correlations in RDH12-associated retinal degeneration. Adv Exp Med Biol. 2019;1185:209–13.
24. Lorenz B, Wabbels B, Wegscheider E, et al. Lack of fundus autofluorescence to 488 nanometers from childhood on in patients with early-onset severe retinal dystrophy associated with mutations in RPE65. Ophthalmology. 2004;111(8):1585–94.
25. Jacobson SG, Aleman TS, Cideciyan AV, et al. Identifying photoreceptors in blind eyes caused by RPE65 mutations: prerequisite for human gene therapy success. Proc Natl Acad Sci U S A. 2005;102(17):6177–82.
26. den Hollander AI, van Lith-Verhoeven JJ, Arends ML, vtions in a family with severe early-onset retinitis pigmentosa. Arch Ophthalmol. 2007;125(7):932–5.
27. Mataftsi A, Schorderet DF, Chachoua L, et al. Novel TULP1 mutation causing leber congenital amaurosis or early onset retinal degeneration. Invest Ophthalmol Vis Sci. 2007;48(11):5160–7.
28. Kumaran N, Robson AG, Michaelides M. A novel case series of nmnat1-associated early-onset retinal dystrophy: extending the phenotypic spectrum. Retin Cases Brief Rep. 2018; https://doi.org/10.1097/ICB.0000000000000754.
29. Falk MJ, Zhang Q, Nakamaru-Ogiso E, et al. NMNAT1 mutations cause Leber congenital amaurosis. Nat Genet. 2012;44(9):1040–5.
30. Aboshiha J, Dubis AM, van der Spuy J, et al. Preserved outer retina in AIPL1 Leber's congenital amaurosis: implications for gene therapy. Ophthalmology. 2015;122(4):862–4.
31. Sacristan-Reviriego A, Bellingham J, Prodromou C, et al. The integrity and organization of the human AIPL1 functional domains is critical for its role as a HSP90-dependent co-chaperone for rod PDE6. Hum Mol Genet. 2018;27(7):1309.

7 Congenital Stationary Night Blindness

Bum-Joo Cho

7.1 Introduction

Congenital stationary night blindness (CSNB) is a disease group including congenital non-progressive retinal disorders characterized by reduced night vision and impaired dark adaptation [1]. This disease group is quite rare, and the prevalence of CSNB has been estimated at 0.34 per 100,000 in Northern Europe [2]. The prevalence might have been underestimated because night blindness symptom decreases due to the expansion of night lighting in urban cities, and night vision is not routinely measured [1]. Like the name of the disease, night blindness is typical which is generally not progressing [3]. Other associated abnormalities are color vision defect, nystagmus, photophobia, strabismus, refractive error, and fundus abnormality [4, 5]. Clinical presentation may appear differently depending on the causative gene.

CSNB is associated with genetic abnormalities in several steps of the intraretinal visual pathway, involving signal processing of photoreceptors, retinoid recycling of retinal pigment epithelium (RPE), or signal transmission of retinal bipolar cells [1]. In the past, the classification of CSNB mainly relied on clinical features and electroretinography (ERG) findings. Recent advances in genetics have provided an advanced understanding of the causative genes of CSNB and their pathogenesis [6]. In addition to 17 genes reported for CSNB by 2015 [1], four genes were newly identified for autosomal recessive CSNB [7].

B.-J. Cho (✉)
Hallym University Sacred Heart Hospital,
Anyang, Korea

7.2 CSNB with Normal Fundus Appearance

CSNB with a normal fundus appearance is more common than CSNB with an abnormal fundus. This group can be divided into three subtypes according to the full-field ERG findings: the complete form of Schubert–Bornschein type, the incomplete form of Schubert–Bornschein type, and Riggs type [8]. Miyake et al. subdivided the Schubert–Bornschein type according to the results of electrophysiologic tests, dark adaptation curve, and refractive error into a complete form and an incomplete form [9].

7.2.1 Schubert–Bornschein Type CSNB, Complete Form

Schubert–Bornschein type CSNB is the most commonly reported type of CSNB [1] and is caused by ON- or both ON- and OFF-bipolar cell pathway dysfunction [10]. The typical ERG finding shows a normal or minimally reduced scotopic ERG a-wave and a severely reduced b-wave, thus giving an electronegative waveform [11]. This ERG pattern means abnormalities in the

H.-G. Yu (ed.), *Inherited Retinal Disease*, https://doi.org/10.1007/978-981-16-7337-5_7

signaling process from the photoreceptor cell to the bipolar cell. Of Schubert–Bornschein type CSNB, the complete form (cCSNB) is caused by ON-bipolar cell dysfunction, while the OFF-bipolar cell function is preserved [10]

7.2.1.1 Clinical Presentation

In cCSNB, night vision is significantly reduced in nearly all patients [12], and day vision is also moderately reduced [13]. The patients with cCSNB are mostly myopic, showing a mean refractive error of –7.4 D in a Dutch study [13]. No significant difference is reported for refractive error and visual acuity between different cCSNB genotypes [13]. Nystagmus and strabismus are frequent [13], and nystagmus may decrease over time [1]. Color vision defects may occur in 14% of the patients [13]. However, visual field is usually within normal limits [13].

7.2.1.2 Electrophysiology

In dark-adapted (DA) 0.01 ERG, the ERG response completely disappears, and in DA 3.0 ERG, the a-wave is normal or minimally subnormal, but the b-wave is severely reduced or lost [9]. This implies that the rod response does not appear, and the cone response is greatly reduced. The oscillatory potential usually does not appear, suggesting an abnormality in the retinal middle layer [9]. The ERG of S-cone cells, which has connections only to the ON-bipolar cells, also appears markedly abnormal [14, 15].

7.2.1.3 Genetics and Pathogenesis

The main associated genes for cCSNB include NYX, TRPM1, GRM6, GPR179, and LRIT3 [1, 13]. NYX gene is located on the X chromosome (Xp11.4), so the mutation of NYX gene usually results in an X-linked recessive inheritance pattern [16]. GRM6, TRPM1, GPR179, and LRIT3 genes are related to the proteins present in the dendrite of ON-bipolar cells and associated with the autosomal recessive inheritance pattern [17–20]. Specifically, the TRPM1 (the transient receptor potential cation channel, subfamily M, member 1) encodes a receptor potential cation channel in ON-bipolar cells [21], and its mutation is reported to cause CSNB in Japanese and Korean patients [10, 22]. Histopathological studies also suggested that the abnormality of Schubert–Bornschein type CSNB is in the bipolar cell layer of the retina [23].

7.2.2 Schubert–Bornschein Type CSNB, Incomplete Form

The incomplete form CSNB (icCSNB) is a subtype of Schubert–Bornschein CSNB, which has an abnormality in both the ON- and OFF-bipolar cell pathways [1].

7.2.2.1 Clinical Presentation

In icCSNB, night vision problem is relatively less prevalent (54%) compared to cCSNB [13], and the subjective discomfort was also much lower [12]. Nevertheless, these patients had nystagmus (66%) and strabismus (38%) quite frequently [13]. Day vision of the patients was much worse (logMAR, 0.52) than that of cCSNB patients (logMAR 0.30) [13]. icCSNB showed less myopic refractive error (–4.8D), having 22% of hyperopic patients [13]. Color vision defect is also quite frequent (47%), but visual fields are normal [13]. The clinical presentation of icCSNB appears variable especially when associated with the CACNA1F mutation [24]. Fundus appearance is usually normal, the thinning of the ganglion cell layer, inner plexiform layer, inner nuclear layer, and RPE/photoreceptor outer segment complex may be observed in the nasal area to the fovea [25].

7.2.2.2 Electrophysiology

Unlike the ERG of cCSNB, the response to the scotopic dim flash ERG, or DA 0.01 ERG, is decreased, but not completely diminished ("incomplete") [9]. In the scotopic bright flash ERG, or DA 3.0 ERG, the a-wave appears nearly normal, but the b-wave is significantly reduced, giving an electronegative waveform [9] The normal a-wave may imply normal rod phototransduction [1]. On the other hand, the LA 3.0 ERG is significantly reduced, with a much decreased b/a ratio [1]. The LA 3.0 flicker is markedly delayed having a bifid peak [1].

7.2.2.3 Genetics and Pathogenesis

The most common genetic cause is the mutation in CACNA1F, which shows an X-linked recessive inheritance [1, 25, 26]. The CACNA1F encodes a calcium-channel α1-subunit gene in Xp11.23 [26]. In a patient having frameshift mutation in CACNA1F, the synapses in the outer nuclear layer were abnormal [27]. Thus far, the associated genes with icCSNB are known to affect the presynaptic proteins, thus disturbing both ON- and OFF-bipolar cell pathways [1]. In addition, the mutations in CABP4 and CACNA2D4 may present icCSNB with an autosomal recessive inheritance pattern [13, 28, 29]. Most of the patients having CABP4 mutation presented hyperopia [13, 30].

7.2.3 Riggs Type CSNB

The Riggs-type CSNB is known to be caused by the dysfunction of the phototransduction of the rod cells [7].

7.2.3.1 Clinical Presentation

As in the first-reported family having Riggs type of CSNB in 1838, the patients usually have a normal visual function other than decreased night vision [31]. The symptoms include mild night blindness, but no high myopia or nystagmus, and normal day vision [1, 32]. Visual fields and color vision are also within normal limits [1]. Fundus appearance is also normal [32].

7.2.3.2 Electrophysiology

The ERG of Riggs type shows a scotopic a-wave reduction and preserved photopic responses [1, 10]. The DA 0.01 ERG is usually undetectable implying severe rod cell dysfunction [8]. The amplitude of a-wave in DA 3.0 ERG is also significantly reduced, which means rod cell dysfunction [33]. The significantly reduced a-wave is a distinguished feature from Schubert–Bornschein type CSNB [8]. In DA 3.0 ERG, the b/a ratio may be also reduced, but the electronegative ERG may sometimes occur [1]. On the other hand, dark-adapted cone cell function is preserved or slightly reduced [1, 32]. The scotopic red flash ERG also shows a preserved x-wave showing a normal cone function [8].

7.2.3.3 Genetics and Pathogenesis

The implicated genes in Riggs type CSNB include RHO, GNAT1 (G protein subunit alpha transducin 1), and PDE6B (cGMP-phosphodiesterase) of the rod cells [8]. These genes are believed to be involved in the phototransduction process of rod cells, and the mutation may cause the rod cells to act as if they were exposed to a constant background light [1]. The Nougaret family had their mutation in p. Gly38Asp mutation in GNAT1 [34], and the Danish Rambusch family also showed a p. Gln200Glu mutation in the GNAT1 gene [35]. The GNAT1 mutation usually presents an autosomal recessive inheritance or autosomal dominant pattern [1, 36]. A heterozygous missense mutation in cGMP-phosphodiesterase, p.His258Asn, was also reported in autosomal dominant CSNB [37], and the truncating mutation in PDE6B was reported in a Riggs-type of CSNB [38]. The autosomal dominant inheritance pattern usually presents with the mutation in the RHO (rhodopsin) gene, such as Ala292Glu or Thr94Ile [39, 40]. The Gly90Asp mutation in RHO may also induce a CSNB with the fundus appearance of bony spicules [41].

7.3 CSNB with Abnormal Fundus Appearance

7.3.1 Oguchi Disease

Oguchi disease is a very rare type of CSNB having characteristic golden sheen fundus with normal visual acuity and visual fields [8].

7.3.1.1 Clinical Presentation

Patients with Oguchi disease complain of congenital night blindness, but visual acuity, color vision, and visual field are usually normal [8]. The fundus was discolored to a peculiar gold or gray-yellowish color and was accompanied by a metallic luster [42]. The golden sheen may change depending on the intensity or angle of incident light during examination [43]. After prolonged dark adaptation, the golden sheen recovers to normal, showing time differences between areas of the retina [44]. The recovery of the golden color of the fundus was named as "Mizuo–Nakamura phenomenon" or just "Mizuo phenomenon" [43, 44]. When exposed to light again, the retina slowly reverts back to its original gold color [44]. In the optical coherence tomography (OCT), the length of the rod cell outer segment is shortened in the light adaptation state and recovers after prolonged dark adaptation, which may explain the restoration of fundus discoloration [45, 46]. Oguchi's disease generally does not progress but may progress with photoreceptor degeneration [1].

7.3.1.2 Electrophysiology

The scotopic ERG response after 20 min of dark adaptation is similar to those of Riggs-type of CSNB, fundus albipunctatus and vitamin A deficiency showing severe and selective rod photoreceptor dysfunction [1]. DA 0.01 ERG response does not appear [47], and DA 3.0 ERG shows a significantly reduced a-wave and a decreased b/a ratio having a shortened b-wave peak time [8]. An electronegative waveform may appear, but the dark-adapted cone response is not affected [47]. The light-adapted ERG responses are normal for both ON- and OFF-responses [8, 48]. The appearance of cone-rod break point on the dark adaptation curve is delayed [49].

After prolonged dark adaptation, the rod cell function recovers, and the ERG response to a single flash show normalized a- and b-waves [50]. However, after that, the scotopic ERG responses turn to be abnormal and need another prolonged dark adaptation to be normalized [50].

7.3.1.3 Genetics and Pathogenesis

The implicated genes in Oguchi disease include SAG and GRK1 [51–54]. The GRK1 (G protein-coupled receptor kinase) and the SAG (arrestin) genes are associated with the deactivation process of the phototransduction cascade, and the continued activation of the phototransduction gives rise to the abnormal desensitization of the rod cells [1, 55]. Oguchi disease shows an autosomal recessive inheritance pattern [1].

7.3.2 Fundus Albipunctatus

Fundus albipunctatus is a subtype of CSNB showing multiple yellow-white dots in the retina with macular sparing [8].

7.3.2.1 Clinical Presentation

Patients with Fundus albipunctatus usually have night blindness and delayed dark adaptation [1]. Visual acuity and color vision are generally normal [1]. Visual fields are usually normal in fundus albipunctatus [56], but adult-onset central visual loss may occur [57]. Fundus examination reveals multiple small white or yellowish dots in the posterior pole and mid-periphery, while the macula is spared [58]. The characteristic dots are densely distributed around the lateral vascular arcades, but the number decreases toward the periphery [1] There is usually no optic nerve pallor, retinal vessel attenuation, or pigmentary bone spicules [1]. The flecks in childhood may become in the form of fine punctuate dots, may fade, and may increase in number [59, 60]. Those white dots are presumed to have 11-cis-retinal precursors [61]. The fundus appearance may be similar to retinitis punctata albescens, but the latter is progressive and has a worse visual prognosis [1]. However, fundus albipunctatus may sometimes progress with macular atrophy and cone dystrophy [62, 63].

The white dots may be hyperautofluorescent in young patients but maybe iso- or hypoautofluorescent in old patients [1, 57]. The background autofluorescence is severely reduced implying the disruption of retinoid recycling [61]. In the OCT, white dots appear as deep hyperreflective lesions around the external limiting membrane and the ellipsoid zone [57, 58]. In adaptive optics, a lower macular cone density with disrupted macular cone mosaic arrangement is observed [64].

7.3.2.2 Electrophysiology

In the ISCEV-standard DA 0.01 ERG, the a-wave and b-wave are nearly diminished, resembling the result of Riggs type CSNB or vitamin A deficiency [65]. On the other hand, the scotopic red flash ERG presents a preserved cone function [8]. The DA 3.0 ERG shows a reduced a-wave with or without a decreased b/a ratio [57]. In less than half of the patients, the b-wave of the light-adapted cone ERG is decreased [66], but the majority may show normal light-adapted ERG responses [8, 65]. The delay of the LA flicker ERG may be presented [1]. The abnormal rod and cone ERGs may occur in childhood [67].

ISCEV-standard ERG cannot make a diagnosis alone because recovery should be demonstrated after extended dark adaptation. After prolonged dark adaptation, the rod cell response recovers significantly or becomes normal [57]. It usually takes several hours and varies from patient to patient [65].

7.3.2.3 Genetics and Pathogenesis

Most of the patients have the mutation in the RDH5 (11-cis retinol dehydrogenase 5) gene [65]. RDH5 encodes retinol dehydrogenase, which is responsible for converting 11-cis-retinol to 11-cis-retinal in RPE [1]. RDH5 is associated with the recycling of rhodopsin in RPE, and its dysfunction causes delayed rhodopsin regeneration [68]. In most patients, the rhodopsin level normalizes after prolonged dark adaptation, which may require overnight time [1]. The RDH5 mutation of fundus albipunctatus shows an autosomal recessive inheritance pattern [65, 69]. Some of non-Asian cases have not reported the RDH5 mutation [70, 71]. The association with compound heterozygous mutation in RPE65 is also reported, which induced a more severe form of early-onset rod-cone dystrophy [67].

References

1. Zeitz C, Robson AG, Audo I. Congenital stationary night blindness: an analysis and update of genotype-phenotype correlations and pathogenic mechanisms. Prog Retin Eye Res. 2015;45:58–110.
2. Haim M. Congenital stationary night blindness. Acta Ophthalmol (Copenh). 1986;64:192–8.
3. Carr RE. Congenital stationary nightblindness. Trans Am Ophthalmol Soc. 1974;72:448–87.
4. Zeitz C. Molecular genetics and protein function involved in nocturnal vision. Expert Rev Ophthalmol. 2007;2:467–85.
5. Tan X, Aoki A, Yanagi Y. Color vision abnormality as an initial presentation of the complete type of congenital stationary night blindness. Clin Ophthalmol. 2013;7:1587–90.
6. Koenekoop RK. Revisiting congenital stationary night blindness in the molecular era. JAMA Ophthalmol. 2018;136:398–9.
7. Almutairi F, Almeshari N, Ahmad K, Magliyah MS, Schatz P. Congenital stationary night blindness: an update and review of the disease spectrum in Saudi Arabia. Acta Ophthalmol. 2020; https://doi.org/10.1111/aos.14693.
8. Baldwin AN, Robson AG, Moore AT, Duncan JL. Abnormalities of rod and cone function. In: Schachat A, editor. Ryan's retina. 6th ed. Edinburgh: Elsevier; 2017. p. 1006–17.
9. Miyake Y, Yagasaki K, Horiguchi M, Kawase Y, Kanda T. Congenital stationary night blindness with negative electroretinogram. A new classification. Arch Ophthalmol. 1986;104:1013–20.
10. Lee YJ, Joo K, Seong MW, Park KH, Park SS, Woo SJ. Congenital stationary night blindness due to novel TRPM1 gene mutations in a Korean patient. Korean J Ophthalmol. 2020;34:170–2.
11. Schubert G, Bornschein H. [Analysis of the human electroretinogram]. Ophthalmologica. 1952;123:396–413.
12. Bijveld MM, van Genderen MM, Hoeben FP, et al. Assessment of night vision problems in patients with congenital stationary night blindness. PLoS One. 2013;8:e62927.
13. Bijveld MM, Florijn RJ, Bergen AA, et al. Genotype and phenotype of 101 Dutch patients with congenital stationary night blindness. Ophthalmology. 2013;120:2072–81.
14. Kamiyama M, Yamamoto S, Nitta K, Hayasaka S. Undetectable S cone electroretinogram b-wave in complete congenital stationary night blindness. Br J Ophthalmol. 1996;80:637–9.
15. Kolb H, Goede P, Roberts S, McDermott R, Gouras P. Uniqueness of the S-cone pedicle in the human retina and consequences for color processing. J Comp Neurol. 1997;386:443–60.
16. Pusch CM, Zeitz C, Brandau O, et al. The complete form of X-linked congenital stationary night blindness is caused by mutations in a gene encoding a leucine-rich repeat protein. Nat Genet. 2000;26:324–7.
17. Dryja TP, McGee TL, Berson EL, et al. Night blindness and abnormal cone electroretinogram ON responses in patients with mutations in the GRM6 gene encoding mGluR6. Proc Natl Acad Sci U S A. 2005;102:4884–9.

18. Audo I, Kohl S, Leroy BP, et al. TRPM1 is mutated in patients with autosomal-recessive complete congenital stationary night blindness. Am J Hum Genet. 2009;85:720–9.
19. Audo I, Bujakowska K, Orhan E, et al. Whole-exome sequencing identifies mutations in GPR179 leading to autosomal-recessive complete congenital stationary night blindness. Am J Hum Genet. 2012;90:321–30.
20. Zeitz C, Jacobson SG, Hamel CP, et al. Whole-exome sequencing identifies LRIT3 mutations as a cause of autosomal-recessive complete congenital stationary night blindness. Am J Hum Genet. 2013;92:67–75.
21. Miraldi Utz V, Pfeifer W, Longmuir SQ, Olson RJ, Wang K, Drack AV. Presentation of TRPM1-associated congenital stationary night blindness in children. JAMA Ophthalmol. 2018;136:389–98.
22. Nakamura M, Sanuki R, Yasuma TR, et al. TRPM1 mutations are associated with the complete form of congenital stationary night blindness. Mol Vis. 2010;16:425–37.
23. Watanabe I, Taniguchi Y, Morioka K, Kato M. Congenital stationary night blindness with myopia: a clinico-pathologic study. Doc Ophthalmol. 1986;63:55–62.
24. Boycott KM, Pearce WG, Bech-Hansen NT. Clinical variability among patients with incomplete X-linked congenital stationary night blindness and a founder mutation in CACNA1F. Can J Ophthalmol. 2000;35:204–13.
25. Chen RW, Greenberg JP, Lazow MA, et al. Autofluorescence imaging and spectral-domain optical coherence tomography in incomplete congenital stationary night blindness and comparison with retinitis pigmentosa. Am J Ophthalmol. 2012;153:143–54.e2.
26. Bech-Hansen NT, Naylor MJ, Maybaum TA, et al. Loss-of-function mutations in a calcium-channel alpha1-subunit gene in Xp11.23 cause incomplete X-linked congenital stationary night blindness. Nat Genet. 1998;19:264–7.
27. Vincent A, Héon E. Outer retinal structural anomaly due to frameshift mutation in CACNA1F gene. Eye (Lond). 2012;26:1278–80.
28. Zeitz C, Kloeckener-Gruissem B, Forster U, et al. Mutations in CABP4, the gene encoding the Ca2+-binding protein 4, cause autosomal recessive night blindness. Am J Hum Genet. 2006;79:657–67.
29. Wycisk KA, Zeitz C, Feil S, et al. Mutation in the auxiliary calcium-channel subunit CACNA2D4 causes autosomal recessive cone dystrophy. Am J Hum Genet. 2006;79:973–7.
30. Khan AO, Alrashed M, Alkuraya FS. Clinical characterisation of the CABP4-related retinal phenotype. Br J Ophthalmol. 2013;97:262–5.
31. Cunier F. Hemeralopie hereditaire depuis deux siecles dans une famille de la commune de Vendemian, a cinq lieues de Montpellier. Ann d'Ocul. 1838;1:32–4.
32. Riggs LA. Electroretinography in cases of night blindness. Am J Ophthalmol. 1954;38:70–8.
33. Sandberg MA, Pawlyk BS, Dan J, Arnaud B, Dryja TP, Berson EL. Rod and cone function in the Nougaret form of stationary night blindness. Arch Ophthalmol. 1998;116:867–72.
34. Dryja TP, Hahn LB, Reboul T, Arnaud B. Missense mutation in the gene encoding the alpha subunit of rod transducin in the Nougaret form of congenital stationary night blindness. Nat Genet. 1996;13:358–60.
35. Szabo V, Kreienkamp HJ, Rosenberg T, Gal A. p.Gln200Glu, a putative constitutively active mutant of rod alpha-transducin (GNAT1) in autosomal dominant congenital stationary night blindness. Hum Mutat. 2007;28:741–2.
36. Nettleship E. A history of congenital stationary night blindness in nine consecutive generations. Trans Ophthalmol Soc UK. 1907;27:269.
37. Gal A, Orth U, Baehr W, Schwinger E, Rosenberg T. Heterozygous missense mutation in the rod cGMP phosphodiesterase beta-subunit gene in autosomal dominant stationary night blindness. Nat Genet. 1994;7:64–8.
38. Manes G, Cheguru P, Majumder A, et al. A truncated form of rod photoreceptor PDE6 beta-subunit causes autosomal dominant congenital stationary night blindness by interfering with the inhibitory activity of the gamma-subunit. PLoS One. 2014;9:e95768.
39. Dryja TP, Berson EL, Rao VR, Oprian DD. Heterozygous missense mutation in the rhodopsin gene as a cause of congenital stationary night blindness. Nat Genet. 1993;4:280–3.
40. al-Jandal N, Farrar GJ, Kiang AS, et al. A novel mutation within the rhodopsin gene (Thr-94-Ile) causing autosomal dominant congenital stationary night blindness. Hum Mutat. 1999;13:75–81.
41. Sieving PA, Richards JE, Naarendorp F, Bingham EL, Scott K, Alpern M. Dark-light: model for nightblindness from the human rhodopsin Gly-90-->Asp mutation. Proc Natl Acad Sci U S A. 1995;92:880–4.
42. Oguchi C. Ueber einen Fall von eigenartiger Hemeralopie. Nippon Ganka Gakkai Zasshi. 1907;11:123–34.
43. Mizuo G. On a new discovery in the dark adaptation of Oguchi's disease. Acta Societatis Ophthalmologicae Japonicae. 1913;17:1854–9.
44. Mizuo G, Nakamura B. On new discovery in dark adaptation in Oguchi's disease. Acta Societatis Ophthalmologicae Japonicae. 1914;18:73–127.
45. Hashimoto H, Kishi S. Shortening of the rod outer segment in Oguchi disease. Graefes Arch Clin Exp Ophthalmol. 2009;247:1561–3.
46. Takada M, Otani A, Ogino K, Yoshimura N. Spectral-domain optical coherence tomography findings in the Mizuo-Nakamura phenomenon of Oguchi disease. Retina. 2011;31:626–8.
47. Carr RE, Gouras P. Oguchi's disease. Arch Ophthalmol. 1965;73:646–56.
48. Miyake Y, Horiguchi M, Suzuki S, Kondo M, Tanikawa A. Electrophysiological findings in patients with Oguchi's disease. Jpn J Ophthalmol. 1996;40:511–9.

49. Nakamura B. Ueber ein neues Phanomen der Farbenveranderung des menschlichen Augenhintergrundes im Zusammenhang mit der fortschreitenden Dunkeladaptation. Klin Monatsbl Augenheilkd. 1920;65:883.
50. Gouras P. Electroretinography: some basic principles. Invest Ophthalmol. 1970;9:557–69.
51. Fuchs S, Nakazawa M, Maw M, Tamai M, Oguchi Y, Gal A. A homozygous 1-base pair deletion in the arrestin gene is a frequent cause of Oguchi disease in Japanese. Nat Genet. 1995;10:360–2.
52. Yamamoto S, Sippel KC, Berson EL, Dryja TP. Defects in the rhodopsin kinase gene in the Oguchi form of stationary night blindness. Nat Genet. 1997;15:175–8.
53. Hayashi T, Gekka T, Takeuchi T, Goto-Omoto S, Kitahara K. A novel homozygous GRK1 mutation (P391H) in 2 siblings with Oguchi disease with markedly reduced cone responses. Ophthalmology. 2007;114:134–41.
54. Hayashi T, Tsuzuranuki S, Kozaki K, Urashima M, Tsuneoka H. Macular dysfunction in oguchi disease with the frequent mutation 1147delA in the SAG gene. Ophthalmic Res. 2011;46:175–80.
55. Paskowitz DM, LaVail MM, Duncan JL. Light and inherited retinal degeneration. Br J Ophthalmol. 2006;90:1060–6.
56. Lauber H. Die sogenannte Retinitis punctata albescens. Klin Monatasbl Augenheilkd. 1910;48:133.
57. Sergouniotis PI, Sohn EH, Li Z, et al. Phenotypic variability in RDH5 retinopathy (Fundus Albipunctatus). Ophthalmology. 2011;118:1661–70.
58. Wang NK, Chuang LH, Lai CC, et al. Multimodal fundus imaging in fundus albipunctatus with RDH5 mutation: a newly identified compound heterozygous mutation and review of the literature. Doc Ophthalmol. 2012;125:51–62.
59. Marmor MF. Long-term follow-up of the physiologic abnormalities and fundus changes in fundus albipunctatus. Ophthalmology. 1990;97:380–4.
60. Sekiya K, Nakazawa M, Ohguro H, Usui T, Tanimoto N, Abe H. Long-term fundus changes due to Fundus albipunctatus associated with mutations in the RDH5 gene. Arch Ophthalmol. 2003;121:1057–9.
61. Schatz P, Preising M, Lorenz B, et al. Lack of autofluorescence in fundus albipunctatus associated with mutations in RDH5. Retina. 2010;30:1704–13.
62. Hotta K, Nakamura M, Kondo M, et al. Macular dystrophy in a Japanese family with fundus albipunctatus. Am J Ophthalmol. 2003;135:917–9.
63. Nakamura M, Hotta Y, Tanikawa A, Terasaki H, Miyake Y. A high association with cone dystrophy in Fundus albipunctatus caused by mutations of the RDH5 gene. Invest Ophthalmol Vis Sci. 2000;41:3925–32.
64. Makiyama Y, Ooto S, Hangai M, et al. Cone abnormalities in fundus albipunctatus associated with RDH5 mutations assessed using adaptive optics scanning laser ophthalmoscopy. Am J Ophthalmol. 2014;157:558–70.e1–4.
65. Skorczyk-Werner A, Pawlowski P, Michalczuk M, et al. Fundus albipunctatus: review of the literature and report of a novel RDH5 gene mutation affecting the invariant tyrosine (p.Tyr175Phe). J Appl Genet. 2015;56:317–27.
66. Niwa Y, Kondo M, Ueno S, Nakamura M, Terasaki H, Miyake Y. Cone and rod dysfunction in fundus albipunctatus with RDH5 mutation: an electrophysiological study. Invest Ophthalmol Vis Sci. 2005;46:1480–5.
67. Schatz P, Preising M, Lorenz B, Sander B, Larsen M, Rosenberg T. Fundus albipunctatus associated with compound heterozygous mutations in RPE65. Ophthalmology. 2011;118:888–94.
68. Yamamoto H, Simon A, Eriksson U, Harris E, Berson EL, Dryja TP. Mutations in the gene encoding 11-cis retinol dehydrogenase cause delayed dark adaptation and fundus albipunctatus. Nat Genet. 1999;22:188–91.
69. Carr RE, Ripps H, Siegel IM. Visual pigment kinetics and adaptation in fundus albipunctatus. Doc Ophthalmol. 1974;4:193–204.
70. Driessen CA, Janssen BP, Winkens HJ, et al. Null mutation in the human 11-cis retinol dehydrogenase gene associated with fundus albipunctatus. Ophthalmology. 2001;108:1479–84.
71. Marmor MF, Haeseleer F, Palczewski K. Albipunctate retinopathy with cone dysfunction and no abnormality in the RDH5 or RLBP1 genes. Retina. 2003;23:543–6.

8 Vitelliform Macular Dystrophy

Min Kim and Hyeong-Gon Yu

Abstract

Vitelliform macular dystrophy (VMD) is a group of macular dystrophy characterized by the subretinal accumulation of yellow yolk-like materials, which predominantly affects the macula. Best vitelliform macular dystrophy is among the most common autosomal dominant (AD) retinal dystrophy caused by mutations in the *BEST1* gene. Since first identification of *BEST1* gene in 1998, molecular biology and pathophysiology of *BEST1* gene and vitelliform macular dystrophy were studied. Recent advances in genetic analysis have described over 200 different human *BEST1* mutations to date, associated with a broad spectrum of ocular diseases, called bestrophinopathy. However, the genotype-phenotype correlation in VMD is largely unexplored. Genetic test is clinically important in the diagnosis of VMD because the clinical features of VMD are similar to those of exudative age-related macular degeneration (AMD), choroidal neovascularization (CNV), or central serous chorioretinopathy (CSC). Here, in addition to describing the clinical characteristics of VMD, this chapter focuses on the clinical genetics of *BEST1* gene in VMD.

Keywords

Vitelliform macular dystrophy · Bestrophin-1 · Best vitelliform macular dystrophy · Adult-onset vitelliform macular dystrophy · *BEST1* gene mutation · Genome editing

M. Kim
Department of Ophthalmology, College of Medicine, Yonsei University, Seoul, Republic of Korea

H.-G. Yu (✉)
Department of Ophthalmology, College of Medicine, Seoul National University, Seoul, Republic of Korea

Retinal Degeneration Research Lab, Seoul National University Hospital Biomedical Research Institute, Seoul, Republic of Korea
e-mail: hgonyu@snu.ac.kr

8.1 Introduction

Macular dystrophy is a group of heritable disorders that cause ophthalmoscopically visible macular abnormalities. Vitelliform macular dystrophy (VMD) is a group of macular dystrophy characterized by the subretinal accumulation of yellow yolk-like materials, which predominantly affects the macula. Best vitelliform macular dystrophy (BVMD) is named after Friedrich Best, who described a family with a history of early-onset macular degeneration in 1905 [1]. BVMD is among the most common autosomal dominant (AD) retinal dystrophy caused by mutations in the *BEST1* gene. Since the first identification of *BEST1* gene in 1998 [2], molecular biology and

H.-G. Yu (ed.), *Inherited Retinal Disease*, https://doi.org/10.1007/978-981-16-7337-5_8

pathophysiology of *BEST1* gene in VMD have been studied. Recent advances in genetic analysis have described over 200 different human *BEST1* mutations to date, associated with a broad spectrum of ocular diseases, called bestrophinopathy [3, 4]. Bestrophinopathy includes five clinically distinct categories: BVMD, adult-onset vitelliform macular dystrophy (AVMD), autosomal recessive bestrophinopathy (ARB), autosomal dominant vitreoretinochoroidopathy (ADVIRC), and retinitis pigmentosa. AVMD was first described by Gass in 1974, who initially termed it peculiar foveomacular dystrophy [5]. AVMD is one of the most common forms of macular dystrophy as well [6]. Many investigators suggested that AVMD is a mild form of BVMD within the same spectrum because the clinical features of AVMD were similar to those of early-stage BVMD, and the age of onset was highly variable [7–9]. Clinically, BVMD is distinguished from AVMD by an earlier age of onset, larger lesion size, and an abnormal electrooculogram (EOG). Clinical features of VMD are similar to those of exudative age-related macular degeneration (AMD), choroidal neovascularization (CNV), or central serous chorioretinopathy (CSC). Thus, a genetic test is clinically important in the diagnosis of VMD. Here, in addition to describing the clinical characteristics of VMD, this chapter focuses on the clinical genetics of the *BEST1* gene in VMD (BVMD and AVMD).

8.2 Epidemiology and Asian Perspective

VMD is an autosomal dominant macular dystrophy with an estimated prevalence of 1 in 10,000 in USA [10], 2/10,000 in Sweden [11], 1.5/100,000 in Denmark [12], and 1 in 16,500 to 1 in 21,000 in Olmsted County, Minnesota, USA [13]. Males are more affected than females (3:1) [11, 12]. Despite the update of novel mutations of *BEST1* in Asian VMD patients, there was no report of the prevalence of VMD in Asian countries. Thus, a study of the prevalence of VMD with genetic analysis in Asian countries is necessary.

8.3 Molecular Biology

The *BEST1* gene consists of 11 exons, including non-coding exon 1, which encode the bestrophin-1 protein (585 amino acids). The functional bestrophin/UPF0187 domain is located at exon 2–9. Bestrophin-1 is a retinal pigment epithelium (RPE) protein hypothesized to function as a Ca^{2+}-activated Cl^- channel (CaCC), or a regulator of ion transport [14]. Bestrophin-1 is predominantly expressed in the basolateral membrane of the RPE [15]. X-ray structure of chicken BEST1-Fab complexes indicates that Bestrophin-1 forms a homo-pentamer and functions as a CaCC [16]. Disease-causing mutations are prevalent within the gating apparatus. In addition, Bestrophin-1 functions as a regulator of intracellular calcium signaling and influences transepithelial electrical properties [17]. Recently, patient stem cell-derived RPE used for the function of bestrophin-1 reveals that bestrophin-1 assembles into a key calcium-sensing chloride channel in human RPE [18]. Further study using RPE cells from patient-derived induced pluripotent stem cells (iPSc) harboring *BEST1* mutations is required to elucidate the exact functional role of bestrophin-1.

Recently, a novel perspective on the role of *BEST-1* mutation in the pathogenesis of BVMD was reported by Gao et al. [19] In this study, apoptotic markers caspase-3 and PARP expression were significantly increased in *BEST1*-pcDNA3.1 p.S142G and p.A146T group. Also, flow cytometry showed that the apoptosis rates were significantly increased in the *BEST1*-pcDNA3.1 p.V143F, p.S142G, and p.A146T group compared with the wild-type group, suggesting that BEST1 mutations does not only affect CaCC function but also may have a role in apoptosis and degenerative changes of RPE.

8.4 Clinical Features

8.4.1 BVMD

BVMD is an early-onset autosomal dominant disorder showing extremely variable penetrance and expressivity. The diagnosis of BVMD shows a bimodal age distribution, the first maximum peak was made during childhood, but the second peak was made following puberty and extending into the sixth decade of life [20]. Before the era of genetic analysis, the diagnosis of BVMD was based on typical fundus findings, family history, and a decreased Arden ratio (light peak/dark trough) of EOG with a normal electroretinogram (ERG), which may contribute to the variability of penetrance, expressivity, and onset age.

BVMD is caused by dysfunction of Bestrophin-1 protein, a CaCC protein located on the basolateral membrane of RPE, causes abnormal fluid and ion exchange that decrease pumping the fluid from the subretinal space, resulting in swelling of RPE and subretinal lipofuscin accumulation [21]. Histopathologically, autofluorescent material was accumulated in the outer retina and the subretinal space in BVMD, which is considered as indigestible components of photoreceptor outer segments that accumulate due to the lack of direct apposition of the outer segments and the RPE [22]. Eventual phagocytosis of these older materials over time would load the RPE cells and may account for excessive accumulation of abnormal lipofuscin in RPE cells across the entire fundus [23]. These findings coincide with the decreased Arden ratio of EOG, less than 1.5, seen in BVMD, which suggest generalized dysfunction of the RPE. Even otherwise, asymptomatic carriers of *BEST1* mutations will exhibit an altered EOG [24]. Full-field ERG is generally normal, but the multifocal ERG amplitudes of the central and pericentral responses were significantly reduced in the majority of patients [25]. However, the photoreceptor structure evaluated by cellular imaging with adaptive optics scanning light ophthalmoscopy was retained within active BVMD lesions, even in apparently advanced disease [26, 27].

Five progressive stages can be defined based on fundus examination [21, 28]. However, these stages are not observed in all patients, nor do they occur consecutively. The first previtelliform stage is characterized by the absence of symptoms and subtle RPE changes such as RPE mottling and a small yellow spot. On optical coherence tomography (OCT), RPE and ellipsoid zone (EZ) disruption was detectable in a small fraction of eyes [29, 30]. A slight thickening of the interdigitation zone was also observed [31]. EOG is abnormal, and fluorescein angiogram (FA) shows window defects. Visual acuity remains intact in most patients. The previtelliform lesions are characterized by absence or only slight autofluorescence on fundus autofluorescence (FAF) imaging.

The second vitelliform shows a well circumscribed, circular, homogeneous, yellow-opaque, 0.5 to 3-disc diameter sized, yolk-like macular lesions. The remaining part of the fundus usually has a normal appearance, but multifocal lesions also can be seen. The accumulation of hyperreflective vitelliform material is clearly visible on OCT below the neurosensory retina, located between the EZ and the RPE. The disruption of outer retinal layers and neurosensory retinal detachment with subretinal fluid can be seen in many cases [29, 30]. The yellowish subretinal material is intensely hyperautofluorescent in FAF imaging. FA shows marked hypofluorescence in the zone covered by blockage of fluorescence. Metamorphopsia, blurred vision and a decrease of central vision can occur.

In the third pseudohypopyon stage, the vitelliform material accumulates inferiorly and develops a fluid level. On OCT, the upper part of the lesion is observed as hyporeflective area located between RPE and EZ, with clumping of hyperreflective material on the posterior retinal surface. The lower part of the lesion, where the vitelliform material is still accumulated, shows a highly reflective area located in the subretinal space. FA shows hypofluorescence in the lower part resulting from the blockage by the vitelliform material. The superior part shows hyperfluorescent due to transmission defects linked to RPE and chorioretinal atrophy in the early phase. FAF shows a loss of autofluorescence, particularly in the upper part.

The fourth vitelliruptive stage is characterized by the partial reabsorption of the vitelliform material. This vitelliform material becomes less homogeneous to develop a "scrambled-egg" appearance. OCT shows an optically empty lesion between EZ and RPE, with clumping of hyperreflective material on the posterior retinal surface like the upper part of the pseudohypopyon. The areas of focal RPE hypertrophy can be observed as hyperreflective mottling on the RPE layer on some parts. FAF shows decreased autofluorescence centrally but increased autofluorescence at the outer border of the lesion.

In the last atrophic/fibrotic stage, RPE atrophy and loss of central vision occur after rupture and reabsorption of the cystic lesion. FA shows hyperfluorescence without leakage. OCT reveals thinning of all the retinal layers and diffuse disappearance of outer retinal layers within the macular area, with highly hyperreflective thickening at the RPE level [30, 32]. Atrophic lesions are characterized by decreased autofluorescence on FAF.

Choroidal neovascularization (CNV) may develop and can lead to form a disciform scar. Patients usually experience sudden visual disturbance with central scotoma and/or metamorphopsia, showing a macular hemorrhage on fundus examination. In that case, FA shows hyperfluorescence because of CNV and leakage. Intravitreal anti-vascular endothelial growth (VEGF) injection was effective in treating CNV complicated with BVMD and safe even in children [33–35].

Patients with BVMD undergo a progressive decrease of vision over time. In a study that evaluated the course of visual decline of 53 patients in BVMD with *BEST1* mutation [36], the median age at the onset of visual symptoms was 33 years. Twenty-five percent of patients retained visual acuity of 20/40 or better at the age of 66 years. Another study evaluated 47 patients with BVMD, and 74% of patients older than 30 years old had a visual acuity of 20/100 or worse in at least one eye [37].

Along with the recent developments in multimodal imaging, many studies have demonstrated some parameters that would account for the prognosis of BVMD. Several studies demonstrated that ellipsoid zone (EZ) status represents a valuable functional marker in VMD. While larger EZ alterations resulted in worse BCVA, optically preserved islet resulted in better BCVA [38–40]. In addition, outer nuclear layer (ONL) thickness was negatively correlated with BCVA and the stage progression of BVMD [40]. Interestingly, Parodi et al. have identified intraretinal hyperreflective foci in OCT images of BVMD patients. The number of these intraretinal lesions increased as the stage of the disease progressed and was negatively correlated with BCVA [41]. Although the origin of these lesions is still unclear, histopathologic studies suggest that these originate from the RPE cells that have been detached from Bruch's membrane and have migrated into the vitelliform material, eventually arriving into the neurosensory retina [42]. By using polarization-sensitive OCT, a novel imaging technique that provides tissue-specific contrast, RPE cells were found in the vitelliform material and the neurosensory retina, which supplements the results from previous studies [43].

OCT angiography (OCTA) also served to provide a novel insight into the pathophysiology and prognosis of BVMD. In a cross-sectional case series, OCTA revealed that superficial capillary plexus (SCP) and deep capillary plexus (DCP) were significantly impaired in stage 3–5 compared to normal controls [44]. The foveal avascular zone (FAZ) at DCP was enlarged as stage progressed. The vessel density of DCP was significantly correlated with the patients' stage and BCVA. In another prospective case series, OCTA detected non-exudative macular neovascularization in 96% of patients in stages 4 and 5 [45]. Interestingly, these new vessels were not detected by conventional FA and ICGA. Most macular neovascularization with exudative manifestations was seen in stages 2 and 3 and rarely in stages 4 and 5, which implies that new vessels arise in early stages and tend to stabilize later on at the end stages of the disease.

8.4.2 AVMD

Gass reported a 3-generation family and six sporadic patients characterized by one-third disc diameter sized bilateral subfoveal vitelliform lesions with onset between the ages of 30 and 50 years accompanied by slowly progressive visual loss as "peculiar foveomacular dystrophy" [5]. They also showed occasional paracentral drusen, normal to slightly subnormal response on EOG but normal ERG and color vision [5]. AVMD shows a variable genetic inheritance, although most cases are sporadic [46]. Patients with AVMD may be asymptomatic but become symptomatic in the fourth or fifth decade of life with blurred vision, metamorphopsia or scotoma and typically have a slow progression of vision loss [47]. Patients with AVMD typically presents with a round, yellowish subretinal deposit in one-third to one disc diameter size within the macular area, similar fundus finding to the vitelliform stage of BVMD.

The initial yellow lesion may present in only one eye and appear as small yellow flecks in the paracentral area. EOG shows a normal or slight reduction in the Arden ratio, which is obviously abnormal in BVMD. The macular lesion appears as hyperautofluorescent in FAF. The vitelliform deposit usually appears as initially hypofluorescent but gradually becomes hyperfluorescent on the edges by staining of the dye in FA [48] and appears hypofluorescent on indocyanine green angiography (ICGA). OCT reveals a dome-shaped hyperreflective lesion located between the retina and RPE [49]. The foveal thinning and EZ disruption are also observed and probably explain the progressive visual loss [50, 51].

AVMD progression is characterized by fragmentation and reabsorption of the vitelliform material [6]. Macular atrophy progressively replaces the vitelliform deposits at the advanced stages of the disease in most cases [51], but most patients retain reading vision throughout life [52, 53]. CNV may be complicated in a few cases, six out of 51 patients developed CNV after a 6-year follow-up [54]. Anti-VEGF therapies have shown to be effective in the treatment of CNV associated with AVMD [55].

Recently, several AVMD studies based on OCTA have been published. OCTA was more sensitive in detecting CNV than conventional FA in AVMD patients in pseudohypopyon stage [56]. In quantitative analysis, there was a significant reduction of vessel density of SCP in parafoveal and perifoveal zones. The vessel density of DCP was higher in the parafoveal zone. The foveal avascular zone area was larger in DCP, and choriocapillaris vessel density was lower in the parafoveal zone [57, 58].

8.5 Genetic Aspects

8.5.1 BVMD

Currently, only genetic test for mutation analysis of the *BEST1* gene leads to confirmation of a clinical diagnosis of BVMD. Note that Individuals with clinical findings of BVMD occasionally have a normal EOG, turning out to have a pathogenic variant of *BEST1* [59]. In case of atypical BVMD [3], genetic test for confirmation should be performed. Over 300 *BEST1* mutations with significant clinical heterogeneity require a thorough genetic analysis and clinical examinations to a better understanding of genotype-phenotype correlations in BVMD. Most mutations of *BEST1* gene in BVMD and AVMD are missense mutations. Table 8.1 shows a list of missense mutations of *BEST1* gene in BVMD and AVMD.

Most genetic studies were performed in Western countries, including USA, England, Sweden, Denmark, Germany, Netherlands, Italy, and France. *BEST1* mutations are extremely heterogenous, but several mutations have been frequently found (Thr6Pro, Arg25Trp, Arg218Cys, Tyr227Asn, Arg243Val, Ile295del, Gle300Asp, Asp301Glu, and Asp302Asn). Interestingly, these frequent mutations are ethnic specific (44.4% of Asp302Asn in Danish [12] and 36.8% of Arg25Trp in Italian [103]).

Currently, only limited reports are available in Asian genetic studies of BEST1 from Chinese [62, 68, 84, 86, 92, 97, 104, 105], Japanese [60, 100], and Korean [9]. The mutation spectrum of the *BEST1* gene in Asian patients of BVMD is different from those in Western patients [105]. Six novel missense mutations (Thr2Asn, Leu75Phe, Ser144Asn, Arg255Trp, Pro297Thr, and Asp301Gly) and one previously reported mutation (Arg218Cys) were identified [62].

Table 8.1 *BEST1* missense mutations in BVMD and AVMD

	Mutations a.a	Mutations nucleotide	Associated disease	Inheritance	Ethnicity	Reference
1	Thr2Ala	c.4A>G	BVMD	AD	Japanese	Katagiri et al. [60]
			AVMD	AD	Iowa, USA	Kinnick et al. [61]
2	Thr2Asn	c.5C>A	BVMD	AD	Chinese	Wong et al. [62]
3	Thr2Ile	c.5C>T	AVMD	AD	Iowa, USA	Kinnick et al. [61]
4	Thr2Ser	c.5C>G	BVMD	AD	European	Guo et al. [63]
						Shah et al. [64]
5	Ile3Asn	c.8T>A	Atypical BVMD	AD	USA	Matson et al. [65]
6	Ile3Thr	c.8T>C	BVMD	AD	Dutch	Boon et al. [66]
7	Thr4Ala	c.10A>G	BVMD	AD	French	Querques et al. [67]
8	Thr4Ile	c.11C>T	AVMD	AD	Chinese	Tian et al. [68]
					Iowa, USA	Kinnick et al. [61]
9	Tyr5His	c.13T>C	AVMD	AD	Iowa, USA	Kinnick et al. [61]
10	Tyr5Term	c.15C>A	Multifocal BVMD	AD	French	Lacassagne et al. [69]
11	Thr6Ala	c.16A>G	BVMD	De novo	USA	Apushkin et al. [70]
12	Thr6Arg	c.17C>G	BVMD	AD	Iowa, USA	Mullins et al. [71]
				AD	USA or Swiss	Lotery et al. [72]
13	Thr6Lys	c.17C>A	AVMD	AD	Iowa, USA	Kinnick et al. [61]
14	Thr6Pro	c.16A>C	BVMD	AD	Dutch	Booij et al. [73]
			BVMD	AD	Dutch	Boon et al. [66]
			Multifocal BVMD	AD	Dutch	Boon et al. [74]
			AVMD	AD	German	Kramer et al. [75]
			BVMD	AD	Dutch	Bakall et al. [76]
			BVMD	AD	Dutch	Petrukhin et al. [2]
15	Ser7Asn	c.20G>A	BVMD	AD	Japanese	Katagiri et al. [60]
16	Val9Ala	c.26T>C	AVMD	AD	French	Querques et al. [67]
					Swedish	Petrukhin et al. [2]
17	Val9Glu	c.26T>A	BVMD	Unknown	Portuguese	Maia-Lopes et al. [77]
18	Val9Leu	c.25G>C	BVMD	AD	USA	Meunier et al. [78]
			AVMD	AD	Iowa, USA	Kinnick et al. [61]

	Mutations a.a	Mutations nucleotide	Associated disease	Inheritance	Ethnicity	Reference
19	Val9Met	c.25G>A	BVMD	AD	German	Renner et al. [79]
			BVMD	AD	German	Kramer et al. [75]
			BVMD	AD	German	Marquardt et al. [80]
20	Ala10Thr	c.28G>A	BVMD	AD	German	Kramer et al. [75]
			BVMD	AD	German	Marquardt et al. [80]
21	Ala10Val	c.29C>T	BVMD	AD	Dutch	Booij et al. [73]
			BVMD	AD	Dutch	Bakall et al. [76]
22	Asn11Ile	c.32A>T	BVMD	AD	German	Kramer et al. [81]
23	Arg13Cys	c.37C>T	AVMD	AD	Iowa, USA	Kinnick et al. [61]
24	Arg13His	c.38G>A	BVMD	AD	Chinese	Tian et al. [68]
			BVMD	AD	USA	Caldwell et al. [82]
25	Arg13Pro	c.38G>C	AVMD	AD	Iowa, USA	Kinnick et al. [61]
26	Gly15Arg	c.43G>C	BVMD	AD	Slovenian	Glavac et al. [83]
27	Gly15Asp	c.44G>A	BVMD	AD	Italian	Querques et al. [67]
28	Ser16Phe	c.47C>T	BVMD	AD	Chinese	Liu et al. [84]
			BVMD	AD	French	Marchant et al. [85]
29	Ser16Tyr	c.47C>A	BVMD	AD	Dutch	Booij et al. [73]
			Multifocal BVMD	AD	Dutch	Boon et al. [74]
30	Phe17Cys	c.50T>G	BVMD	AD	French	Marchant et al. [85]
				AD	USA or Swiss	Lotery et al. [72]
31	Phe17Ser	c.50T>C	AVMD	AD	Iowa, USA	Kinnick et al. [61]
32	Arg19Cys	c.55C>T	BVMD	AD	Chinese	Tian et al. [86]
33	Arg19Leu	c.56G>T	AVMD	AD	Iowa, USA	Kinnick et al. [61]
34	Leu20Val	c.58C>G	BVMD	AD	Danish	Bitner et al. [12]
35	Leu21Val	c.61C>G	BVMD	AD	German	White et al. [87]
			BVMD	AD	English, Canadian	Kramer et al. [75]
36	Trp24Cys	c.72G>T	BVMD	AD	USA or Swiss	Lotery et al. [72]
			BVMD	AD	German	Marquardt et al. [80]
37	Arg25Gln	c.74G>A	BVMD	AD	German	Marquardt et al. [80]

(continued)

Table 8.1 (continued)

	Mutations a.a	Mutations nucleotide	Associated disease	Inheritance	Ethnicity	Reference
38	Arg25Trp	c.73C>T	BVMD	AD	Japanese	Katagiri et al. [60]
			BVMD	AD	French	Querques et al. [67]
			BVMD	AD	Italian	Sodi et al. [88]
			BVMD	AD	USA or Swiss	Lotery et al. [72]
			BVMD	AD	German	Kramer et al. [75]
39	Gly26Arg	c.76G>C	BVMD	AD	German	Kramer et al. [81]
40	Gly26Ser	c.76G>A	BVMD	AD	Italian	Campa et al. [89]
41	Ser27Arg	c.81C>G	BVMD	AD	German	Kramer et al. [75]
42	Tyr29His	c.85T>C	BVMD	AD	German	Kramer et al. [81]
43	Lys30Arg	c.89A>G	BVMD	AD	USA or Swiss	Lotery et al. [72]
44	Lys30Asn	c.90G>C	AVMD	AD	Iowa, USA	Kinnick et al. [61]
45	Glu35Lys	c.103G>A	BVMD	Unknown	Portuguese	Maia-Lopes et al. [77]
46	Leu41Pro	c.122T>C	BVMD	AD	German	Kramer et al. [81]
47	Arg47Cys	c.139C>T	AVMD	AR	Iowa, USA	Kinnick et al. [61]
48	Arg47His	c.728C>T	BVMD	AD	Chinese	Liu et al. [84]
			AVMD	AD	German	Kramer et al. [75]
49	Gln58Leu	c.173A>T	BVMD	AD	German	Renner et al. [79]
			BVMD	AD	German	Kramer et al. [75]
50	Tyr72Asp	c.214T>G	AVMD	AD	Iowa, USA	Kinnick et al. [61]
51	Ile73Asn	c.218T>A	BVMD	AD	French	Marchant et al. [85]
52	Ile73Phe	c.217A>T	BVMD	AD	USA	Meunier et al. [78]
53	Leu75Phe	c.223C>T	BVMD	AD	Chinese	Wong et al. [62]
54	Ile76Asn	c.227T>A	AVMD	AD	Iowa, USA	Kinnick et al. [61]
55	Ile76Val	c.226A>G	BVMD	AD	Iowa, USA	Kinnick et al. [61]
56	Phe80Leu	c.240C>A	BVMD	AD	Japanese	Katagiri et al. [60]
			BVMD	AD	USA or Swiss	Lotery et al. [72]
57	Phe80Val	c.238T>G	BVMD	AD	USA	Meunier et al. [78]
58	Val81Met	c.241G>A	BVMD	AD	Japanese	Katagiri et al. [60]
			BVMD	AD	Iowa, USA	Kinnick et al. [61]

	Mutations a.a	Mutations nucleotide	Associated disease	Inheritance	Ethnicity	Reference
59	Leu82Val	c.244C>G	BVMD	AD	Danish	Bitner et al. [12]
			BVMD	AD	German	Schatz et al. [90]
			BVMD	AD	Dutch	Boon et al. [66]
			BVMD	AD	Danish	Bakall et al. [76]
60	Phe84Val	c.250T>G	AVMD	AD	Iowa, USA	Kinnick et al. [61]
61	Tyr85His	c.253T>C	BVMD	AD	Danish	Bitner et al. [12]
			BVMD	AD	Danish	Schatz et al. [90]
			BVMD	AD	Swedish	Petrukhin et al. [2]
62	Val89Ala	c.266T>C	BVMD	AD	Swedish	Eksandh et al. [91]
63	Thr91Ile	c.272C>T	BVMD	AD	French	Querques et al. [67]
				AD	USA or Swiss	Lotery et al. [72]
64	Arg92Cys	c.274C>T	BVMD	AD	Italian, French	Querques et al. [67]
			BVMD	AD	Swedish	Bakall et al. [76]
65	Arg92Gly	c.274C>G	AVMD	AD	Italian	Querques et al. [67]
66	Arg92His	c.275G>A	BVMD	AD	Danish	Bitner et al. [12]
			BVMD	AD	Danish	Schatz et al. [90]
			BVMD	AD	French	Marchant et al. [85]
67	Arg92Ser	c.274C>A	BVMD	AD	German	Renner et al. [79]
			BVMD	AD	German	Kramer et al. [75]
68	Trp93Arg	c.277T>C	AVMD	AD	Iowa, USA	Kinnick et al. [61]
69	Trp93Cys	c.279G>C	BVMD	AD	Swedish	Petrukhin et al. [2]
70	Gln96Arg	c.287A>G	BVMD	AD	Danish	Bitner et al. [12]
71	Gln96Glu	c.286C>G	AVMD	AD	Iowa, USA	Kinnick et al. [61]
72	Gln96His	c.288G>C	BVMD	AD	Dutch	Booij et al. [73]
			BVMD	AD	Dutch	Bakall et al. [76]
73	Asn99Lys	c.297C>A	BVMD	AD	German	Kramer et al. [75]
74	Asn99Tyr	c.295A>T	BVMD	AD	Iowa, USA	Kinnick et al. [61]
75	Leu100Arg	c.299T>G	BVMD	AD	German	Kramer et al. [81]
			BVMD	AD	German	Kramer et al. [75]
76	Pro101Leu	c.302C>T	AVMD	AD	Iowa, USA	Kinnick et al. [61]
77	Pro101Thr	c.301C>A	BVMD	AD	USA or Swiss	Lotery et al. [72]

(continued)

Table 8.1 (continued)

	Mutations a.a	Mutations nucleotide	Associated disease	Inheritance	Ethnicity	Reference
78	Tryp102Arg	c.304T>C	BVMD	AD	German	Kramer et al. [81]
79	Asp104Glu	c.312C>A	BVMD	AD	Swedish	Petrukhin et al. [2]
80	Asp104His	c.301G>C	BVMD	AD	German	Kramer et al. [81]
81	Arg105Gly	c.313G>C	BVMD	AD	Slovenian	Glavac et al. [83]
82	Phe113Leu	c.339C>G	BVMD	AD	Chinese	Li et al. [92]
83	Arg130Ser	c.388C>A	BVMD	AD	USA	Meunier et al. [78]
84	Asn133Lys	c.399C>G	BVMD	AD	USA or Swiss	Lotery et al. [72]
85	Leu134Val	c.400C>G	BVMD	AD	Dutch	Booij et al. [73]
			BVMD	AD	French	Marchant et al. [93]
			Multifocal BVMD	AD	Dutch	Boon et al. [74]
86	Gly135Ser	c.403G>A	BVMD	AD	USA or Swiss	Lotery et al. [72]
			BVMD	AD	Swedish	Bakall et al. [76]
87	Leu140Arg	c.419T>G	BVMD	AD	USA or Swiss	Lotery et al. [72]
88	Arg141His	c.422G>A	BVMD	AD	USA or Swiss	Lotery et al. [72]
				AD	German	Kramer et al. [75]
89	Arg141Ser	c.421C>A	BVMD	AR	Iowa, USA	Kinnick et al. [61]
90	Val143Phe	c.427G>T	AVMD	AD	Iowa, USA	Kinnick et al. [61]
			AVMD	AD	Chinese	Gao et al. [94]
			AVMD	AD	Chinese	Gao et al. [19]
91	Ser144Asn	c.431G>A	BVMD	AD	Chinese	Liu et al. [84]
			BVMD	AD	Chinese	Wong et al. [62]
92	Ser144Gly	c.430A>G	Multifocal BVMD	AD	French	Lacassagne et al. [69]
93	Ala195Val	c.584C>T	BVMD	AD	Japanese	Katagiri et al. [60]
			BVMD	AD	Dutch	Booij et al. [73]
			Multifocal	AD	Dutch	Boon et al. [74]
			BVMD	AD	German	Kramer et al. [81]
			BVMD	AD	USA or Swiss	Lotery et al. [72]
94	Ile201Thr	c.602T>C	BVMD	AD	USA or Swiss	Lotery et al. [72]
95	Ser209Asn	c.626G>A	BVMD	AD	English, Canadian	Kramer et al. [75]
96	Leu211Thr	c.632T>C	BVMD	AD	USA or Swiss	Lotery et al. [72]

	Mutations a.a	Mutations nucleotide	Associated disease	Inheritance	Ethnicity	Reference
97	Arg218Cys	c.652C>T	BVMD	AD	Chinese	Tian et al. [68]
			BVMD	AD	Danish	Bitner et al. [12]
			BVMD	AD	German	Kramer et al. [81]
			BVMD	AD	French	Marchant et al. [85]
			BVMD	AD	Chinese	Wong et al. [62]
			BVMD	AD	USA or Swiss	Lotery et al. [72]
			BVMD	AD	Dutch	Bakall et al. [76]
			BVMD	AD	USA	Caldwell et al. [82]
98	Arg218Gly	c.652C>G	BVMD	AD	Italian	Sodi et al. [88]
99	Arg218His	c.653G>A	BVMD	AD	Japanese	Katagiri et al. [60]
			BVMD	AD	Dutch	Booij et al. [73]
			BVMD	AD	French	Marchant et al. [85]
			BVMD	AD	USA or Swiss	Lotery et al. [72]
100	Arg218Ser	c.652C>A	BVMD	AD	German	Kramer et al. [81]
			BVMD	AD	Swedish	Bakall et al. [76]
101	Arg218Gln	c.654T>G	BVMD	AD	Dutch	Marquardt et al. [80]
102	Gln220Pro	c.659A>C	AVMD	AD	Iowa, USA	Kinnick et al. [61]
103	Cys221Phe	c.662G>T	BVMD	AD	Iowa, USA	Kinnick et al. [61]
104	Cys221Trp	c.663T>G	BVMD	De novo	Italy	Palomba et al. [95]
105	Gly222Glu	c.665G>A	BVMD	AD	Japanese	Katagiri et al. [60]
106	Gly222Val	c.665G>T	BVMD	AD	USA or Swiss	Lotery et al. [72]
107	Leu224Met	c.670C>A	BVMD	AD	German	Kramer et al. [75]
108	Leu224Pro	c.671T>C	BVMD	AD	USA or Swiss	Lotery et al. [72]
109	Tyr227Asn	c.679T>A	BVMD	AD	Dutch	Booij et al. [73]
			BVMD	AD	USA or Swiss	Lotery et al. [72]
			BVMD	AD	Dutch	Marquardt et al. [80]
			BVMD	AD	Dutch	Petrukhin et al. [2]
110	Tyr227Cys	c.680A>G	BVMD	AD	USA or Swiss	Lotery et al. [72]
			BVMD	AD	Dutch	Marquardt et al. [80]
111	Tyr227Phe	c.680A>T	BVMD	AD	German	Wabbels et al. [96]
112	Trp229Gly	c.685T>G	BVMD	AD	Chinese	Lin et al. [97]

(continued)

Table 8.1 (continued)

	Mutations a.a	Mutations nucleotide	Associated disease	Inheritance	Ethnicity	Reference
113	Ile230Asn	c.689T>A	AVMD	AD	Iowa, USA	Kinnick et al. [61]
114	Ile230Trh	c.689T>C	BVMD	AD	French	Querques et al. [67]
115	Ser231Arg	c.693T>G	BVMD	AD	German	Kramer et al. [75]
116	Ser231Thr	c.692G>C	BVMD	AD	French	Marchant et al. [93]
117	Ile232Asn	c.695T>A	BVMD	AD	German	Wabbels et al. [96]
118	Pro233Ala	c.697C>G	BVMD	AD	Swedish	Wittstrom et al. [98]
119	Pro233Gln	c.698C>A	BVMD	AD	French	Marchant et al. [93]
120	Pro233Leu	c.698C>A	AVMD	AD	Iowa, USA	Kinnick et al. [61]
121	Leu234Pro	c.698C>T	BVMD	Unknown	USA	Moshfegh et al. [18]
122	Val235Leu	c.703G>C	BVMD	AD	French	Marchant et al. [85]
123	Val235Met	c.703G>A	BVMD	AD	Dutch	Marquardt et al. [80]
124	Thr237Arg	c.710C>G	BVMD	AD	German	Kramer et al. [81]
			BVMD	AD	German	Kramer et al. [75]
125	Thr237Ser	c.709A>T	BVMD	AD	German	Wabbels et al. [96]
126	Thr241Asn	c.722C>A	BVMD	AD	German	Kramer et al. [81]
127	Val242Met	c.724G>A	BVMD	AD	Japanese	Katagiri et al. [60]
128	Ala243Thr	c.727G>A	BVMD	AD	Danish	Bitner et al. [12]
			BVMD	AD	German	Kramer et al. [75]
			BVMD	AD	USA or Swiss	Lotery et al. [72]
129	Ala243Val	c.728C>T	BVMD	AD	Italian	Querques et al. [67]
			BVMD	AD	German	Kramer et al. [81]
			AVMD	AD	German	Kramer et al. [75]
130	Arg255Trp	c.763C>T	BVMD	AD	Chinese	Wong et al. [62]
131	Pro274Arg	c.821C>G	AVMD	AR	Iowa, USA	Kinnick et al. [61]
132	Phe276Leu	c.828C>G	BVMD	AD	USA or Swiss	Lotery et al. [72]
133	Tyr284Cys	c.851A>G	BVMD	AD	Iowa, USA	Kinnick et al. [61]
134	Arg291Val	c.872C>T	BVMD	AD	Chinese	Tian et al. [68]
135	Glu292Lys	c.874G>A	BVMD	AD	Chinese	Liu et al. [84]
			BVMD	AD	USA	Sohn et al. [99]
136	Gln293His	c.879G>C	BVMD	AD	Chinese	Tian et al. [68]
			BVMD	AD	French	Marchant et al. [93]

	Mutations a.a	Mutations nucleotide	Associated disease	Inheritance	Ethnicity	Reference
137	Gln293Lys	c.877C>A	BVMD	AD	Dutch	Booij et al. [73]
			BVMD	AD	Dutch	Bakall et al. [76]
138	Leu294Val	c.880C>G	BVMD	AD	German	Kramer et al. [81]
139	Ile295Thr	c.884T>C	BVMD	AD	German	Kramer et al. [81]
			BVMD	AD	Japanese	Yanagi et al. [100]
140	Ile295Val	c.883A>G	BVMD	AD	Iowa, USA	Kinnick et al. [61]
141	Asn296His	c.886A>C	BVMD	AD	USA or Swiss	Lotery et al. [72]
142	Asn296Lys	c.891C>A	Multifocal BVMD	AD	Dutch	Boon et al. [74]
143	Asn296Ser	c.887A>G	BVMD	AD	Danish	Bitner et al. [12]
			BVMD	AD	French	Marchant et al. [85]
144	Pro297Ala	c.889C>G	BVMD	AD	USA or Swiss	Lotery et al. [72]
			BVMD	AD	Dutch	Marquardt et al. [80]
145	Pro297Ser	c.889C>T	BVMD	AD	Iowa, USA	Kinnick et al. [61]
146	Pro297Thr	c.889C>T	BVMD	AD	Chinese	Wong et al. [62]
147	Phe298Cys	c.893T>G	BVMD	AD	USA	Meunier et al. [78]
148	Phe298Ser	c.893T>C	BVMD	AD	Dutch	Booij et al. [73]
			Multifocal BVMD	AD	Dutch	Boon et al. [74]
			BVMD	AD	German	Kramer et al. [81]
149	Phe298Val	c.892T>G	BVMD	Unknown	English	Arora et al. [101]
150	Gly299Ala	c.896G>C	BVMD	AD	Dutch	Booij et al. [73]
			BVMD	AD	Dutch	Boon et al. [66]
151	Gly299Arg	c.895G>A	BVMD	AD	French	Marchant et al. [93]
152	Gly299Glu	c.896G>A	BVMD	AD	Swedish	Petrukhin et al. [2]
153	Glu300Asp	c.900G>C	BVMD	AD	Iowa, USA	Kinnick et al. [61]
			BVMD	AD	USA or Swiss	Lotery et al. [72]
			BVMD	AD	USA	Caldwell et al. [82]
154	Glu300Lys	c.898G>A	BVMD	AD	Chinese	Liu et al. [84]
			BVMD	AD	German	Kramer et al. [75]
			BVMD	AD	USA or Swiss	Lotery et al. [72]
155	Asp301Asn	c.901G>A	BVMD	AD	German	Kramer et al. [75]

(continued)

Table 8.1 (continued)

	Mutations a.a	Mutations nucleotide	Associated disease	Inheritance	Ethnicity	Reference
156	Asp301Glu	c.903T>G	BVMD	AD	German	Renner et al. [79]
			BVMD	AD	German	Kramer et al. [81]
			BVMD	AD	German	Kramer et al. [75]
			BVMD	AD	USA	Caldwell et al. [82]
157	Asp301Gly	c.902A>G	BVMD	AD	Chinese	Wong et al. [62]
			BVMD	AD	Chinese	Tian et al. [68]
158	Asp302Ala	c.905A>C	BVMD	AD	Danish	Bitner et al. [12]
			BVMD	AD	USA	Meunier et al. [78]
			BVMD	AD	Dutch	Booij et al. [73]
159	Asp302Asn	c.904G>A	BVMD	AD	Danish	Bitner et al. [12]
160	Asp302Gly	c.905A>G	BVMD	AD	USA or Swiss	Lotery et al. [72]
161	Asp302His	c.904G>C	BVMD	AD	French	Marchant et al. [102]
162	Asp302Val	c.905A>T	BVMD	AD	USA or Swiss	Lotery et al. [72]
163	Asp303Asn	c.907G>A	BVMD	AD	Italian	Sodi et al. [103]
164	Asp303Glu	c.909T>A	BVMD	AD	French	Marchant et al. [102]
165	Asp303Gly	c.908A>G	AVMD	AD	Iowa, USA	Kinnick et al. [61]
166	Asp304Asn	c.910G>A	AVMD	AD	Iowa, USA	Kinnick et al. [61]
167	Asp304Gly	c.911A>G	BVMD	AD	Italian	Sodi et al. [103]
168	Asp304Val	c.911A>T	BVMD	Unknown	Portuguese	Maia-Lopes et al. [77]
169	Phe305Leu	c.915T>A	BVMD	AD	Italian	Testa et al. [59]
170	Phe305Ser	c.914T>C	BVMD	AD	Dutch	Marquardt et al. [80]
171	Phe305Tyr	c.914T>A	AVMD	AD	Iowa, USA	Kinnick et al. [61]
172	Glu306Asp	c.918G>C	BVMD	AD	Japanese	Katagiri et al. [60]
			BVMD	AD	USA or Swiss	Lotery et al. [72]
173	Glu306Gly	c.917A>G	BVMD	AD	USA or Swiss	Lotery et al. [72]
174	Thr307Asp	c.920C>A	BVMD	AD	Chinese	Liu et al. [84]
175	Thr307Ala	c.919A>G	BVMD	AD	USA or Swiss	Lotery et al. [72]
176	Thr307Ile	c.902C>T	BVMD	AD	USA or Swiss	Lotery et al. [72]
				AD	USA	Caldwell et al. [82]
177	Asn308Ser	c.923A>G	BVMD	AD	French	Marchant et al. [102]
178	Trp309Arg	c.925T>C	AVMD	AD	Iowa, USA	Kinnick et al. [61]
179	Ile310Thr	c.929T>C	BVMD	AD	Germany	Kramer et al. [75]

	Mutations a.a	Mutations nucleotide	Associated disease	Inheritance	Ethnicity	Reference
180	Val311Gly	c.932T>G	BVMD	AD	Germany	Kramer et al. [75]
181	Asp312Asn	c.934G>A	AVMD	AD	Germany	Kramer et al. [75]
182	Asp312Glu	c.936C>A	BVMD	AD	Danish	Bitner et al. [12]
			BVMD	AD	Danish	Schatz et al. [90]
183	Gln316His	c.948G>T	AVMD	AR	Iowa, USA	Kinnick et al. [61]
184	Gln316Pro	c.947A>C	AVMD	AD	Iowa, USA	Kinnick et al. [61]
185	Pro346His	c.1037C>A	BVMD	AD	Japanese	Katagiri et al. [60]
186	Val492Ile	c.1474G>A	AVMD	AD	Iowa, USA	Kinnick et al. [61]
187	Glu557Lys	c.1669G>A	AVMD	AD	Iowa, USA	Kinnick et al. [61]

Three novel mutations Tyr4Ile [68], Ala291Val [68], and Phe113Leu [92] in BVMD were reported. Lin [97] reported two novel heterozygous mutations 304delAsp and Trp229Gly, in Chinese BVMD patients. Liu [84] reported four previously reported mutations (Ser16Phe, Ser144Asn, Glu292Lys, and.Glu300Lys) and two novel disease-causing mutations (Thr307Asp, Arg47His) in Chinese patients with BVMD. Recently, 39 distinct disease-causing BEST1 variants, including 13 novel variants, and two reported variants but novel for autosomal recessive bestrophinopathy (ARB) were found in a large Chinese cohort study (n = 92) [106]. Of these 39 mutations, 23 were associated with BVMD, 14 with ARB, and two (c.604C>T and c.898G>A) with both BVMD and AMD. Most BVMD mutations were missense (97.78%), while ARB was associated with more complex mutations. Hot regions for mutation were located in exon 2, 6, and 8 in BVMD patients and in exons 5 and 7 in ARB patients.

In Japanese study [60], 22 patients, including 16 probands from 16 families with BVMD were analyzed. All 16 probands exhibited characteristic BVMD fundus appearances, abnormal EOG, and normal ERG responses with the exception of one diabetic retinopathy proband. Genetic analysis identified 12 BEST1 variants in 13 probands (81%). Of these, ten variants (Tyr2Arg, Arg25Trp, Phe80Leu, Val81Met, Ala195Val, Arg218His, Gly222Glu, Val-242Met, Asp304del, and Glu306Asp) have been previously reported in BVMD, while two variants (Ser7Asn and Pro346His) were novel disease-causing mutations.

In Korea, we reported a BVMD patient (Fig. 8.1) carrying Asn296Lys mutation, which is a causative mutation of multifocal BVMD in German patient [74]. Arg218Leu is a novel disease-causing mutation in BVMD (Fig. 8.2). We also reported a genetically confirmed case of ARB carrying Leu40Pro mutation in the *BEST1* gene(Fig. 8.3). These findings expand the spectrum of *BEST1* genetic variation in Asia and will be valuable for genetic counseling for patients with BVMD [105].

BVMD shows variable expressivity and incomplete penetrance at the clinical level (Fig. 8.4). Disease-causing effect of *BEST1* mutations seems to be cumulative over time [96]. In genotype-phenotype relationship of Dutch study [73], median age of onset of visual symptoms was 33 years (range: 2–78). The cumulative risk of VA below 0.5 (20/40) was 50% at 55 years and 75% at 66 years. The cumulative risk of VA declines less than 0.3 (20/63) was 50% by age 66 years and 75% by age 74 years. Most patients (96%) had missense mutations; the Thr6Pro, Ala10Val, and Tyr227Asn mutations were most common. The visual decline was significantly faster in patients with an Ala10Val mutation than either the Thr6Pro or the Tyr227Asn mutation.

In the recent Chinese study, despite the typical macular appearance of BVMD, no clear genotype-phenotype correlation was observed [105]. In the Asian BVMD cohort, genetic tests should be performed for the diagnosis with thorough clinical examinations to elucidate a genotype-phenotype correlation.

8.5.2 AVMD

In AVMD, several mutations in *BEST1* gene have been identified, including p.Ala146Lys [107], p. Thr6Pro, p.Arg47His, P.Ala243Val, and p. Asp312Asn [75], and p.Ile38Ser [9]. Table 8.1 includes the list of missense mutations in AVMD. In addition, AVMD is associated with mutations in *PRPH2* [108], *IMPG1* [109], *IMPG2* [110].

Age of onset is a major criterion to distinguish BVMD from AVMD [78]. Thus, systematic screening of *BEST1* and *PRPH2* has been suggested in BVMD and AVMD. *BEST1* screening should be recommended to patients with an age of onset less than 40 years, and *PRPH2* screening should be recommended to patients with an age of onset more than 40 years. For an onset between 30 and 40 years, *PRPH2* can be screened if no mutation has been detected in *BEST1*. In this screening approach, we found *PRPH2* mutation of p.Pro219_Pro221delinsPro in a 39-year-old female without *BEST1* mutation (Fig. 8.5).

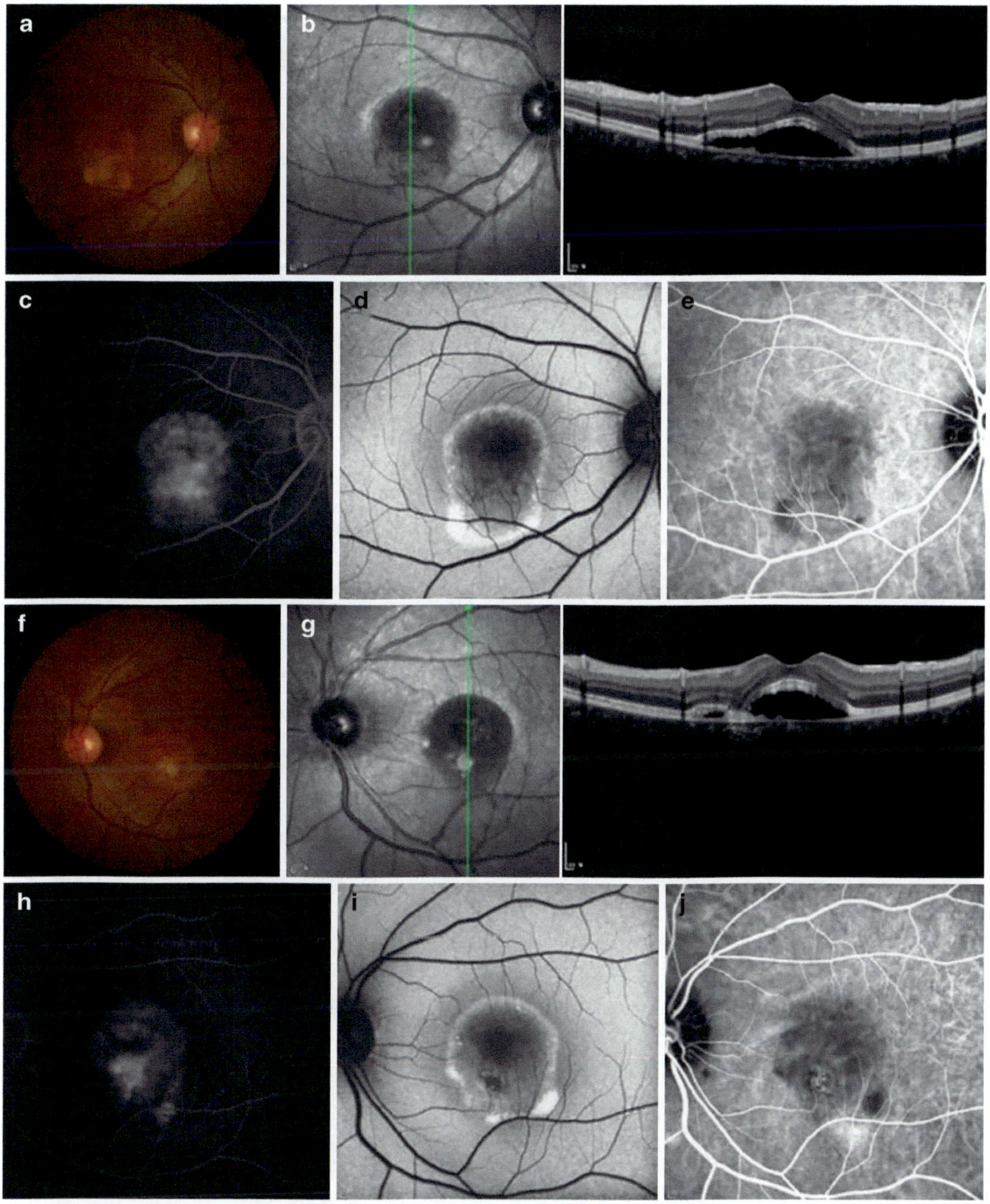

Fig. 8.1 Best vitelliform macular dystrophy (BVMD). A 32-year-old man carrying p.Asn296Lys mutation in the *BEST1* gene was incidentally found on routine fundus examination for a pilot license. The visual acuities (VA) were 20/20 in both eyes. (**a**, **f**) Bilateral BVMD of vitelliruptive stage shows scattered yellow-white vitelliform deposits. (**b**, **g**) Vertical optical coherent tomography (OCT) shows serous retinal detachment and hyperreflective vitelliform materials at RPE in both eyes. (**c**, **h**) Fluorescein angiography (FA) shows the late pooling of fluorescein dye at the vitelliform lesion. (**d**, **i**) Fundus autofluorescent (FAF) image of the vitelliruptive lesion shows increased autofluorescence at the inferior part of ruptured vitelliform lesions and at the border of the serous retinal detachment. (**e**, **j**) Indocyanine green angiography (ICGA) shows hypercyanescence in the left eye

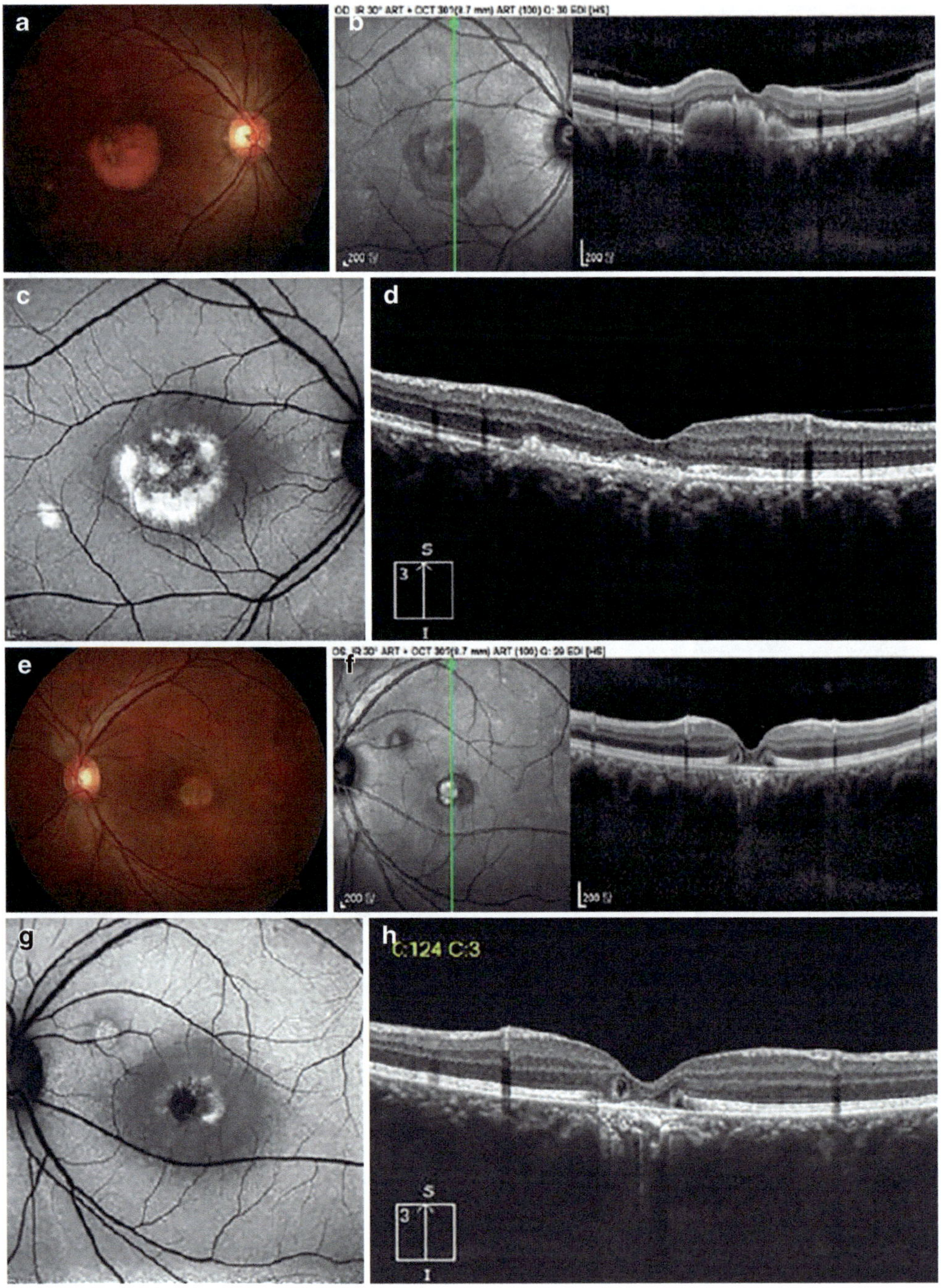

Fig. 8.2 Best vitelliform macular dystrophy (BVMD). A 39-year-old man carrying Arg218Leu mutation in the *BEST1* gene had multiple injections of anti-VEGF agents (10 for right eye and 5 for left eye) in both eyes. At initial presentation, the vitelliform stage of right eye (**a**) reveals a highly reflective subfoveal pillar without surrounding SRF (**b**). Small round vitelliform lesion with central cicatricial change was found in the left eye (**e**). OCT reveals marked RPE loss at the fovea (**f**). Six months later, FAF shows dispersed materials with hyperautofluorescence (**c**), and OCT reveals the disappearance of the subfoveal pillar with a progression to vitelliruptive stage (**d**) in the right eye. FAF shows central hypoautofluorescence and surrounding hyperfluorescent lesions. OCT reveals that hypoautofluorescent lesion corresponds to the enlarged RPE loss (**h**)

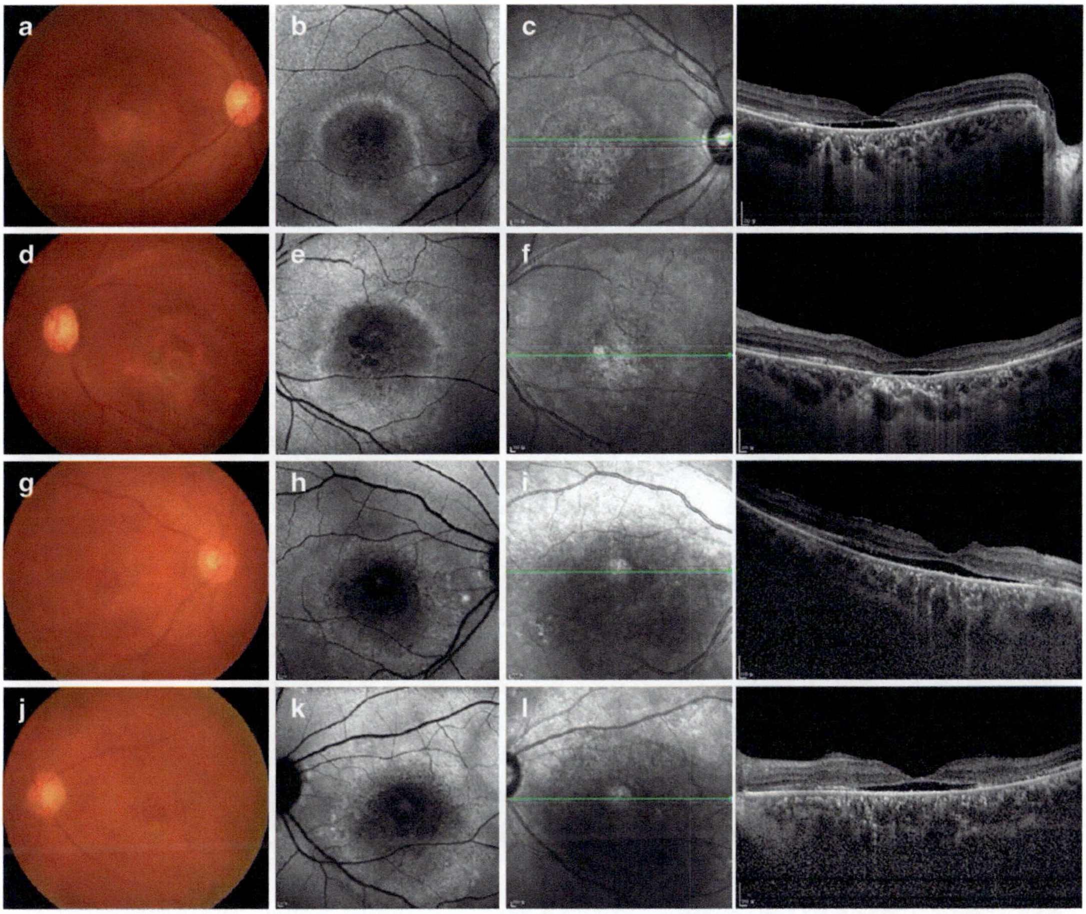

Fig. 8.3 Autosomal recessive bestrophinopathy (ARB). A 52-year-old female visited our clinic with decreased visual acuity of both eyes. Her visual acuity was 20/400 in both eyes. On fundus examination, scar changes at fovea were noted in right eye (**a**). Autofluorescence image shows hypoautofluorescent fovea with hyperautofluorescent ring at perifovea (**b**) OCT exam reveals RPE atrophy with mild subretinal fluid (**c**). Similar changes were seen in her left eye (**d**–**f**). She informed us that out of eight siblings, her brother also had similar symptoms. Genetic study confirmed the diagnosis of ARB carrying Leu40Pro mutation in the *BEST1* gene. Her brother was also examined at our clinic. His visual acuity was 20/125 in both eyes. Fundus examination showed yellowish lesions at the fovea with pigmentary change in his right eye (**g**). Hypoautofluorescent lesions sparing the foveal center were noted (**h**). OCT shows mild SRF (**i**). Similar changes were seen in his left eye (**j**–**l**)

8.6 Future Perspectives for Therapy

The development of gene and cell therapies is promising in various retinal diseases. Indeed, the results of clinical trials using iPSC-derived RPE cells in wet age-related macular degeneration [111] or AAV/RPE65 vectors in Leber's congenital amaurosis [112] were already reported. Therapeutic intervention of inherited retinal dystrophy should be primarily aimed at the restoration of normal gene (i.e., *BEST1* gene in BVMD and AVMD). However, until a decade ago, this therapeutic goal was ideal but unachievable due to the lack of a proper biotechnology. Recent advances in genome editing technology using CRISPR system and gene delivery system are promising and harness the CRISPR-based genome editing for therapeutic applications. Since its first therapeutic applica-

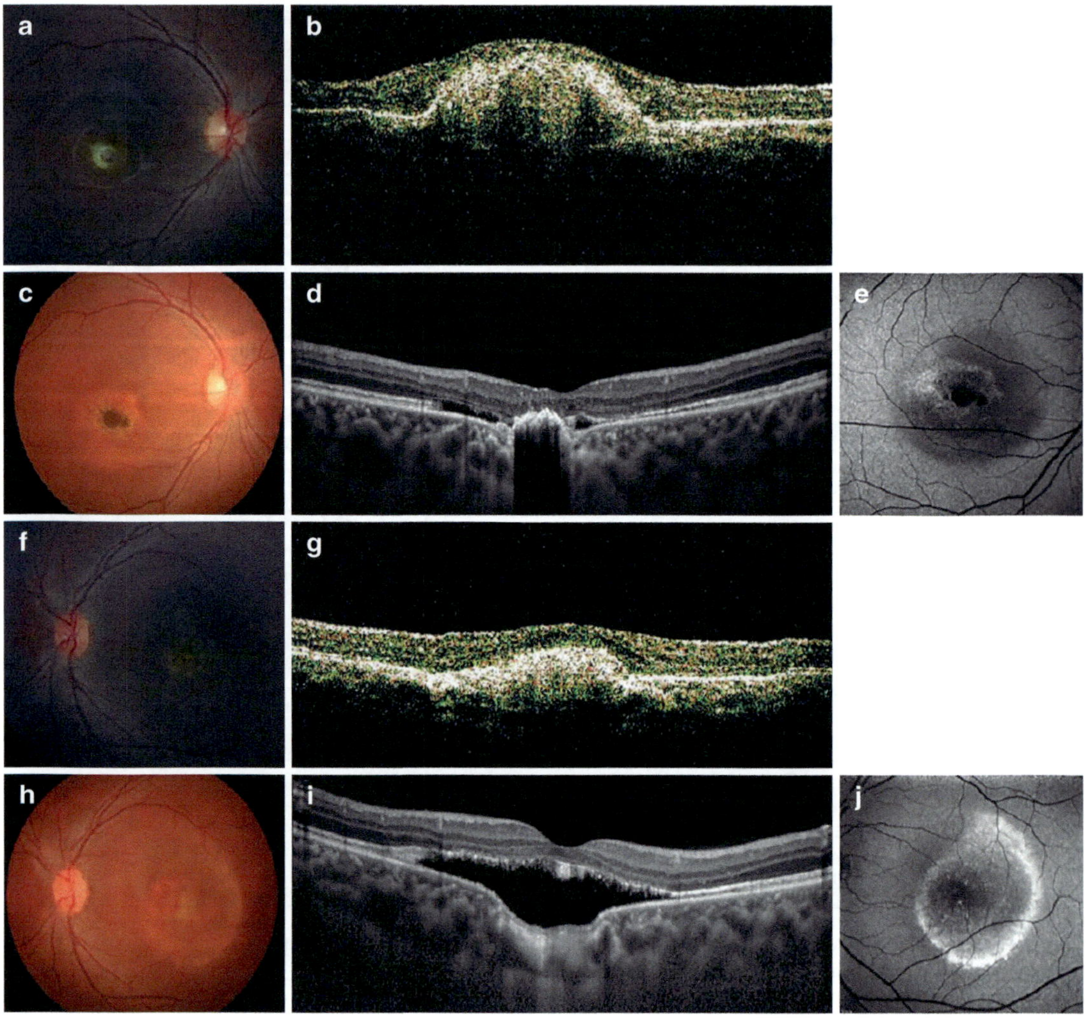

Fig. 8.4 Best vitelliform macular dystrophy (BVMD). A 24-year-old man carrying Leu14Ser mutation in the *BEST1* gene who had received multiple injections of anti-VEGF agents (4 for both eyes) and multiple photodynamic therapies (3 for right eye and 2 for left eye) in both eyes for the treatment of subfoveal choroidal neovascularization visited our clinic for a regular check-up. 11 years ago, the patient's right eye was at vitelliform stage (**a**). Time-domain OCT revealed highly reflective subfoveal vitelliform material without SRF (**b**). After 11 years, scar changes at fovea was noted (**c**) with mild SRF surrounding foveal scar on spectral-domain OCT (D). Macular scar with atrophic changes of RPE was confirmed as hypoautofluorescent lesions on autofluorescence image, confirming stage 5 BVMD (**e**). The left eye of the patient also showed vitelliform lesions on fundus photography 11 years ago (**f**). Time-domain OCT revealed highly reflective vitelliform material without SRF, confirming vitelliform stage of BVMD (**g**). 11 years later, the left eye advanced to vitelliruptive stage (**h**), and spectral-domain OCT showed an optically empty lesion between EZ and RPE, with clumping of hyperreflective material on the posterior retinal surface (**i**). Autofluorescence image showed dispersed hyperautofluorescent lesions at perifovea (**j**)

tions in retinal disease using wet AMD animal models [113, 114], in vivo genome editing using CRISPR-Cas9 enlarged its therapeutic applications both in genetic diseases harboring mutations [115, 116] and non-genetic degenerative diseases [113, 114, 117].

The conventional concept of gene therapy to deliver a normal copy of *BEST1* gene into RPE

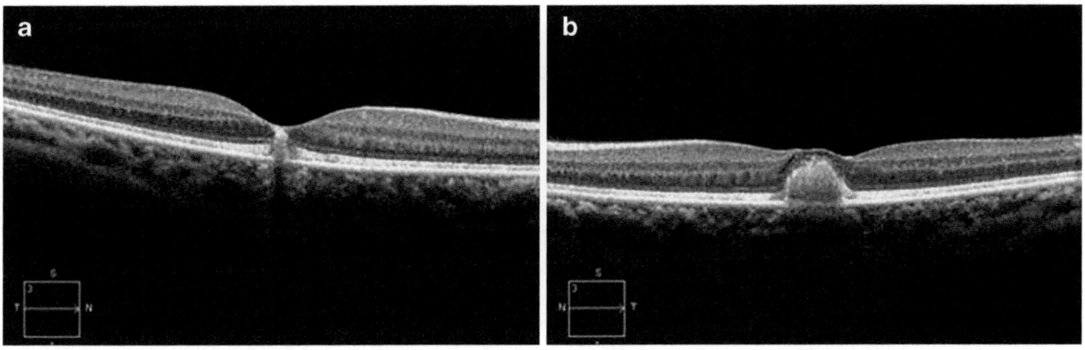

Fig. 8.5 Adult-onset vitelliform macular dystrophy (AVMD). A 39-year-old woman carrying Pro219_Pro221delinsPro in *PRPH2* gene suffered from dysmorphopsia of right eye. OCT reveals subfoveal vitelliform lesion in the right eye (**a**) and left eye (**b**)

would be effective in the treatment of VMD of haploinsufficiency phenotype, which is caused by *BEST1* mutations that exclusively result in a loss of sufficient wild-type protein. In a recent report, Ji et al. have successfully restored Ca^{2+} dependent Cl^- currents in patient-derived RPEs with dominant mutations by WT *BEST1* gene supplementation via adeno-associated virus [118]. In addition, simple destruction of mutant proteins at the DNA level is achievable by genome editing of mutant *BEST1* allele using CRISPR-Cas9.

Currently, many BEST1 mutations cause VMD through dominant-negative effect. In addition, in over 300 mutations of *BEST1* gene, a large number of *BEST1* mutations are missense mutations; thus, a precise base-editing using base-editors enables literally complete recovery of normal gene [119, 120]. According to the recent advances in genome editing technology using CRISPR system, in vivo genome editing has emerged as a potential treatment strategy for inherited retinal dystrophies [121].

There have been efforts to develop alternative treatments to gene-specific therapies, given their costs. A recent study has investigated whether FDA-approved small molecules sodium phenylbutyrate (4PBA) and 2-naphthoxyacetic acid (2-NOAA) would functionally rescue bestrophin 1 function in RPE generated from induced pluripotent stem cells derived from BVMD patients [122]. This study showed that these molecules, acting as a chemical chaperone to enhance protein folding in the endoplasmic reticulum, restore the expression and function of mutant bestrophin 1 proteins.

8.7 Summary

VMD is among the most common autosomal dominant macular dystrophy. Multimodal imaging with SD-OCT, FAF, FA, and ICGA is useful to the diagnosis of VMD. Genetic test is clinically important in the diagnosis of VMD because the clinical features of VMD can be similar to those of exudative AMD, CNV, or CSC. Future studies are needed to identify the prevalence of precise genetic mutations of *BEST1* in Asian VMD patients. This could provide a clear genotype-phenotype correlation in VMD. In vitro studies using RPE cells from patient-derived iPSC help to understand the molecular biology of bestrophin-1 protein. Furthermore, in vivo genome editing using CRISPR-based base-editors might be a potential treatment strategy for the correction of missense mutations in VMD.

All procedures followed were in accordance with the ethical standards of the responsible committee on the institutional review board and with the Helsinki Declaration of 1975, as revised in 2000. Informed consent was obtained from all patients for being included in the study.

References

1. Best F. Uber eine hereditare maculaafektion; Beitrage zur verergslehre. Zschr Augenheilkd. 1905;13:199–212.
2. Petrukhin K, et al. Identification of the gene responsible for Best macular dystrophy. Nat Genet. 1998;19:241–7.
3. Boon CJ, et al. The spectrum of ocular phenotypes caused by mutations in the BEST1 gene. Prog Retin Eye Res. 2009;28:187–205.
4. Johnson AA, et al. Bestrophin 1 and retinal disease. Prog Retin Eye Res. 2017;58:45–69.
5. Gass J. A clinicopathologic study of a peculiar foveomacular dystrophy. Trans Am Ophthalmol Soc. 1974;72:139.
6. Chowers I, Tiosano L, Audo I, Grunin M, Boon CJ. Adult-onset foveomacular vitelliform dystrophy: a fresh perspective. Prog Retin Eye Res. 2015;47:64–85.
7. Johnson AA, et al. Bestrophin 1 and retinal disease. Prog Retin Eye Res. 2017;58:45–69.
8. Boon CJ, et al. The spectrum of ocular phenotypes caused by mutations in the BEST1 gene. Prog Retin Eye Res. 2009;28:187–205.
9. Jun I, et al. Adult-onset vitelliform macular dystrophy caused by best1 p.ile38ser mutation is a mild form of best vitelliform macular dystrophy. Sci Rep. 2017;7:9146.
10. Mohler CW, Fine SL. Long-term evaluation of patients with Best's vitelliform dystrophy. Ophthalmology. 1981;88:688–92.
11. Nordstrom S. Hereditary macular degeneration—a population survey in the country of Vsterbotten, Sweden. Hereditas. 1974;78:41–62.
12. Bitner H, Schatz P, Mizrahi-Meissonnier L, Sharon D, Rosenberg T. Frequency, genotype, and clinical spectrum of best vitelliform macular dystrophy: data from a national center in Denmark. Am J Ophthalmol. 2012;154:403–12 e404.
13. Dalvin LA, Pulido JS, Marmorstein AD. Vitelliform dystrophies: prevalence in Olmsted County, Minnesota, United States. Ophthalmic Genet. 2017;38:143–7.
14. Marmorstein AD, Cross HE, Peachey NS. Functional roles of bestrophins in ocular epithelia. Prog Retin Eye Res. 2009;28:206–26.
15. Marmorstein AD, et al. Bestrophin, the product of the Best vitelliform macular dystrophy gene (VMD2), localizes to the basolateral plasma membrane of the retinal pigment epithelium. Proc Natl Acad Sci U S A. 2000;97:12758–63.
16. Kane Dickson V, Pedi L, Long SB. Structure and insights into the function of a Ca(2+)-activated Cl(-) channel. Nature. 2014;516:213–8.
17. Marmorstein AD, et al. Bestrophin-1 influences transepithelial electrical properties and Ca2+ signaling in human retinal pigment epithelium. Mol Vis. 2015;21:347–59.
18. Moshfegh Y, et al. BESTROPHIN1 mutations cause defective chloride conductance in patient stem cell-derived RPE. Hum Mol Genet. 2016;25:2672–80.
19. Gao T, et al. Disease-causing mutations associated with bestrophinopathies promote apoptosis in retinal pigment epithelium cells. Graefes Arch Clin Exp Ophthalmol. 2020;258:2251–61.
20. Nordstrom S, Barkman Y. Hereditary macular degeneration (HMD) in 246 cases traced to one gene-source in central Sweden. Hereditas. 1977;84:163–76.
21. Mohler CW, Fine SL. Long-term evaluation of patients with Best's vitelliform dystrophy. Ophthalmology. 1981;88:688–92.
22. Zhang Q, Small KW, Grossniklaus HE. Clinicopathologic findings in Best vitelliform macular dystrophy. Graefes Arch Clin Exp Ophthalmol. 2011;249:745–51.
23. O'Gorman S, Flaherty WA, Fishman GA, Berson EL. Histopathologic findings in Best's vitelliform macular dystrophy. Arch Ophthalmol. 1988;106:1261–8.
24. Deutman A. Electro-oculography in families with vitelliform dystrophy of the fovea: detection of the carrier state. Arch Ophthalmol. 1969;81:305–16.
25. Scholl HPN, Schuster AM, Vonthein R, Zrenner E. Mapping of retinal function in Best macular dystrophy using multifocal electroretinography. Vis Res. 2002;42:1053–61.
26. Scoles D, et al. Photoreceptor inner segment morphology in best vitelliform macular dystrophy. Retina (Philadelphia, Pa). 2017;37:741–8.
27. Kay DB, et al. Outer retinal structure in best vitelliform macular dystrophy. JAMA Ophthalmol. 2013;131:1207–15.
28. Deutman AF. Ph.D. thesis, Koninklijke Van Gorcum, Assen; 1971.
29. Battaglia Parodi M, et al. Optical coherence tomography in Best vitelliform macular dystrophy. Eur J Ophthalmol. 2017;27:201–4.
30. Battaglia Parodi M, Iacono P, Romano F, Bandello F. Spectral domain optical coherence tomography features in different stages of best vitelliform macular dystrophy. Retina (Philadelphia, Pa). 2017; https://doi.org/10.1097/IAE.0000000000001634.
31. Qian CX, et al. Optical coherence tomography examination of the retinal pigment epithelium in best vitelliform macular dystrophy. Ophthalmology. 2017;124:456–63.
32. Querques G, et al. High-definition optical coherence tomography features in vitelliform macular dystrophy. Am J Ophthalmol. 2008;146:501–7. e501.
33. Ruiz-Moreno O, Calvo P, Ferrández B, Torrón C. Long-term outcomes of intravitreal ranibizumab for choroidal neovascularization secondary to Best's disease: 3-year follow-up. Acta Ophthalmol. 2012;90:e574–5.
34. Chhablani J, Jalali S. Intravitreal bevacizumab for choroidal neovascularization secondary to Best

vitelliform macular dystrophy in a 6-year-old child. Eur J Ophthalmol. 2012;22:677–9.
35. Leu J, Schrage NF, Degenring RF. Choroidal neovascularisation secondary to Best's disease in a 13-year-old boy treated by intravitreal bevacizumab. Graefes Arch Clin Exp Ophthalmol. 2007;245:1723–5.
36. Booij JC, et al. Course of visual decline in relation to the Best1 genotype in vitelliform macular dystrophy. Ophthalmology. 2010;117:1415–22.
37. Fishman GA, et al. Visual acuity in patients with best vitelliform macular dystrophy. Ophthalmology. 1993;100:1665–70.
38. Romano F, Arrigo A, Leone PP, Bandello F, Battaglia Parodi M. Short-term modifications of ellipsoid zone in best vitelliform macular dystrophy. Retina. 2021;41:1010–7.
39. Romano F, et al. Altered ellipsoid zone reflectivity and deep capillary plexus rarefaction correlate with progression in Best disease. Br J Ophthalmol. 2020;104:461–5.
40. Augstburger E, et al. Outer retinal alterations associated with visual outcomes in best vitelliform macular dystrophy. Am J Ophthalmol. 2019;208:429–37.
41. Parodi MB, et al. Intraretinal hyperreflective foci in best vitelliform macular dystrophy. Retina. 2018;38:2379–86.
42. Chen KC, et al. Intraretinal hyperreflective foci in acquired vitelliform lesions of the macula: clinical and histologic study. Am J Ophthalmol. 2016;164:89–98.
43. Deak GG, et al. Imaging of vitelliform macular lesions using polarization-sensitive optical coherence tomography. Retina J Ret Vit Dis. 2019;39:558–69.
44. Battaglia Parodi M, et al. Retinal vascular impairment in best vitelliform macular dystrophy assessed by means of optical coherence tomography angiography. Am J Ophthalmol. 2018;187:61–70.
45. Parodi MB, Arrigo A, Bandello F. Optical coherence tomography angiography quantitative assessment of macular neovascularization in best vitelliform macular dystrophy. Invest Ophthalmol Vis Sci. 2020;61:61.
46. Brecher R, Bird A. Adult vitelliform macular dystrophy. Eye. 1990;4:210–5.
47. Glacet-Bernard A, Soubrane G, Coscas G. Macular vitelliform degeneration in adults. Retrospective study of a series of 85 patients. Journal francais d'ophtalmologie. 1989;13:407–20.
48. Chowers I, Tiosano L, Audo I, Grunin M, Boon CJ. Adult-onset foveomacular vitelliform dystrophy: a fresh perspective. Prog Retin Eye Res. 2015;47:64–85.
49. Puche N, et al. High-resolution spectral domain optical coherence tomography features in adult onset foveomacular vitelliform dystrophy. Br J Ophthalmol. 2010; https://doi.org/10.1136/bjo.2009.17507.
50. Benhamou N, et al. Adult-onset foveomacular vitelliform dystrophy: a study by optical coherence tomography. Am J Ophthalmol. 2003;135:362–7.
51. Querques G, Forte R, Querques L, Massamba N, Souied EH. Natural course of adult-onset foveomacular vitelliform dystrophy: a spectral-domain optical coherence tomography analysis. Am J Ophthalmol. 2011;152:304–13.
52. Felbor U, Schilling H, Weber BH. Adult vitelliform macular dystrophy is frequently associated with mutations in the peripherin/RDS gene. Hum Mutat. 1997;10:301–9.
53. Yamaguchi K, et al. Adult-onset foveomacular vitelliform dystrophy with retinal folds. Jpn J of Ophthalmol. 2001;45:533–7.
54. Da Pozzo S, Parodi MB, Toto L, Ravalico G. Occult choroidal neovascularization in adult-onset foveomacular vitelliform dystrophy. Ophthalmologica. 2001;215:412–4.
55. Mimoun G, et al. Ranibizumab for choroidal neovascularization associated with adult-onset foveomacular vitelliform dystrophy: one-year results. Retina (Philadelphia, Pa). 2013;33:513–21.
56. Joshi KM, Nesper PL, Fawzi AA, Mirza RG. Optical coherence tomography angiography in adult-onset foveomacular vitelliform dystrophy. Retina. 2018;38:600–5.
57. Battaglia Parodi M, et al. Quantitative analysis of optical coherence tomography angiography in adult-onset foveomacular vitelliform dystrophy. Retina. 2018;38:237–44.
58. Toto L, et al. Adult-onset foveomacular vitelliform dystrophy evaluated by means of optical coherence tomography angiography: a comparison with dry age-related macular degeneration and healthy eyes. Retina. 2018;38:731–8.
59. Testa F, et al. A normal electro-oculography in a family affected by best disease with a novel spontaneous mutation of the BEST1 gene. Br J Ophthalmol. 2008;92:1467–70.
60. Katagiri S, et al. Mutation analysis of BEST1 in Japanese patients with Best's vitelliform macular dystrophy. Br J Ophthalmol. 2015;99:1577–82.
61. Kinnick TR, et al. Autosomal recessive vitelliform macular dystrophy in a large cohort of vitelliform macular dystrophy patients. Retina (Philadelphia, Pa). 2011;31:581–95.
62. Wong RL, et al. Novel and homozygous BEST1 mutations in Chinese patients with Best vitelliform macular dystrophy. Retina (Philadelphia, Pa). 2010;30:820–7.
63. Guo J, et al. Novel Best1 mutations detected by next-generation sequencing in a chinese population with vitelliform macular dystrophy. Retina. 2019;39:1613–22.
64. Shah M, et al. Association of clinical and genetic heterogeneity with BEST1 sequence variations. JAMA Ophthalmol. 2020;138:544–51.
65. Matson ME, Ly SV, Monarrez JL. Novel mutation in BEST1 associated with atypical best vitelliform dystrophy. Optom Vis Sci. 2015;92:e180–9.

66. Boon CJ, et al. Clinical and molecular genetic analysis of best vitelliform macular dystrophy. Retina (Philadelphia, Pa). 2009;29:835–47.
67. Querques G, et al. Functional and clinical data of Best vitelliform macular dystrophy patients with mutations in the BEST1 gene. Mol Vis. 2009;15:2960–72.
68. Tian R, Yang G, Wang J, Chen Y. Screening for BEST1 gene mutations in Chinese patients with bestrophinopathy. Mol Vis. 2014;20:1594–604.
69. Lacassagne E, et al. Phenotypic variability in a French family with a novel mutation in the BEST1 gene causing multifocal best vitelliform macular dystrophy. Mol Vis. 2011;17:309–22.
70. Apushkin MA, Fishman GA, Taylor CM, Stone EM. Novel de novo mutation in a patient with Best macular dystrophy. Arch Ophthalmol. 2006;124:887–9.
71. Mullins RF, Kuehn MH, Faidley EA, Syed NA, Stone EM. Differential macular and peripheral expression of bestrophin in human eyes and its implication for best disease. Invest Ophthalmol Vis Sci. 2007;48:3372–80.
72. Lotery AJ, et al. Allelic variation in the VMD2 gene in best disease and age-related macular degeneration. Invest Ophthalmol Vis Sci. 2000;41:1291–6.
73. Booij JC, et al. Course of visual decline in relation to the Best1 genotype in vitelliform macular dystrophy. Ophthalmology. 2010;117:1415–22.
74. Boon CJ, et al. Clinical and genetic heterogeneity in multifocal vitelliform dystrophy. Arch Ophthalmol. 2007;125:1100–6.
75. Kramer F, et al. Mutations in the VMD2 gene are associated with juvenile-onset vitelliform macular dystrophy (Best disease) and adult vitelliform macular dystrophy but not age-related macular degeneration. Eur J Hum Genet. 2000;8:286–92.
76. Bakall B, et al. The mutation spectrum of the bestrophin protein—functional implications. Hum Genet. 1999;104:383–9.
77. Maia-Lopes S, et al. Gene symbol: BEST1. Disease: best macular dystrophy. Hum Genet. 2008;123(111)
78. Meunier I, et al. Systematic screening of BEST1 and PRPH2 in juvenile and adult vitelliform macular dystrophies: a rationale for molecular analysis. Ophthalmology. 2011;118:1130–6.
79. Renner AB, et al. Late onset is common in best macular dystrophy associated with VMD2 gene mutations. Ophthalmology. 2005;112:586–92.
80. Marquardt A, et al. Mutations in a novel gene, VMD2, encoding a protein of unknown properties cause juvenile-onset vitelliform macular dystrophy (Best's disease). Hum Mol Genet. 1998;7:1517–25.
81. Kramer F, Mohr N, Kellner U, Rudolph G, Weber BH. Ten novel mutations in VMD2 associated with Best macular dystrophy (BMD). Hum Mutat. 2003;22:418.
82. Caldwell GM, et al. Bestrophin gene mutations in patients with Best vitelliform macular dystrophy. Genomics. 1999;58:98–101.
83. Glavac D, et al. Clinical and genetic heterogeneity in Slovenian patients with BEST disease. Acta Ophthalmol. 2016;94:e786–94.
84. Liu J, Zhang Y, Xuan Y, Liu W, Wang M. Novel BEST1 mutations and special clinical features of best vitelliform macular dystrophy. Ophthalmic Res. 2016;56:178–85.
85. Marchant D, et al. Identification of novel VMD2 gene mutations in patients with best vitelliform macular dystrophy. Hum Mutat. 2001;17:235.
86. Tian L, et al. Screening of BEST1 gene in a Chinese cohort with best vitelliform macular dystrophy or autosomal recessive bestrophinopathy. Invest Ophthalmol Vis Sci. 2017;58:3366–75.
87. White K, Marquardt A, Weber BH. VMD2 mutations in vitelliform macular dystrophy (Best disease) and other maculopathies. Hum Mutat. 2000;15:301–8.
88. Sodi A, et al. A novel mutation in the VMD2 gene in an Italian family with Best maculopathy. J Fr Ophtalmol. 2007;30:616–20.
89. Campa C, et al. A novel mutation of BEST1 gene in Best disease. Eur J Ophthalmol. 2020; https://doi.org/10.1177/1120672120920536.
90. Schatz P, et al. Evaluation of macular structure and function by OCT and electrophysiology in patients with vitelliform macular dystrophy due to mutations in BEST1. Invest Ophthalmol Vis Sci. 2010;51:4754–65.
91. Eksandh L, Bakall B, Bauer B, Wadelius C, Andreasson S. Best's vitelliform macular dystrophy caused by a new mutation (Val89Ala) in the VMD2 gene. Ophthalmic Genet. 2001;22:107–15.
92. Li Y, et al. A novel mutation of the VMD2 gene in a Chinese family with best vitelliform macular dystrophy. Ann Acad Med Singapore. 2006;35:408–10.
93. Marchant D, et al. New VMD2 gene mutations identified in patients affected by Best vitelliform macular dystrophy. J Med Genet. 2007;44:e70.
94. Gao T, et al. Clinical and mutation analysis of patients with best vitelliform macular dystrophy or autosomal recessive bestrophinopathy in Chinese population. Biomed Res Int. 2018;2018:4582816.
95. Palomba G, et al. A novel spontaneous missense mutation in VMD2 gene is a cause of a best macular dystrophy sporadic case. Am J Ophthalmol. 2000;129:260–2.
96. Wabbels B, Preising MN, Kretschmann U, Demmler A, Lorenz B. Genotype-phenotype correlation and longitudinal course in ten families with Best vitelliform macular dystrophy. Graefes Arch Clin Exp Ophthalmol. 2006;244:1453–66.
97. Lin Y, et al. Two novel mutations in the bestrophin-1 gene and associated clinical observations in patients with best vitelliform macular dystrophy. Mol Med Rep. 2015;12:2584–8.
98. Wittstrom E, et al. Morphological and functional changes in multifocal vitelliform retinopathy and biallelic mutations in BEST1. Ophthalmic Genet. 2011;32:83–96.

99. Sohn EH, et al. Phenotypic variability due to a novel Glu292Lys variation in exon 8 of the BEST1 gene causing best macular dystrophy. Arch Ophthalmol. 2009;127:913–20.
100. Yanagi Y, Sekine H, Mori M. Identification of a novel VMD2 mutation in Japanese patients with Best disease. Ophthalmic Genet. 2002;23:129–33.
101. Arora R, et al. Unilateral BEST1-Associated Retinopathy. Am J Ophthalmol. 2016;169:24–32.
102. Marchant D, et al. Use of denaturing HPLC and automated sequencing to screen the VMD2 gene for mutations associated with Best's vitelliform macular dystrophy. Ophthalmic Genet. 2002;23:167–74.
103. Sodi A, et al. BEST1 sequence variants in Italian patients with vitelliform macular dystrophy. Mol Vis. 2012;18:2736–48.
104. Lin Y, et al. Bestrophin 1 gene analysis and associated clinical findings in a Chinese patient with Best vitelliform macular dystrophy. Mol Med Rep. 2017;16:4751–5.
105. Lin Y, et al. Genetic variations in Bestrophin1 and associated clinical findings in two Chinese patients with juvenile onset and adult onset best vitelliform macular dystrophy. Mol Med Rep. 2017; https://doi.org/10.3892/mmr.2017.7927.
106. Gao FJ, et al. Mutation spectrum of the bestrophin-1 gene in a large Chinese cohort with bestrophinopathy. Br J Ophthalmol. 2020;104:846–51.
107. Allikmets R, et al. Evaluation of the Best disease gene in patients with age-related macular degeneration and other maculopathies. Hum Genet. 1999;104:449–53.
108. Wells J, et al. Mutations in the human retinal degeneration slow (RDS) gene can cause either retinitis pigmentosa or macular dystrophy. Nat Genet. 1993;3:213–8.
109. Manes G, et al. Mutations in IMPG1 cause vitelliform macular dystrophies. Am J Hum Genet. 2013;93:571–8.
110. Meunier I, et al. Frequency and clinical pattern of vitelliform macular dystrophy caused by mutations of interphotoreceptor matrix IMPG1 and IMPG2 genes. Ophthalmology. 2014;121:2406–14.
111. Mandai M, et al. Autologous induced stem-cell-derived retinal cells for macular degeneration. N Engl J Med. 2017;376:1038–46.
112. Maguire AM, et al. Safety and efficacy of gene transfer for Leber's congenital amaurosis. N Engl J Med. 2008;358:2240–8.
113. Kim E, et al. In vivo genome editing with a small Cas9 orthologue derived from Campylobacter jejuni. Nat Commun. 2017;8:14500.
114. Kim K, et al. Genome surgery using Cas9 ribonucleoproteins for the treatment of age-related macular degeneration. Genome Res. 2017;27:419–26.
115. Suzuki K, et al. In vivo genome editing via CRISPR/Cas9 mediated homology-independent targeted integration. Nature. 2016;540:144–9.
116. Ruan GX, et al. CRISPR/Cas9-mediated genome editing as a therapeutic approach for leber congenital amaurosis 10. Mol Ther. 2017;25:331–41.
117. Huang X, et al. Genome editing abrogates angiogenesis in vivo. Nat Commun. 2017;8:112.
118. Ji C, et al. Investigation and restoration of BEST1 activity in patient-derived RPEs with dominant mutations. Sci Rep. 2019;9:19026.
119. Gaudelli NM, et al. Programmable base editing of A*T to G*C in genomic DNA without DNA cleavage. Nature. 2017; https://doi.org/10.1038/nature24644.
120. Komor AC, Kim YB, Packer MS, Zuris JA, Liu DR. Programmable editing of a target base in genomic DNA without double-stranded DNA cleavage. Nature. 2016;533:420–4.
121. Yanik M, et al. In vivo genome editing as a potential treatment strategy for inherited retinal dystrophies. Prog Retin Eye Res. 2017;56:1–18.
122. Liu J, et al. Small molecules restore bestrophin 1 expression and function of both dominant and recessive bestrophinopathies in patient-derived retinal pigment epithelium. Invest Ophthalmol Vis Sci. 2020;61:28.

Stargardt Macular Dystrophy

9

Kaoru Fujinami, Yu Fujinami-Yokokawa, Lizhu Yang, Xiao Liu, Gavin Arno, Nikolas Pontikos, and East Asia Inherited Retinal Disease Society (EAIRDs) Study Group

Abstract

Stargardt disease 1 (STGD1; MIM 248200), which is the most prevalent inherited macular dystrophy, is an autosomal recessive condition caused by pathogenic variants in the *ABCA4* gene (ATP-binding cassette subfamily A member 4; MIM 601691). Over the last two decades, clinical and molecular genetic studies of STGD1/*ABCA4* have been intensively conducted worldwide and an understanding of the pathophysiology promotes clinical therapeutic trials. In this review, we describe clinical manifestations, genetic characteristics, pathophysiology, and treatment approaches.

Keywords

Stargardt macular dystrophy · Stargardt disease · *ABCA4* · Macular dystrophy Cone-rod dystrophy · Retinitis pigmentosa Genetics · Electroretinogram

9.1 Introduction

Stargardt macular dystrophy or Stargardt disease (STGD1: OMIM; 248200), first described in detail by Karl Bruno Stargardt of the University of Strasbourg in 1909, is one of the most common macular dystrophies [1–7]. The prevalence

East Asia Inherited Retinal Disease Society (EAIRDs) Study Group

K. Fujinami (✉)
Laboratory of Visual Physiology, Division of Vision Research, National Institute of Sensory Organs, National Hospital Organization, Tokyo Medical Center, Tokyo, Japan

Department of Ophthalmology, Keio University School of Medicine, Tokyo, Japan

UCL Institute of Ophthalmology, London, UK

Moorfields Eye Hospital, London, UK
e-mail: k.fujinami@ucl.ac.uk

Y. Fujinami-Yokokawa
Laboratory of Visual Physiology, Division of Vision Research, National Institute of Sensory Organs, National Hospital Organization, Tokyo Medical Center, Tokyo, Japan

UCL Institute of Ophthalmology, London, UK

Graduate School of Health Management, Keio University, Tokyo, Japan

Division of Public Health, Yokokawa Clinic, Suita, Osaka, Japan

L. Yang · X. Liu
Laboratory of Visual Physiology, Division of Vision Research, National Institute of Sensory Organs, National Hospital Organization, Tokyo Medical Center, Tokyo, Japan

Department of Ophthalmology, Keio University School of Medicine, Tokyo, Japan

G. Arno · N. Pontikos
Laboratory of Visual Physiology, Division of Vision Research, National Institute of Sensory Organs, National Hospital Organization, Tokyo Medical Center, Tokyo, Japan

UCL Institute of Ophthalmology, London, UK

Moorfields Eye Hospital, London, UK

H.-G. Yu (ed.), *Inherited Retinal Disease*, https://doi.org/10.1007/978-981-16-7337-5_9

of STGD1 has been estimated to be 10–12.5 per 100,000; however, scientific evidence for this is lacking [3, 4, 8, 9].

Most cases present with central visual loss (visual acuity decline or central scotoma), which often begins within the first or second decades of life [10, 11]. Patients typically show macular atrophy with yellow-white flecks at the level of the retinal pigment epithelium (RPE) of the posterior pole on ophthalmoscopy (Fig. 9.1) [12–14]. However, there is vast heterogeneity in clinical manifestations, resulting in a large spectrum of clinical presentations, onset, progression, psychophysical and electrophysiological findings, and variable prognosis [10, 11, 14–53].

In the 1990s, the genetic locus responsible was mapped to 1p13 [54–56], and causative mutations in the *ABCA4* (ATP-binding cassette subfamily A member 4: Online Mendelian Inheritance in Man identifier; 601691) gene were first reported by Allikmets et al. in patients with autosomal recessive Stargardt macular dystrophy [57, 58]. The carrier frequency for a disease-associated *ABCA4* variant may be as high as 1:20, and the true prevalence of retinopathy caused by disease-causing *ABCA4* variants is likely much higher than that of STGD1 [8, 59]. The vast allelic heterogeneity of *ABCA4* is illustrated clearly by the number of reported sequence variations (>1200) in the *ABCA4* gene [4, 60–74].

Clinical and molecular genetic investigations of STGD1/*ABCA4* have documented a highly variable phenotype, including macular dystrophy, cone dystrophy, cone-rod dystrophy, and "retinitis pigmentosa". Currently, the term "*ABCA4*-associated retinal disease" refers to the broad range and variability of clinical manifesta-

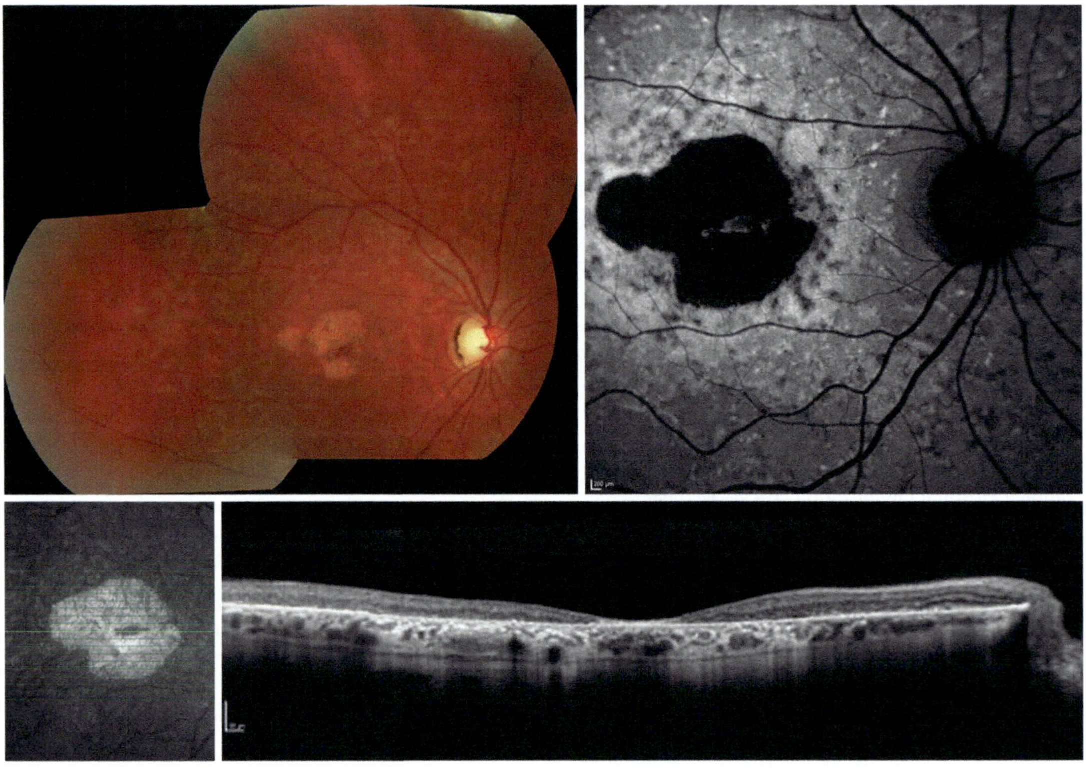

Fig. 9.1 Typical findings of Stargardt macular dystrophy (STGD1). Fundus photographs of the right eye showed macular atrophy with yellow-white flecks at the level of the retinal pigment epithelium (RPE). Fundus autofluorescence (FAF) imaging identified an area of decreased autofluorescence (DAF) at the macula and multiple foci of abnormal AF. Spectral-domain optical coherent tomography (SD-OCT) demonstrated the thinned sensory retina and RPE at the macula, with multiple hyperrefractive foci corresponding to flecks

tions of retinopathy due to pathogenic *ABCA4* variants [10, 11, 17, 26, 64].

In general, knowledge of the underlying pathophysiology of *ABCA4*-associated retinal disease promotes ongoing and planned human therapeutic trials [3, 75, 76]. We herein describe clinical manifestations, genetic characteristics, pathophysiology, and treatment approaches.

9.2 Clinical Presentations

Patients with *ABCA4*-associated retinal disease commonly present with progressive central vision loss, often in the first/second decades of life, but though time of onset can vary [10, 11, 14, 20]. In addition, onset is associated with disease severity, whereby earlier-onset disease is frequently related to more deleterious *ABCA4* variants compared with adult-onset disease, which is more frequently associated with missense variants [14, 26].

For the clinical diagnosis and monitoring of *ABCA4*-associated retinal disease, comprehensive investigations are crucial, including fundus photography, fundus autofluorescence (FAF) imaging, spectral-domain optical coherence tomography (SD-OCT), kinetic and static visual field testing, microperimetry, adaptive optics imaging, and electrophysiological findings (including pattern, full-field, and multifocal electroretinograms; PERG, ffERG, mfERG), as recorded according to the international standard of International Society for Clinical Electrophysiology of Vision (ISCEV) [77–81] (Figs. 9.2, 9.3, 9.4 and 9.5, Tables 9.1, 9.2, 9.3, 9.4, 9.5 and 9.6) [3, 4]. Clinical classifications are useful for assessing disease severity and are associated with genotypic severity [10, 11, 13–15, 22, 26, 31, 33, 40, 66].

At an early stage, ophthalmoscopy reveals normal or minimal retinal changes, including foveal reflex abnormality and RPE disturbance, with or without vision loss [14, 20, 25]. Retinal imaging with FAF, SD-OCT, and electrophysiological assessment are useful for diagnosis [3, 14, 25, 36, 82]. Notably, paediatric patients with *ABCA4*-associated retinal disease may not have flecks on fundoscopy or FAF at the early stage but may develop them in association with increasing macular atrophy in the natural course (Fig. 9.2) [14]. In the very early phase of childhood-onset disease with relatively preserved vision, macular atrophy involves the parafovea with spared foveola and these changes are preceded by tiny, foveal, yellow, hyperautofluorescent dots in some cases [14, 20, 25]. Hyperreflectivity at the base of the outer nuclear layer, described as "thickening of the external limiting membrane", may represent a structural change at the level of the foveal cone nuclei [20].

The clinical and genetic features of *ABCA4*-associated retinal disease with late onset have been increasingly studied recently [26, 27, 83–86]. Patients with late-onset *ABCA4*-associated retinal disease frequently show the foveal-sparing (FS) phenotype (Fig. 9.5) [26, 84]. Additionally, patients with *ABCA4*-associated retinal disease often maintain foveal structure/function associated with preserved visual acuity [26]. SD-OCT identifies outer retinal tabulation at the edge of atrophy in approximately half of cases, suggesting primal damage of the RPE/choroid in this phenotype [26]. In contrast, patients with primal "foveal atrophy" exhibit the sensory retinal atrophy at the early stage [26]. The presence of two distinct phenotypes (non-FS and FS *ABCA4*-associated retinal disease) suggests more than one disease mechanism in *ABCA4*-associated retinal disorder [26]. The different distribution of disease-causing *ABCA4* variants between these two phenotypes also supports this hypothesis, with a relatively high proportion of c.5882G>A (p.Gly1961Glu) for the no-FS phenotype and a high proportion of c.6089G>A (p.Arg2030Gln) for the FS phenotype [26].

FAF is a noninvasive imaging modality that uses the autofluorescence properties of lipofuscin and related fluorophores to provide valuable information on the distribution of lipofuscin in the RPE [11]. FAF subtypes have been characterized in a longitudinal cohort of 68 patients, as follows: type 1—a decreased autofluorescence (DAF) signal at the fovea surrounded by a homogeneous background; type 2—a localized DAF signal at the macula surrounded by a heterogeneous background with numerous foci of abnormal signal; and type 3—multiple low

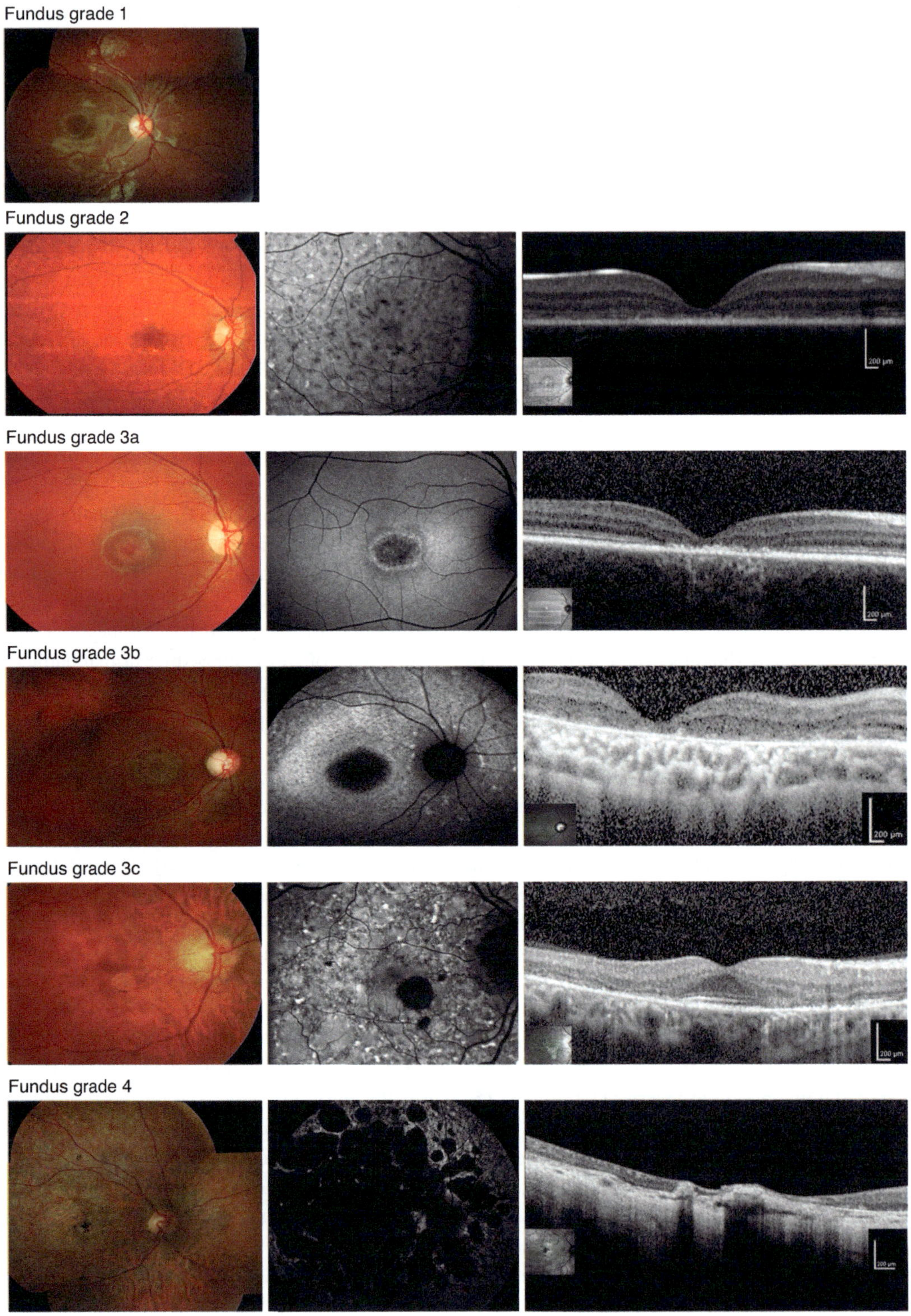

Fig. 9.2 Classification of fundus appearance in *ABCA4*-associated retinal disorder. Fundus grading is performed based on the presence of macular atrophy, flecks, foveal sparing, and peripheral atrophy in patients with *ABCA4*-associated retinal disorder. Detailed descriptions are provided in Table 9.2 (Fujinami et al. Clinical and Molecular Characteristics of Childhood-Onset Stargardt Disease. Ophthalmology 2015)

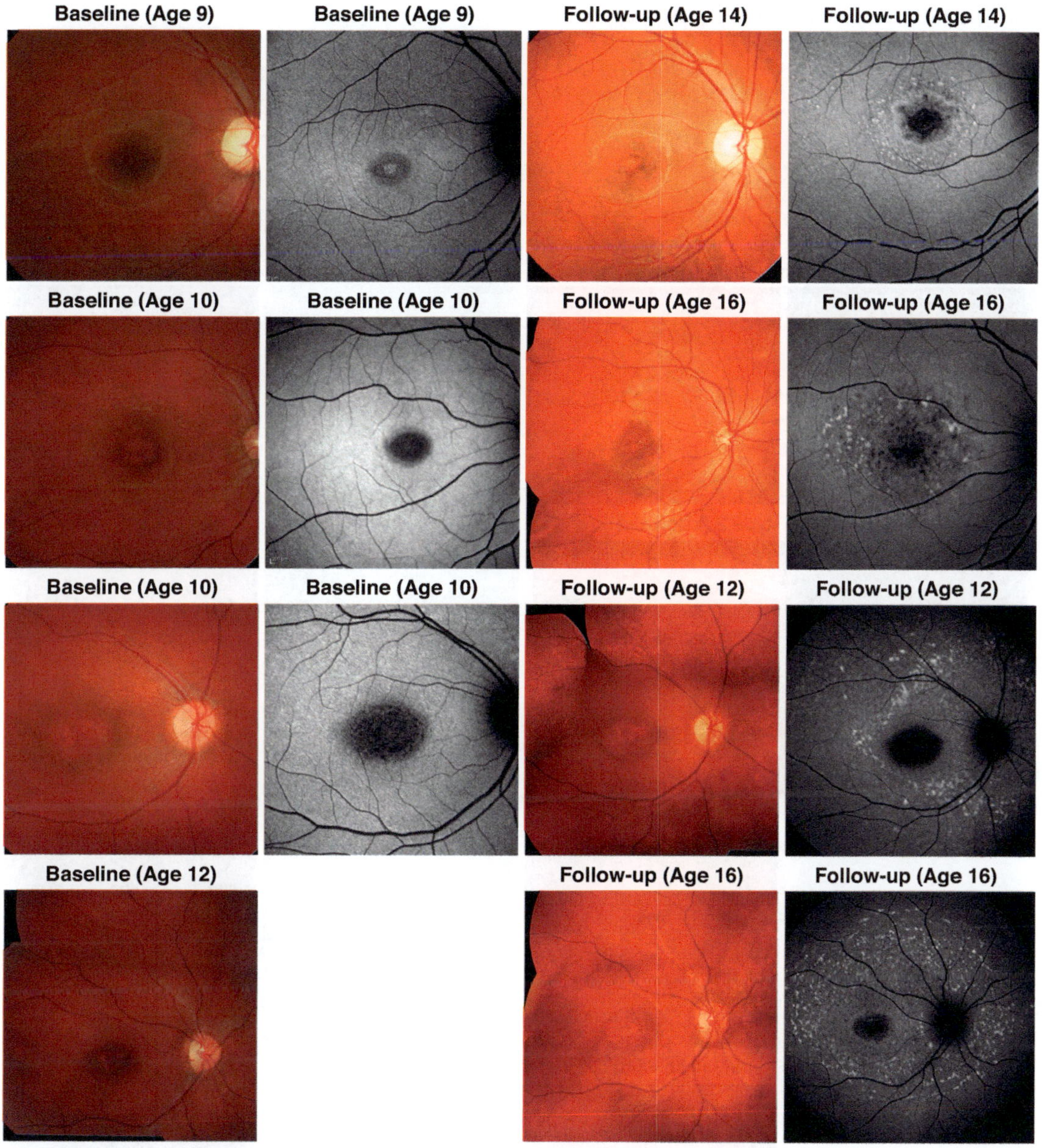

Fig. 9.3 Development of macular atrophy and flecks in childhood-onset *ABCA4*-associated retinal disorder. At baseline, fundus photography showed normal or minimal macular abnormalities with evidence of macular abnormality detected by FAF. Over the follow-up period, remarkable macular atrophy and macular and/or peripheral flecks developed, which were more evident by both fundus photography and FAF imaging

signal areas at the posterior pole with a heterogeneous background (Fig. 9.4, Table 9.6) [11]. The rate of atrophy enlargement (mm^2/year) was significantly different, at 0.06 in type 1, 0.67 in type 2, and 4.37 in type 3. Moreover, it was concluded that the AF type at baseline influences atrophy progression during the median follow-up of 9.1 years, which showed an association with genotypic severity (Table 9.6) [11]. Consequently, a prospective longitudinal study of children and adults with *ABCA4*-associated retinal disease ($n = 90$) was conducted [22]. The DAF area was symmetric between eyes, and the mean rate of progression was 0.69, 0.78, and 0.40 (0.36) mm^2/year for children, adults with childhood-onset disease, and adults with adult-onset disease,

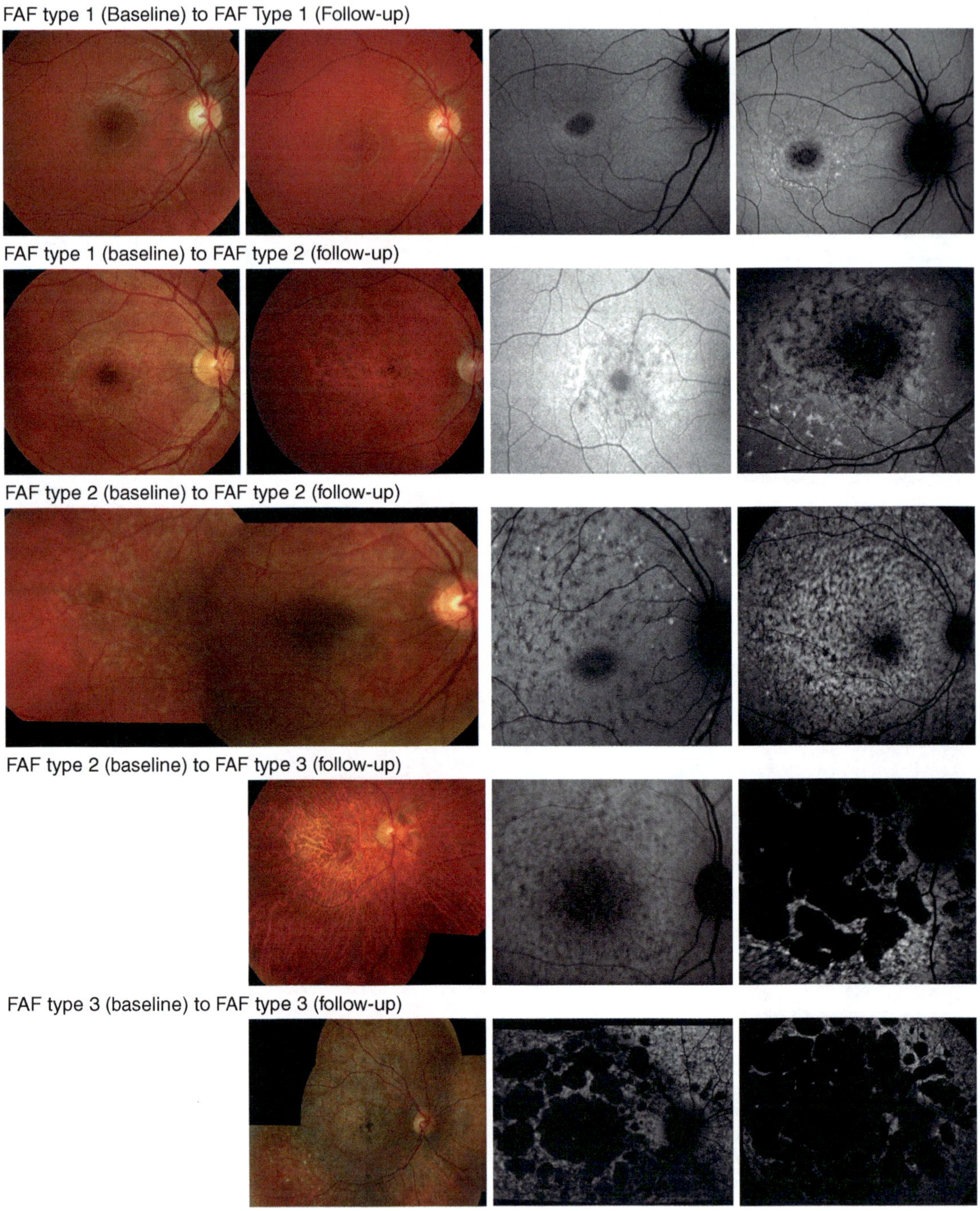

Fig. 9.4 Fundus autofluorescence (FAF) patterns and progression in *ABCA4*-associated retinal disorder. FAF classification was performed based on the size of the DAF area and background features (heterogeneous/homogeneous). A severe type (type 3) exhibited rapid progression associated with deleterious *ABCA4* variants. Detailed descriptions are provided in Table 9.3 (Fujinami et al. A longitudinal study of Stargardt disease: quantitative assessment of fundus autofluorescence, progression, and genotype correlations. Invest Ophthalmol Vis Sci. 2013)

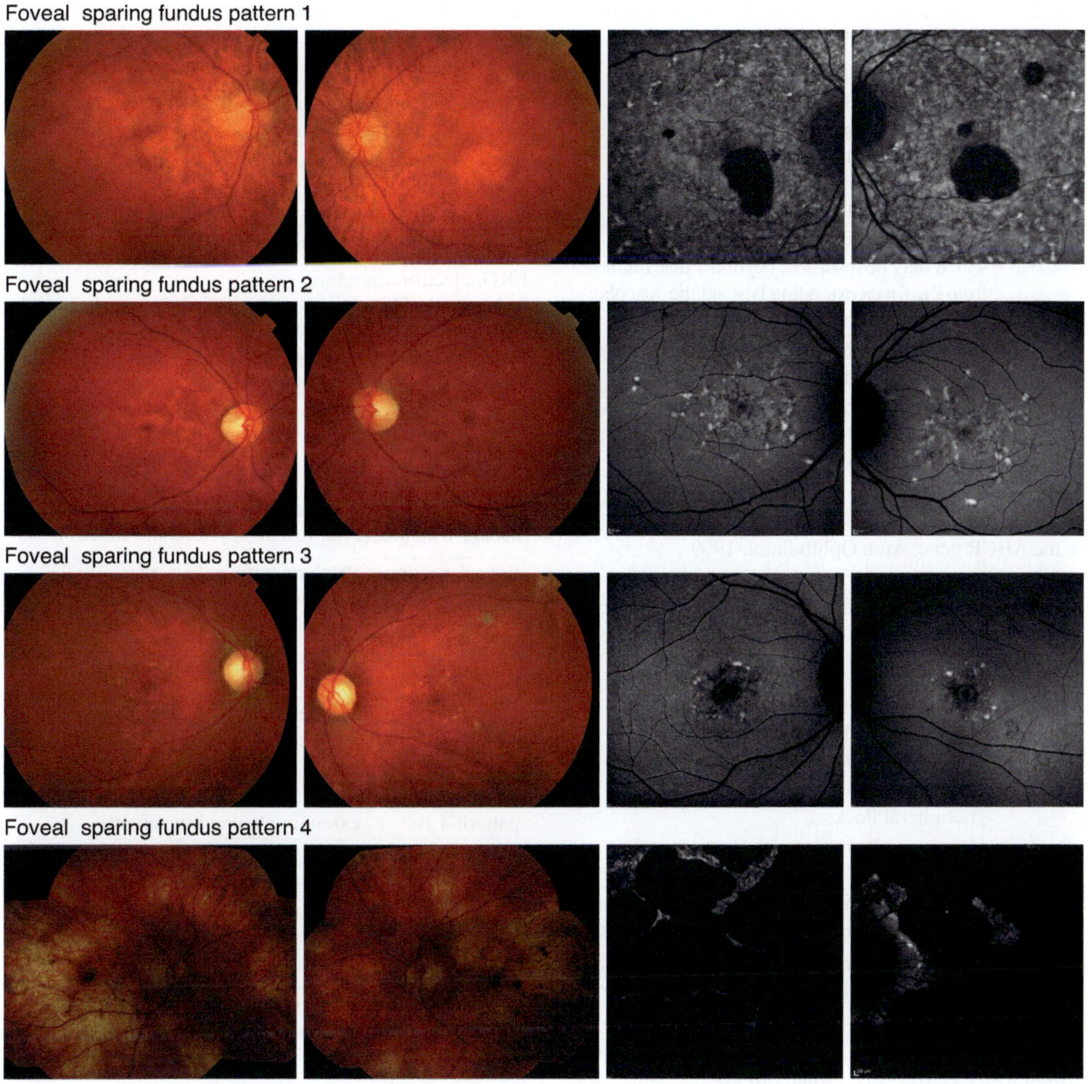

Fig. 9.5 Fundus appearance, FAF images, and spectral-domain optical coherent tomography of the foveal-sparing phenotype. In patients with foveal-sparing *ABCA4*-associated retinal disorder, visual acuity was maintained, and foveal structure and function was relatively preserved. Outer retinal tabulation, as shown with an arrow at the edge of atrophy, is often observed, suggesting the primal damage of RPE/choroid in this late-onset phenotype. Detailed descriptions of the classification are provided in Table 9.5 (Fujinami K et al. Clinical and molecular analysis of Stargardt disease with preserved foveal structure and function. Am J Ophthalmol. 2013.)

respectively [22]. Quantification of the DAF area was highly reliable and should be a robust structural endpoint in clinical trials [22].

Electrophysiological assessment is important for confirming the diagnosis of *ABCA4*-associated retinal disease and providing better informed advice on disease prognosis [10]. A classification of three functional phenotypes based on electrophysiological findings has been well established: Group 1—dysfunction confined to the macula; Group 2—macular and generalized cone system dysfunction; Group 3—macular and both generalized cone and rod system dysfunction (Fig. 9.6, Table 9.4) [10, 15]. A longitudinal study in a large cohort of 59 patients with a mean follow-up interval of 10.5 years has been reported [10]. A total of

Table 9.1 Classical classification of clinical findings in Stargardt macular dystrophy

Stage 1	Confined central macular lesions ranging from irregular pigmentary mottling to well-defined lesions of RPE atrophy with a characteristic "beaten-bronze" or "snail-slime" appearance underlying central or paracentral scotomas
Stage 2	Presence of yellow fundus flecks, some of which may be resorbed, beyond 1 disc diameter from the fovea extending beyond the vascular arcades and regions nasal to the optic disc
Stage 3	Diffusely resorbed flecks and choriocapillaris atrophy within the macula
Stage 4	Extensive choriocapillaris atrophy throughout the posterior pole resulting in moderate to severe restriction of peripheral fields

Fishman, G. A. et al. Variation of clinical expression in patients with Stargardt dystrophy and sequence variations in the ABCR gene. Arch Ophthalmol. 1999

Table 9.2 Classification of fundus appearance in *ABCA4*-associated retinal disease

Grade 1	Normal fundus
Grade 2	Macular and/or peripheral flecks without central atrophy
Grade 3a	Central atrophy without flecks
Grade 3b	Central atrophy with macular and/or peripheral flecks
Grade 3c	Paracentral atrophy with macular and/or peripheral flecks, without a central atrophy
Grade 4	Multiple extensive atrophic changes of the RPE, extending beyond the vascular arcades

Fujinami et al. Clinical and Molecular Characteristics of Childhood-Onset Stargardt Disease. Ophthalmology. 2015

Table 9.3 Classification of fundus autofluorescence pattern in *ABCA4*-associated retinal disease

Pattern 1	Localized low AF signal at the fovea surrounded by a homogeneous background with/without perifoveal foci of high or low signal
Pattern 2	Localized low AF signal at the macula surrounded by a heterogeneous background and widespread foci of high or low AF signal extending anterior to the vascular arcades
Pattern 3	Multiple areas of low AF signal at posterior pole with a heterogeneous background and/or foci of high or low signal

Fujinami et al. A longitudinal study of Stargardt disease: quantitative assessment of fundus autofluorescence, progression, and genotype correlations. Invest Ophthalmol Vis Sci. 2013.; Georgiou M et al. Prospective Cohort Study of Childhood-Onset Stargardt Disease: Fundus Autofluorescence Imaging, Progression, Comparison With Adult-Onset Disease, and Disease Symmetry. Am J Ophthalmol. 2020

Table 9.4 Classification of functional phenotypes based on electrophysiological findings in *ABCA4*-associated retinal disease

Group 1	Confined macular dysfunction (normal full-field ERG)
Group 2	Macular dysfunction with generalized cone dysfunction
Group 3	Macular dysfunction with generalized cone and rod dysfunction

ERG, electroretinogram
Lois et al. Phenotypic subtypes of Stargardt macular dystrophy-fundus flavimaculatus. Arch Ophthalmol 2001; Fujinami et al. A longitudinal study of Stargardt disease: clinical and electrophysiologic assessment, progression, and genotype correlations. Am J Ophthalmol. 2013

Table 9.5 Fundus pattern of *ABCA4*-associated retinal disease with preserved foveal structure and function

Foveal-sparing pattern 1	Patchy parafoveal atrophy surrounded by numerous yellow-white flecks
Foveal-sparing pattern 2	Numerous yellow-white flecks at the posterior pole without atrophy
Foveal-sparing pattern 3	Mottled RPE changes and/or localized parafoveal yellow-white flecks
Foveal-sparing pattern 4	Multiple patchy atrophic lesions, extending beyond the arcades

Fujinami et al. Clinical and Molecular Analysis of Stargardt Disease with Preserved Foveal Structure and Function. Am J Ophthalmol. 2013

Table 9.6 Classification of genotypes based on the presence of deleterious variants in *ABCA4*-associated retinal disease

Genotype A	Two or more likely deleterious variants
Genotype B	One deleterious variant and one or more missense or in-frame insertion/deletion variant(s)
Genotype C	Two or more missense or in-frame insertion/deletion variants

Fujinami et al. Clinical and Molecular Characteristics of Childhood-Onset Stargardt Disease. Ophthalmology 2015; Fujinami et al. Clinical and Detailed Genetic Characteristics of an International Large Cohort of Patients With Stargardt Disease: ProgStar Study Report 8. Br J Ophthalmol. 2019

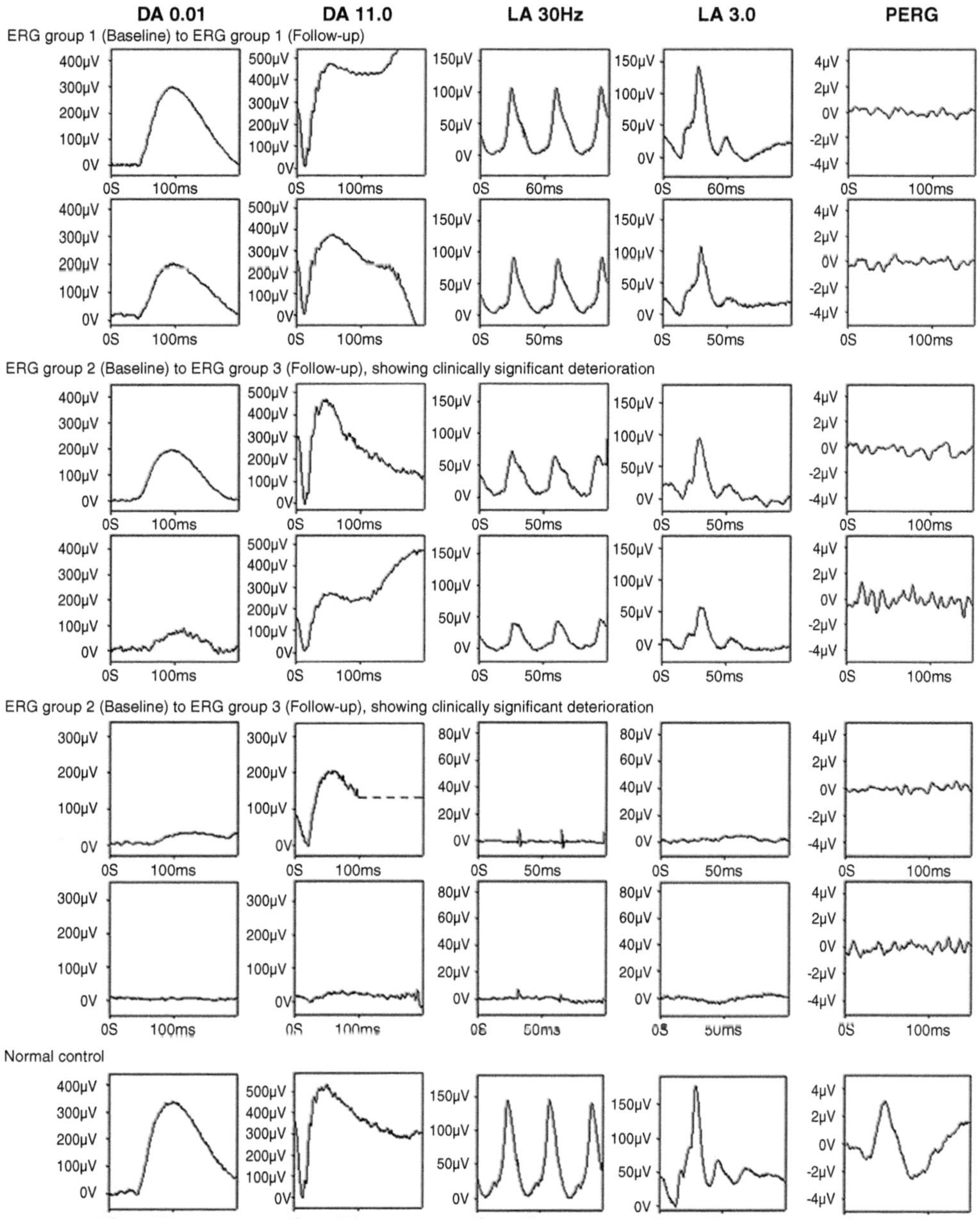

Fig. 9.6 Functional phenotype based on electrophysiological findings and progression in *ABCA4*-associated retinal disorder. Full-field electroretinograms (ffERGs) and pattern ERG (PERG) of three representative cases of each functional phenotype (ERG group) and a normal subject are presented. ERG group classification is performed based on the presence of macular dysfunction (abnormal PERG, mfERG, or focal macular ERG), generalized cone dysfunction (abnormal light-adapted (LA) ffERG responses), and generalized rod dysfunction (abnormal dark-adapted (DA) ffERG responses). Detailed descriptions are provided in Table 9.4. All patients with initial DA ffERG abnormalities demonstrated clinically significant electrophysiological deterioration over 10 years; only 20% of patients with normal ffERGs at baseline showed clinically significant progression (Fujinami et al. A longitudinal study of Stargardt disease: clinical and electrophysiological assessment, progression, and genotype correlations. Am J Ophthalmol 2013)

22% of cases from Group 1 at baseline showed ERG group transition during the follow-up term, with 11% progressing to Group 2 and 11% to Group 3. Forty-seven percent of the cases in Group 2 progressed to Group 3. There was clinically significant ERG deterioration, at 22% for Group 1, 65% for Group 2, and 100% for Group 3 [10]. In a consequent prospective study, patients with a Group 3 ERG functional phenotype showed a significantly greater progression rate [22]. Such data are supported by an association with genotype grouping and are helpful in designing the protocols, selecting patients, and assessing the efficacy of potential therapeutic interventions [10].

Recently, multicentral international large-cohort studies have been conducted [70, 72]. The retrospective and prospective multicentre Natural History of the Progression of Atrophy Secondary to Stargardt Disease (ProgStar) studies were launched to characterize the natural history of STGD1 and identify sensitive, reliable, and clinically relevant outcome measures, which are needed for clinical trials [40]. ProgStar studies investigated demographics, visual acuity, FAF, microperimetry, and genetics in detail in a large cohort (>250 subjects) [28–40, 66]. In a ProgStar retrospective study of a subset of 224 eyes (mean age, 33.0 ± 15.1 years), the total mean area of DAF at the first visit was 2.6 mm^2, and the mean progression was 0.35 mm^2/year [33]. In a prospective study with 12 months of observation, the mean total area of DAF at baseline was 4.07 mm^2, and the estimated progression of DAF was 0.64 mm^2/year [30]. The rate of progression depended on the initial size of the lesion in both these retrospective and prospective studies, as previously reported by other longitudinal studies [11, 87, 88]. The data obtained in the ProgStar studies are helpful for identifying outcome measures in clinical trials.

9.3 Molecular Genetics

The *ABCA4* gene located at chromosome 1p22.1 is a large and highly polymorphic gene [4]. The estimated size of *ABCA4* is 6819 bp, including 50 exons, that encode a 2273-amino acid protein [57, 58]. Over 1200 disease-associated variants in the *ABCA4* gene have been identified in macular dystrophy, cone dystrophy, cone-rod dystrophy, and retinitis pigmentosa [4, 7, 8, 17, 22]. This allelic heterogeneity makes it challenging to establish genotype–phenotype correlations [17]. In general, deleterious variants are associated with earlier-onset disease with a more severe phenotype and missense variants with later-onset disease with a milder phenotype; certain missense variants can have severe functional effects similar to deleterious ones (e.g. c.1622T>C (p. Leu541Pro)/c.3113C>T (p.Ala1038Val) (complex), c.3064G>A (p.Glu1022Lys), c.4469G>A (p.Cys1490Tyr), c.3259G>A (p.Glu1087Lys), c.4577C>T (p.Thr1526Met), c.4918C>T (p. Arg1640Trp), and c.6449G>A (p.Cys2150Tyr) [16–19, 60].

A recent study aiming to identify *ABCA4* pre-mRNA splicing defects utilizing in vitro splice assays in human embryonic kidney 293T cells detected a number of putative disease-causing noncanonical splice site variants, including deep-intronic *ABCA4* variants [4, 67, 70, 89–91]. Although structural variants in the *ABCA4* gene/locus are thought to be relatively rare based on previous reports [4, 65, 67, 92–94], over 40 variants have been reported to date [4]. Interestingly, hypomorphic and modifier alleles have been intensively studied recently. One popular variant is c.5603A>T (p.Asn1868Ile) with high allele frequencies of approximately 7% in the European population [95]. The pathogenicity of this hypomorphic variant c.5603A>T (p.Asn1868Ile) under a specific condition (in trans with a deleterious ABCA4 variant) has been reported and patients harbouring this variant present late-onset disease [95, 96].

Furthermore, *ABCA4* founder variants have been identified in several populations. Most of the reported founder variants are present in European populations; c.2588G>C (p. Gly863Ala/p.Gly863del) in the West European; [92] c.1622T>C (p.Leu541Pro)/c.3113C>T (p. Ala1038Val) in the German; [97] c.3386G>T (p.Arg1129Leu) in the Spanish; and [98] c.2894A>G (p.Asn965Ser) in the Danish [99]. In contrast, a limited number of *ABCA4* founder variants have been reported in non-European populations, including c.6320G>A (p. Arg2107His) in the African population [99]. Regional differences due to ethnic background were also identified in the United States in the ProgStar genetics study [66].

Further studies are required to understand the genetic causes for the disease in the non-European population. To solve these problems, international collaborative studies have been ongoing in the East Asia Inherited Retinal Disease Society (EAIRDs; https://www.eairds.org/) [100], aiming to understand ethnicity-based disease characteristics and develop/apply therapeutic approaches in Asian populations.

9.4 Disease Mechanism

ABCA4, previously described as ABCR, is a member of the ABC transporter gene superfamily that encodes a retinal-specific transmembrane protein, is a member of the ATP-binding cassette transporter superfamily [101, 102]. ABCA4 is localized to the rim of the outer segment discs of both cone and rod photoreceptors and plays a role in the active transport of retinoids from the photoreceptor to the RPE in the retinoid cycle [101–104]. ABCA4 includes two transmembrane domains (TMD), two glycosylated extracellular domains (ECD), and two nucleotide-binding domains (NBD) (Fig. 9.7) [102].

The retinoid cycle involves enzyme-catalysed reactions converting all-trans-retinal, which is generated by photobleaching of rhodopsin or cone opsin, to 11-cis retinal [101–103, 105, 106]. All-trans-retinal is released from the light-activated rhodopsin or cone opsin into the outer segments to form a complex with phosphatidylethanolamine (PE), resulting in N-retinylidene-phosphatidylethanolamine (N-ret-PE); this complex is transported actively to the disc surface by ABCA4.

Failure of active transport due to ABCA4 dysfunction/mislocalization leads to inefficient removal of N-ret-PE from the photoreceptor outer segments and causes accumulation of bisretinoid compounds in the outer segment discs, and ultimately toxic levels of bisretinoid A2PE in the photoreceptor membranes [102, 104, 107]. A2PE is hydrolyzed to form the highly toxic metabolite N-retinylidene-N-retinyl-ethanolamine (A2E), which accumulates as a major component of lipofuscin in RPE cells and eventually causes RPE dysfunction and death with subsequent photoreceptor dysfunction/loss [105, 108]. Previous studies of ABCA4-knockout mice support the aforementioned pathogenesis, though there are limitations such as the lack of a macula in mice and the mild phenotype in a mouse model showing later-onset disease with slower degeneration than that of typical human patients with STGD1 [103, 109].

9.5 Therapeutic Approaches

ABCA4-associated retinal disease is an attractive target for therapeutic interventions, considering the high prevalence and well-studied disease course [4, 75, 76, 110]. Moreover, the retina has several advantages for the development and implementation of novel therapies: accessibility, compartmentalization, and an immune-privileged nature, as well as the possibility of measuring potential therapeutic outcome noninvasively [110].

In addition, several treatment approaches have been developed for *ABCA4*-associated retinal disease, ranging from variant-specific approaches to more generally applicable cell replacement, as based on the primary genetic abnormality and disease stage at the time of treatment [75, 76, 110]. Therapeutic trials of compounds, gene augmentation, and cell transplantation are ongoing (Table 9.7; https://clinicaltrials.gov/).

In addition, several therapeutic trials with compounds that target different aspects of the retinoid cycle have been specifically developed, and these treatments are potentially beneficial for slowing or preventing progression in *ABCA4*-associated retinal disease [111]. The aims of these agents are either (1) to reduce the formation of toxic products of the retinoid cycle by reducing the delivery of vitamin A or to inhibit various enzymes participating in the cycle or (2) to

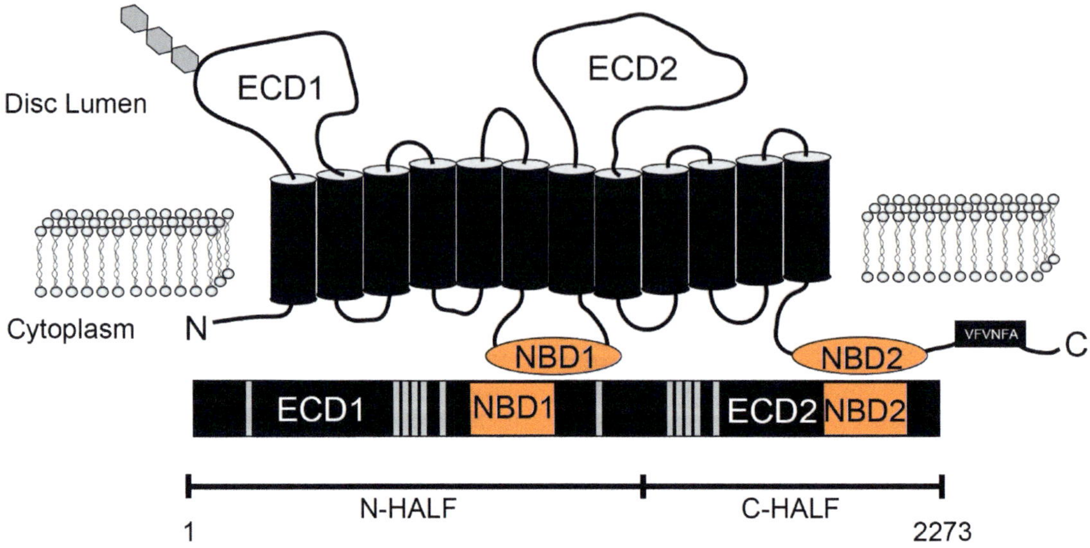

Fig. 9.7 A schematic of *ABCA4* protein structure. The *ABCA4* gene transcribes a large retina-specific ABCA4 protein with two transmembrane domains (TMD), two glycosylated extracellular domains (ECD), and two nucleotide-binding domains (NBD)

Table 9.7 Clinical trials for *ABCA4*-associated retinal disease

ID	Intervention	Phase	Status
Compound administration			
NCT00346853	4-Methylpyrazole (alcohol dehydrogenase inhibitor)	Phase 1	Completed
NCT02402660	ALK-001 (chemically modified vitamin A)	Phase 2	Recruiting
NCT00060749	DHA (omega-3 fatty acid)	Phase 1	Completed
NCT03033108	Emixustat (inhibitor of *RPE65*)	Phase 2	Completed
NCT03772665	Emixustat (inhibitor of *RPE65*)	Phase 3	Recruiting
NCT03297515	MADEOS (omega-3 fatty acid)	NA	Recruiting
NCT01278277	Saffron (neuroprotectant)	Phase 1/2	Unknown
2018-001496-20	Soraprazan (H^+,K^+-ATPase inhibitor)	Phase 2	Active
NCT03364153	Zimura (inhibitor of complement factor C5)	Phase 2	Active, not recruiting
Gene augmentation			
NCT01367444	SAR422459 (lentiviral delivery *ABCA4* cDNA)	Phase 1/2	Terminated
NCT01736592	SAR422459 (lentiviral delivery *ABCA4* cDNA)	Phase 1/2	Active, not recruiting
Cell transplantation			
NCT01920867	Bone marrow-derived stem cells	NA	Enrolling by invitation
NCT03011541	Bone marrow-derived stem cells	NA	Recruiting
NCT02903576	hESC-derived RPE cells	Phase 1/2	Unknown
NCT01345006	hESC-derived RPE cells (MA09-hRPE)	Phase 1/2	Completed
NCT01469832	hESC-derived RPE cells (MA09-hRPE)	Phase 1/2	Completed
NCT03772938	Stem/progenitor cells	Phase 1/2	Enrolling by invitation

hESC, human embryonic stem cell
The information has been provided on the public database (https://clinicaltrials.gov/)

directly target toxic metabolites such as A2E. Visual cycle modulators are candidates for the former treatment [112–116]. A phase II clinical trial with chemically modified vitamin A, which does not dimerize and stops N-ret-PE and A2E formation, is ongoing [117, 118].

Gene augmentation has been increasingly applied to photoreceptor diseases, with the goal of slowing or preventing further retinal degeneration [75, 76, 110]. To this end, adeno-associated virus (AAV) vectors have been the major choice for the gene transfer system of human gene therapy. However, there is a size limitation; that is, the *ABCA4* gene is larger than the current AAV vector capacity [119]. Considering the larger cargo capacity of lentiviruses, subretinal injection of a lentivirus vector delivering *ABCA4* has been developed, which is in an ongoing Phase I/II clinical trial [120].

A phase I/II stem cell therapy trial with subretinal transplantation of human embryonic stem cell (hESC)-derived RPE cells has also been ongoing in patients with severe and advanced *ABCA4*-associated retinal disease, given that RPE cell dysfunction/loss is believed to precede photoreceptor cell dysfunction/loss [121, 122].

9.6 Conclusion

ABCA4-associated retinal disease is one of the most common causes of inherited retinal disease and is highly heterogeneous both phenotypically and genetically. A number of clinical and genetic investigations have been performed to understand the underlying disease mechanisms, allowing several therapeutic trials to be conducted.

Acknowledgements We are grateful to Prof Michel Michaelides, Prof Anthony T. Moore, Prof Graham E. Holder, Prof Andrew R. Webster, Prof Anthony G. Robson, Prof Yozo Miyake, Prof Kazushige Tsunoda, Prof Takeshi Iwata, Prof Hendrik P. N. Scholl, Dr Rupert W Strauss, Dr Michalis Georgiou, Dr Kamron N. Khan, Dr Preena Tanna, Dr Ana Fakin, Prof Se Joon Woo, Prof Ruifang Sui, Prof Shiying Li, Kwangsic Joo, Dr. Panagiotis Sergouniotis, Dr Eva Lenassi, Dr Toshihide Kurihara, and Prof Kazuo Tsubota for their great guidance.

Funding Kaoru Fujinami is supported by grants from Grant-in-Aid for Young Scientists (A) of the Ministry of Education, Culture, Sports, Science and Technology, Japan (16H06269), grants from Grant-in-Aid for Scientists to support international collaborative studies of the Ministry of Education, Culture, Sports, Science and Technology, Japan (16KK01930002), grants from National Hospital Organization Network Research Fund (H30-NHO-Sensory Organs-03), grants from FOUNDATION FIGHTING BLINDNESS ALAN LATIES CAREER DEVELOPMENT PROGRAM (CF-CL-0416-0696-UCL), grants from Health Labour Sciences Research Grant, The Ministry of Health Labour and Welfare (201711107A), and grants from Great Britain Sasakawa Foundation Butterfield Awards.

Yu Fujinami-Yokokawa was supported by grants from Grant-in-Aid for Young Scientists of the Ministry of Education, Culture, Sports, Science and Technology, Japan (18K16943).

The sponsor or funding organization had no role in the design or conduct of this research.

Conflict of Interest Disclosures All authors have completed Disclosure of Potential Conflicts of Interest. Individual investigators who participate in the sponsored project(s) are not directly compensated by the sponsor but may receive salary or other support from the institution to support their effort on the project(s).

Kaoru Fujinami is a paid consultant of Astellas Pharma Inc, Kubota Pharmaceutical Holdings Co., Ltd, Acucela Inc., Janssen Pharm, Sanofi Genzyme, and NightstaRx Limited. Kaoru Fujinami reports personal fees from Astellas Pharma Inc, personal fees from Kubota Pharmaceutical Holdings Co., Ltd., personal fees from Acucela Inc., personal fees from NightstaRx Limited., personal fees from SANTEN Company Limited, personal fees from Foundation Fighting Blindness, personal fees from Foundation Fighting Blindness Clinical Research Institute, personal fees from Japanese Ophthalmology Society, personal fees from Japan Retinitis Pigmentosa Society. Laboratory of Visual Physiology, Division for Vision Research, National Institute of Sensory Organs, National Hospital Organization, Tokyo Medical Center, Tokyo, Japan is supported by grants from Astellas Pharma Inc (NCT03281005), outside the submitted work.

Yu Fujinami-Yokokawa was supported by grants from Grant-in-Aid for Young Scientists of the Ministry of Education, Culture, Sports, Science and Technology, Japan (18K16943).

Role of the Funder/Sponsor The funding sources had no role in the design and conduct of the study; collection, management, analysis, and interpretation of the data; preparation, review, or approval of the manuscript; and decision to submit the manuscript for publication.

References

1. Stargardt K. Über familiäre, progressive Degeneration in der Maculagegend des Auges. Graefes Arch Clin Exp Ophthalmol. 1909;71:534–50.
2. Michaelides M, Hunt DM, Moore AT. The genetics of inherited macular dystrophies. J Med Genet. 2003;40(9):641–50.
3. Tanna P, Strauss RW, Fujinami K, Michaelides M. Stargardt disease: clinical features, molecular genetics, animal models and therapeutic options. Br J Ophthalmol. 2017;101(1):25–30.
4. Cremers FPM, Lee W, Collin RWJ, Allikmets R. Clinical spectrum, genetic complexity and therapeutic approaches for retinal disease caused by ABCA4 mutations. Prog Retin Eye Res. 2020;79:100861.
5. Pontikos N, Arno G, Jurkute N, Schiff E, Ba-Abbad R, Malka S, et al. Genetic basis of inherited retinal disease in a molecularly characterized cohort of more than 3000 families from the United Kingdom. Ophthalmology. 2020;127(10):1384–94.
6. Stone EM, Andorf JL, Whitmore SS, DeLuca AP, Giacalone JC, Streb LM, et al. Clinically focused molecular investigation of 1000 consecutive families with inherited retinal disease. Ophthalmology. 2017;124(9):1314–31.
7. Liu X, Fujinami YY, Yang L, Arno G, Fujinami K. Stargardt disease in asian population. Advances in vision research, vol. II. Singapore: Springer; 2019. p. 279–95.
8. Burke TR, Tsang SH. Allelic and phenotypic heterogeneity in ABCA4 mutations. Ophthalmic Genet. 2011;32(3):165–74.
9. Blacharski P. Retinal dystrophies and degenerations. New York: Raven; 1988.
10. Fujinami K, Lois N, Davidson AE, Mackay DS, Hogg CR, Stone EM, et al. A longitudinal study of Stargardt disease: clinical and electrophysiologic assessment, progression, and genotype correlations. Am J Ophthalmol. 2013;155(6):1075–88.e13.
11. Fujinami K, Lois N, Mukherjee R, McBain VA, Tsunoda K, Tsubota K, et al. A longitudinal study of Stargardt disease: quantitative assessment of fundus autofluorescence, progression, and genotype correlations. Invest Ophthalmol Vis Sci. 2013;54(13):8181–90.
12. Fishman GA. Fundus flavimaculatus. A clinical classification. Arch Ophthalmol. 1976;94(12):2061–7.
13. Fishman GA, Stone EM, Grover S, Derlacki DJ, Haines HL, Hockey RR. Variation of clinical expression in patients with Stargardt dystrophy and sequence variations in the ABCR gene. Arch Ophthalmol. 1999;117(4):504–10.
14. Fujinami K, Zernant J, Chana RK, Wright GA, Tsunoda K, Ozawa Y, et al. Clinical and molecular characteristics of childhood-onset Stargardt disease. Ophthalmology. 2015;122(2):326–34.
15. Lois N, Holder GE, Bunce C, Fitzke FW, Bird AC. Phenotypic subtypes of Stargardt macular dystrophy-fundus flavimaculatus. Arch Ophthalmol. 2001;119(3):359–69.
16. Yatsenko AN, Shroyer NF, Lewis RA, Lupski JR. Late-onset Stargardt disease is associated with missense mutations that map outside known functional regions of ABCR (ABCA4). Hum Genet. 2001;108(4):346–55.
17. Fujinami K, Sergouniotis PI, Davidson AE, Mackay DS, Tsunoda K, Tsubota K, et al. The clinical effect of homozygous ABCA4 alleles in 18 patients. Ophthalmology. 2013;120(11):2324–31.
18. Fakin A, Robson AG, Chiang JP, Fujinami K, Moore AT, Michaelides M, et al. The effect on retinal structure and function of 15 specific ABCA4 Mutations: a detailed examination of 82 hemizygous patients. Invest Ophthalmol Vis Sci. 2016;57(14):5963–73.
19. Fakin A, Robson AG, Fujinami K, Moore AT, Michaelides M, Pei-Wen Chiang J, et al. Phenotype and progression of retinal degeneration associated with nullizigosity of ABCA4. Invest Ophthalmol Vis Sci. 2016;57(11):4668–78.
20. Khan KN, Kasilian M, Mahroo OAR, Tanna P, Kalitzeos A, Robson AG, et al. Early patterns of macular degeneration in ABCA4-associated retinopathy. Ophthalmology. 2018;125(5):735–46.
21. Mahroo OA, Fujinami K, Moore AT, Webster AR. Retinal findings in a patient with mutations in ABCC6 and ABCA4. Eye (Lond). 2018;32(9):1542–3.
22. Georgiou M, Kane T, Tanna P, Bouzia Z, Singh N, Kalitzeos A, et al. Prospective cohort study of childhood-onset Stargardt disease: fundus autofluorescence imaging, progression, comparison with adult-onset disease, and disease symmetry. Am J Ophthalmol. 2020;211:159–75.
23. Tanna P, Georgiou M, Strauss RW, Ali N, Kumaran N, Kalitzeos A, et al. Cross-sectional and longitudinal assessment of the ellipsoid zone in childhood-onset Stargardt disease. Transl Vis Sci Technol. 2019;8(2):1.
24. Singh R, Fujinami K, Chen LL, Michaelides M, Moore AT. Longitudinal follow-up of siblings with a discordant Stargardt disease phenotype. Acta Ophthalmol. 2014;92(4):e331–2.
25. Fujinami K, Singh R, Carroll J, Zernant J, Allikmets R, Michaelides M, et al. Fine central macular dots

associated with childhood-onset Stargardt disease. Acta Ophthalmol. 2014;92(2):e157–9.
26. Fujinami K, Sergouniotis PI, Davidson AE, Wright G, Chana RK, Tsunoda K, et al. Clinical and molecular analysis of Stargardt disease with preserved foveal structure and function. Am J Ophthalmol. 2013;156(3):487–501. e1
27. Fujinami K, Akahori M, Fukui M, Tsunoda K, Iwata T, Miyake Y. Stargardt disease with preserved central vision: identification of a putative novel mutation in ATP-binding cassette transporter gene. Acta Ophthalmol. 2011;89(3):e297–8.
28. Schonbach EM, Strauss RW, Munoz B, Wolfson Y, Ibrahim MA, Birch DG, et al. Longitudinal microperimetric changes of macular sensitivity in Stargardt disease after 12 months: ProgStar Report No. 13. JAMA Ophthalmol. 2020;138(7):772–9.
29. Schonbach EM, Strauss RW, Ibrahim MA, Janes JL, Birch DG, Cideciyan AV, et al. Faster sensitivity loss around dense scotomas than for overall macular sensitivity in Stargardt disease: ProgStar Report No. 14. Am J Ophthalmol. 2020;216:219–25.
30. Strauss RW, Kong X, Ho A, Jha A, West S, Ip M, et al. Progression of Stargardt disease as determined by fundus autofluorescence over a 12-month period: ProgStar Report No. 11. JAMA Ophthalmol. 2019;137(10):1134–45.
31. Kong X, Fujinami K, Strauss RW, Munoz B, West SK, Cideciyan AV, et al. Visual acuity change over 24 months and its association with foveal phenotype and genotype in individuals with Stargardt disease: ProgStar Study Report No. 10. JAMA Ophthalmol. 2018;136(8):920–8.
32. Schonbach EM, Strauss RW, Kong X, Munoz B, Ibrahim MA, Sunness JS, et al. Longitudinal changes of fixation location and stability within 12 months in Stargardt disease: ProgStar Report No. 12. Am J Ophthalmol. 2018;193:54–61.
33. Strauss RW, Munoz B, Ho A, Jha A, Michaelides M, Cideciyan AV, et al. Progression of Stargardt disease as determined by fundus autofluorescence in the retrospective progression of Stargardt Disease Study (ProgStar Report No. 9). JAMA Ophthalmol. 2017;135(11):1232–41.
34. Kong X, Strauss RW, Cideciyan AV, Michaelides M, Sahel JA, Munoz B, et al. Visual Acuity change over 12 months in the prospective progression of atrophy secondary to Stargardt Disease (ProgStar) Study: ProgStar Report Number 6. Ophthalmology. 2017;124(11):1640–51.
35. Strauss RW, Munoz B, Ho A, Jha A, Michaelides M, Mohand-Said S, et al. Incidence of atrophic lesions in Stargardt disease in the progression of atrophy secondary to Stargardt Disease (ProgStar) Study: Report No. 5. JAMA Ophthalmol. 2017;135(7):687–95.
36. Schonbach EM, Wolfson Y, Strauss RW, Ibrahim MA, Kong X, Munoz B, et al. Macular sensitivity measured with microperimetry in Stargardt disease in the progression of atrophy secondary to Stargardt Disease (ProgStar) Study: Report No. 7. JAMA Ophthalmol. 2017;135(7):696–703.
37. Kong X, West SK, Strauss RW, Munoz B, Cideciyan AV, Michaelides M, et al. Progression of visual acuity and fundus autofluorescence in recent-onset Stargardt disease: ProgStar Study Report #4. Ophthalmol Retina. 2017;1(6):514–23.
38. Schonbach EM, Ibrahim MA, Strauss RW, Birch DG, Cideciyan AV, Hahn GA, et al. Fixation location and stability using the MP-1 microperimeter in Stargardt disease: ProgStar Report No. 3. Ophthalmol Retina. 2017;1(1):68–76.
39. Kong X, Strauss RW, Michaelides M, Cideciyan AV, Sahel JA, Munoz B, et al. Visual Acuity loss and associated risk factors in the retrospective progression of Stargardt Disease Study (ProgStar Report No. 2). Ophthalmology. 2016;123(9):1887–97.
40. Strauss RW, Ho A, Munoz B, Cideciyan AV, Sahel JA, Sunness JS, et al. The natural history of the progression of atrophy secondary to Stargardt disease (ProgStar) Studies: design and baseline characteristics: ProgStar Report No. 1. Ophthalmology. 2016;123(4):817–28.
41. Tanaka K, Lee W, Zernant J, Schuerch K, Ciccone L, Tsang SH, et al. The rapid-onset chorioretinopathy phenotype of ABCA4 disease. Ophthalmology. 2018;125(1):89–99.
42. Lee W, Zernant J, Nagasaki T, Tsang SH, Allikmets R. Deep scleral exposure: a degenerative outcome of end-stage Stargardt disease. Am J Ophthalmol. 2018;195:16–25.
43. Jauregui R, Cho A, Lee W, Zernant J, Allikmets R, Sparrow JR, et al. Progressive choriocapillaris impairment in ABCA4 maculopathy is secondary to retinal pigment epithelium atrophy. Invest Ophthalmol Vis Sci. 2020;61(4):13.
44. Michaelides M, Chen LL, Brantley MA Jr, Andorf JL, Isaak EM, Jenkins SA, et al. ABCA4 mutations and discordant ABCA4 alleles in patients and siblings with bull's-eye maculopathy. Br J Ophthalmol. 2007;91(12):1650–5.
45. Huang L, Xiao X, Li S, Jia X, Wang P, Sun W, et al. Molecular genetics of cone-rod dystrophy in Chinese patients: new data from 61 probands and mutation overview of 163 probands. Exp Eye Res. 2016;146:252–8.
46. Oishi M, Oishi A, Gotoh N, Ogino K, Higasa K, Iida K, et al. Next-generation sequencing-based comprehensive molecular analysis of 43 Japanese patients with cone and cone-rod dystrophies. Mol Vis. 2016;22:150–60.
47. Lee W, Schuerch K, Zernant J, Collison FT, Bearelly S, Fishman GA, et al. Genotypic spectrum and phenotype correlations of ABCA4-associated disease in patients of south Asian descent. Eur J Hum Genet. 2017;25(6):735–43.
48. Jiang F, Pan Z, Xu K, Tian L, Xie Y, Zhang X, et al. Screening of ABCA4 gene in a chinese cohort with

Stargardt disease or cone-rod dystrophy with a report on 85 novel mutations. Invest Ophthalmol Vis Sci. 2016;57(1):145–52.
49. Fukui T, Yamamoto S, Nakano K, Tsujikawa M, Morimura H, Nishida K, et al. ABCA4 gene mutations in Japanese patients with Stargardt disease and retinitis pigmentosa. Invest Ophthalmol Vis Sci. 2002;43(9):2819–24.
50. Nakao T, Tsujikawa M, Sawa M, Gomi F, Nishida K. Foveal sparing in patients with Japanese Stargardt's disease and good visual acuity. Jpn J Ophthalmol. 2012;56(6):584–8.
51. Song WK, Park KM, Kim HJ, Lee JH, Choi J, Chong SY, et al. Treatment of macular degeneration using embryonic stem cell-derived retinal pigment epithelium: preliminary results in Asian patients. Stem Cell Rep. 2015;4(5):860–72.
52. Battu R, Verma A, Hariharan R, Krishna S, Kiran R, Jacob J, et al. Identification of novel mutations in ABCA4 gene: clinical and genetic analysis of indian patients with Stargardt disease. Biomed Res Int. 2015;2015:940864.
53. Koyanagi Y, Akiyama M, Nishiguchi KM, Momozawa Y, Kamatani Y, Takata S, et al. Genetic characteristics of retinitis pigmentosa in 1204 Japanese patients. J Med Genet. 2019;56(10):662–70.
54. Anderson KL, Baird L, Lewis RA, Chinault AC, Otterud B, Leppert M, et al. A YAC contig encompassing the recessive Stargardt disease gene (STGD) on chromosome 1p. Am J Hum Genet. 1995;57(6):1351–63.
55. Gerber S, Rozet JM, Bonneau D, Souied E, Camuzat A, Dufier JL, et al. A gene for late-onset fundus flavimaculatus with macular dystrophy maps to chromosome 1p13. Am J Hum Genet. 1995;56(2):396–9.
56. Kaplan J, Gerber S, Larget-Piet D, Rozet JM, Dollfus H, Dufier JL, et al. A gene for Stargardt's disease (fundus flavimaculatus) maps to the short arm of chromosome 1. Nat Genet. 1993;5(3):308–11.
57. Allikmets R. A photoreceptor cell-specific ATP-binding transporter gene (ABCR) is mutated in recessive Stargardt macular dystrophy. Nat Genet. 1997;17(1):122.
58. Allikmets R, Singh N, Sun H, Shroyer NF, Hutchinson A, Chidambaram A, et al. A photoreceptor cell-specific ATP-binding transporter gene (ABCR) is mutated in recessive Stargardt macular dystrophy. Nat Genet. 1997;15(3):236–46.
59. Jaakson K, Zernant J, Kulm M, Hutchinson A, Tonisson N, Glavac D, et al. Genotyping microarray (gene chip) for the ABCR (ABCA4) gene. Hum Mutat. 2003;22(5):395–403
60. Briggs CE, Rucinski D, Rosenfeld PJ, Hirose T, Berson EL, Dryja TP. Mutations in ABCR (ABCA4) in patients with Stargardt macular degeneration or cone-rod degeneration. Invest Ophthalmol Vis Sci. 2001;42(10):2229–36.
61. Klevering BJ, Yzer S, Rohrschneider K, Zonneveld M, Allikmets R, van den Born LI, et al. Microarray-based mutation analysis of the ABCA4 (ABCR) gene in autosomal recessive cone-rod dystrophy and retinitis pigmentosa. Eur J Hum Genet. 2004;12(12):1024–32.
62. Ernest PJ, Boon CJ, Klevering BJ, Hoefsloot LH, Hoyng CB. Outcome of ABCA4 microarray screening in routine clinical practice. Mol Vis. 2009;15:2841–7.
63. Zernant J, Schubert C, Im KM, Burke T, Brown CM, Fishman GA, et al. Analysis of the ABCA4 gene by next-generation sequencing. Invest Ophthalmol Vis Sci. 2011;52(11):8479–87.
64. Fujinami K, Zernant J, Chana RK, Wright GA, Tsunoda K, Ozawa Y, et al. ABCA4 gene screening by next-generation sequencing in a British cohort. Invest Ophthalmol Vis Sci. 2013;54(10):6662–74.
65. Zernant J, Xie YA, Ayuso C, Riveiro-Alvarez R, Lopez-Martinez MA, Simonelli F, et al. Analysis of the ABCA4 genomic locus in Stargardt disease. Hum Mol Genet. 2014;23(25):6797–806.
66. Fujinami K, Strauss RW, Chiang JP, Audo IS, Bernstein PS, Birch DG, et al. Detailed genetic characteristics of an international large cohort of patients with Stargardt disease: ProgStar study report 8. Br J Ophthalmol. 2019;103(3):390–7.
67. Bauwens M, Garanto A, Sangermano R, Naessens S, Weisschuh N, De Zaeytijd J, et al. ABCA4-associated disease as a model for missing heritability in autosomal recessive disorders: novel noncoding splice, cis-regulatory, structural, and recurrent hypomorphic variants. Genet Med. 2019;21(8):1761–71.
68. Sangermano R, Garanto A, Khan M, Runhart EH, Bauwens M, Bax NM, et al. Deep-intronic ABCA4 variants explain missing heritability in Stargardt disease and allow correction of splice defects by antisense oligonucleotides. Genet Med. 2019;21(8):1751–60.
69. Webster AR, Heon E, Lotery AJ, Vandenburgh K, Casavant TL, Oh KT, et al. An analysis of allelic variation in the ABCA4 gene. Invest Ophthalmol Vis Sci. 2001;42(6):1179–89.
70. Khan M, Cornelis SS, Pozo-Valero MD, Whelan L, Runhart EH, Mishra K, et al. Resolving the dark matter of ABCA4 for 1054 Stargardt disease probands through integrated genomics and transcriptomics. Genet Med. 2020;22(7):1235–46.
71. Cornelis SS, Bax NM, Zernant J, Allikmets R, Fritsche LG, den Dunnen JT, et al. In silico functional meta-analysis of 5,962 ABCA4 variants in 3,928 retinal dystrophy cases. Hum Mutat. 2017;38(4):400–8.
72. Schulz HL, Grassmann F, Kellner U, Spital G, Ruther K, Jagle H, et al. Mutation spectrum of the ABCA4 gene in 335 Stargardt disease patients from a multicenter German cohort-impact of selected deep intronic variants and common SNPs. Invest Ophthalmol Vis Sci. 2017;58(1):394–403.
73. Joo K, Seong MW, Park KH, Park SS, Woo SJ. Genotypic profile and phenotype correlations of ABCA4-associated retinopathy in Koreans. Mol Vis. 2019;25:679–90.

74. Fujinami-Yokokawa Y, Pontikos N, Yang L, Tsunoda K, Yoshitake K, Iwata T, et al. Prediction of causative genes in inherited retinal disorders from spectral-domain optical coherence tomography utilizing deep learning techniques. J Ophthalmol. 2019;2019:1691064.
75. Scholl HP, Strauss RW, Singh MS, Dalkara D, Roska B, Picaud S, et al. Emerging therapies for inherited retinal degeneration. Sci Transl Med. 2016;8(368):368rv6.
76. Smith J, Ward D, Michaelides M, Moore AT, Simpson S. New and emerging technologies for the treatment of inherited retinal diseases: a horizon scanning review. Eye (Lond). 2015;29(9):1131–40.
77. Hood DC, Bach M, Brigell M, Keating D, Kondo M, Lyons JS, et al. ISCEV standard for clinical multifocal electroretinography (mfERG) (2011 edition). Doc Ophthalmol. 2012;124(1):1–13.
78. Bach M, Brigell MG, Hawlina M, Holder GE, Johnson MA, McCulloch DL, et al. ISCEV standard for clinical pattern electroretinography (PERG): 2012 update. Doc Ophthalmol. 2013;126(1):1–7.
79. McCulloch DL, Marmor MF, Brigell MG, Hamilton R, Holder GE, Tzekov R, et al. Erratum to: ISCEV Standard for full-field clinical electroretinography (2015 update). Doc Ophthalmol. 2015;131(1):81–3.
80. McCulloch DL, Marmor MF, Brigell MG, Hamilton R, Holder GE, Tzekov R, et al. ISCEV Standard for full-field clinical electroretinography (2015 update). Doc Ophthalmol. 2015;130(1):1–12.
81. Robson AG, Nilsson J, Li S, Jalali S, Fulton AB, Tormene AP, et al. ISCEV guide to visual electrodiagnostic procedures. Doc Ophthalmol. 2018;136(1):1–26.
82. Lambertus S, van Huet RA, Bax NM, Hoefsloot LH, Cremers FP, Boon CJ, et al. Early-onset Stargardt disease: phenotypic and genotypic characteristics. Ophthalmology. 2015;122(2):335–44.
83. van Huet RA, Bax NM, Westeneng-Van Haaften SC, Muhamad M, Zonneveld-Vrieling MN, Hoefsloot LH, et al. Foveal sparing in Stargardt disease. Invest Ophthalmol Vis Sci. 2014;55(11):7467–78.
84. Westeneng-van Haaften SC, Boon CJ, Cremers FP, Hoefsloot LH, den Hollander AI, Hoyng CB. Clinical and genetic characteristics of late-onset Stargardt's disease. Ophthalmology. 2012;119(6):1199–210.
85. Lambertus S, Lindner M, Bax NM, Mauschitz MM, Nadal J, Schmid M, et al. Progression of late-onset Stargardt disease. Invest Ophthalmol Vis Sci. 2016;57(13):5186–91.
86. Runhart EH, Valkenburg D, Cornelis SS, Khan M, Sangermano R, Albert S, et al. Late-onset Stargardt disease due to mild, deep-intronic ABCA4 alleles. Invest Ophthalmol Vis Sci. 2019;60(13):4249–56.
87. McBain VA, Townend J, Lois N. Progression of retinal pigment epithelial atrophy in Stargardt disease. Am J Ophthalmol. 2012;154(1):146–54.
88. Chen B, Tosha C, Gorin MB, Nusinowitz S. Analysis of autofluorescent retinal images and measurement of atrophic lesion growth in Stargardt disease. Exp Eye Res. 2010;91(2):143–52.
89. Sangermano R, Bax NM, Bauwens M, van den Born LI, De Baere E, Garanto A, et al. Photoreceptor progenitor mrna analysis reveals exon skipping resulting from the ABCA4 c.5461-10T-->C mutation in Stargardt disease. Ophthalmology. 2016;123(6):1375–85.
90. Sangermano R, Khan M, Cornelis SS, Richelle V, Albert S, Garanto A, et al. ABCA4 midigenes reveal the full splice spectrum of all reported noncanonical splice site variants in Stargardt disease. Genome Res. 2018;28(1):100–10.
91. Fadaie Z, Khan M, Del Pozo-Valero M, Cornelis SS, Ayuso C, Cremers FPM, et al. Identification of splice defects due to noncanonical splice site or deep-intronic variants in ABCA4. Hum Mutat. 2019;40(12):2365–76.
92. Maugeri A, van Driel MA, van de Pol DJ, Klevering BJ, van Haren FJ, Tijmes N, et al. The 2588G-->C mutation in the ABCR gene is a mild frequent founder mutation in the Western European population and allows the classification of ABCR mutations in patients with Stargardt disease. Am J Hum Genet. 1999;64(4):1024–35.
93. Yatsenko AN, Shroyer NF, Lewis RA, Lupski JR. An ABCA4 genomic deletion in patients with Stargardt disease. Hum Mutat. 2003;21(6):636–44.
94. Bax NM, Sangermano R, Roosing S, Thiadens AA, Hoefsloot LH, van den Born LI, et al. Heterozygous deep-intronic variants and deletions in ABCA4 in persons with retinal dystrophies and one exonic ABCA4 variant. Hum Mutat. 2015;36(1):43–7.
95. Zernant J, Lee W, Collison FT, Fishman GA, Sergeev YV, Schuerch K, et al. Frequent hypomorphic alleles account for a significant fraction of ABCA4 disease and distinguish it from age-related macular degeneration. J Med Genet. 2017;54(6):404–12.
96. Runhart EH, Sangermano R, Cornelis SS, Verheij J, Plomp AS, Boon CJF, et al. The common ABCA4 variant p.Asn1868Ile shows nonpenetrance and variable expression of Stargardt disease when present in trans with severe variants. Invest Ophthalmol Vis Sci. 2018;59(8):3220–31.
97. Rivera A, White K, Stohr H, Steiner K, Hemmrich N, Grimm T, et al. A comprehensive survey of sequence variation in the ABCA4 (ABCR) gene in Stargardt disease and age-related macular degeneration. Am J Hum Genet. 2000;67(4):800–13.
98. Valverde D, Riveiro-Alvarez R, Bernal S, Jaakson K, Baiget M, Navarro R, et al. Microarray-based mutation analysis of the ABCA4 gene in Spanish patients with Stargardt disease: evidence of a prevalent mutated allele. Mol Vis. 2006;12:902–8.
99. Rosenberg T, Klie F, Garred P, Schwartz M. N965S is a common ABCA4 variant in Stargardt-related retinopathies in the Danish population. Mol Vis. 2007;13:1962–9.

100. Fujinami K, Yang L, Joo K, Tsunoda K, Kameya S, Hanazono G, et al. Clinical and genetic characteristics of East Asian patients with occult macular dystrophy (Miyake disease): East Asia occult macular dystrophy studies report number 1. Ophthalmology. 2019;126(10):1432–44.
101. Cideciyan AV, Aleman TS, Swider M, Schwartz SB, Steinberg JD, Brucker AJ, et al. Mutations in ABCA4 result in accumulation of lipofuscin before slowing of the retinoid cycle: a reappraisal of the human disease sequence. Hum Mol Genet. 2004;13(5):525–34.
102. Tsybovsky Y, Molday RS, Palczewski K. The ATP-binding cassette transporter ABCA4: structural and functional properties and role in retinal disease. Adv Exp Med Biol. 2010;703:105–25.
103. Charbel Issa P, Barnard AR, Singh MS, Carter E, Jiang Z, Radu RA, et al. Fundus autofluorescence in the Abca4(-/-) mouse model of Stargardt disease—correlation with accumulation of A2E, retinal function, and histology. Invest Ophthalmol Vis Sci. 2013;54(8):5602–12.
104. Sun H, Nathans J. ABCR: rod photoreceptor-specific ABC transporter responsible for Stargardt disease. Methods Enzymol. 2000;315:879–97.
105. Sparrow JR, Boulton M. RPE lipofuscin and its role in retinal pathobiology. Exp Eye Res. 2005;80(5):595–606.
106. Radu RA, Mata NL, Bagla A, Travis GH. Light exposure stimulates formation of A2E oxiranes in a mouse model of Stargardt's macular degeneration. Proc Natl Acad Sci U S A. 2004;101(16):5928–33.
107. Smith RT, Gomes NL, Barile G, Busuioc M, Lee N, Laine A. Lipofuscin and autofluorescence metrics in progressive STGD. Invest Ophthalmol Vis Sci. 2009;50(8):3907–14.
108. Sparrow JR, Fishkin N, Zhou J, Cai B, Jang YP, Krane S, et al. A2E, a byproduct of the visual cycle. Vision Res. 2003;43(28):2983–90.
109. Weng J, Mata NL, Azarian SM, Tzekov RT, Birch DG, Travis GH. Insights into the function of Rim protein in photoreceptors and etiology of Stargardt's disease from the phenotype in abcr knockout mice. Cell. 1999;98(1):13–23.
110. Vazquez-Dominguez I, Garanto A, Collin RWJ. Molecular therapies for inherited retinal diseases-current standing, opportunities and challenges. Genes (Basel). 2019;10(9).
111. Travis GH, Golczak M, Moise AR, Palczewski K. Diseases caused by defects in the visual cycle: retinoids as potential therapeutic agents. Annu Rev Pharmacol Toxicol. 2007;47:469–512.
112. Dugel PU, Novack RL, Csaky KG, Richmond PP, Birch DG, Kubota R. Phase ii, randomized, placebo-controlled, 90-day study of emixustat hydrochloride in geographic atrophy associated with dry age-related macular degeneration. Retina. 2015;35(6):1173–83.
113. Kubota R, Al-Fayoumi S, Mallikaarjun S, Patil S, Bavik C, Chandler JW. Phase 1, dose-ranging study of emixustat hydrochloride (ACU-4429), a novel visual cycle modulator, in healthy volunteers. Retina. 2014;34(3):603–9.
114. Kubota R, Boman NL, David R, Mallikaarjun S, Patil S, Birch D. Safety and effect on rod function of ACU-4429, a novel small-molecule visual cycle modulator. Retina. 2012;32(1):183–8.
115. Rosenfeld PJ, Dugel PU, Holz FG, Heier JS, Pearlman JA, Novack RL, et al. Emixustat hydrochloride for geographic atrophy secondary to age-related macular degeneration: a randomized clinical trial. Ophthalmology. 2018;125(10):1556–67.
116. Kubota R, Calkins DJ, Henry SH, Linsenmeier RA. Emixustat reduces metabolic demand of dark activity in the retina. Invest Ophthalmol Vis Sci. 2019;60(14):4924–30.
117. Kaufman Y, Ma L, Washington I. Deuterium enrichment of vitamin A at the C20 position slows the formation of detrimental vitamin A dimers in wild-type rodents. J Biol Chem. 2011;286(10):7958–65.
118. Charbel Issa P, Barnard AR, Herrmann P, Washington I, MacLaren RE. Rescue of the Stargardt phenotype in Abca4 knockout mice through inhibition of vitamin A dimerization. Proc Natl Acad Sci U S A. 2015;112(27):8415–20.
119. Allocca M, Doria M, Petrillo M, Colella P, Garcia-Hoyos M, Gibbs D, et al. Serotype-dependent packaging of large genes in adeno-associated viral vectors results in effective gene delivery in mice. J Clin Invest. 2008;118(5):1955–64.
120. Dalkara D, Goureau O, Marazova K, Sahel JA. Let there be light: gene and cell therapy for blindness. Hum Gene Ther. 2016;27(2):134–47.
121. Schwartz SD, Regillo CD, Lam BL, Eliott D, Rosenfeld PJ, Gregori NZ, et al. Human embryonic stem cell-derived retinal pigment epithelium in patients with age-related macular degeneration and Stargardt's macular dystrophy: follow-up of two open-label phase 1/2 studies. Lancet. 2015;385(9967):509–16.
122. Mehat MS, Sundaram V, Ripamonti C, Robson AG, Smith AJ, Borooah S, et al. Transplantation of human embryonic stem cell-derived retinal pigment epithelial cells in macular degeneration. Ophthalmology. 2018;125(11):1765–75.

Cone Dystrophy/Cone-Rod Dystrophy

10

Jung Hyun Park

Abstract

Cone dystrophy is a rare genetic retinal disorder characterized by primary cone degeneration and secondary rod involvement, with a variable fundus appearance. The loss of cones leads to predominant symptoms such as decreased visual acuity, color vision defects and day blindness. Cone dystrophies are genetically heterogeneous and can be inherited by autosomal recessive, autosomal dominant or X-linked recessive patterns.

Keywords

Cone dystrophy · Cone-rod dystrophy · ERG · Genetic counseling · Day blindness · Color vision defects

10.1 Introduction

Cone dystrophy or cone-rod dystrophy is a rare genetic retinal disorder characterized by primary cone degeneration and secondary rod involvement or concomitant loss of both cones and rods (cone-rod dystrophy), with a variable fundus appearance. The prevalence of cone/cone-rod dystrophy is estimated at 1/40,000 [1].

Cone dystrophies usually present in childhood or early adult life, with many patients developing rod photoreceptor involvement in later life, thereby leading to considerable overlap between cone and cone-rod dystrophies.

10.2 Clinical Feature and Diagnosis

Cone dystrophies are characterized by retinal pigment deposits visible on fundus examination, predominantly localized to the macular region. In contrast to typical retinitis pigmentosa (RP), also called the rod-cone dystrophy which is caused by primary loss in rod photoreceptors and later followed by the secondary loss in cone photoreceptors, cone dystrophy reflects the opposite sequence of the events.

The predominant symptoms are decreased visual acuity, central scotoma, color vision defects, hemeralopia (day blindness), photoaversion (avoidance of light due to decreased visual acuity) and decreased sensitivity in the central visual field, later followed by progressive loss in peripheral vision and night blindness. The age of onset of vision loss may be from the late teens to the sixties.

The clinical course of cone dystrophy is generally more severe and rapid than RPs, leading to earlier central vision loss. At the end stage, however, cone dystrophies do not differ from RPs.

J. H. Park (✉)
Department of Ophthalmology, Seoul Paik Hospital, Inje University, Seoul, Korea

H.-G. Yu (ed.), *Inherited Retinal Disease*, https://doi.org/10.1007/978-981-16-7337-5_10

Early color vision abnormality appears even when visual acuity is still not significantly affected in patients with cone dystrophy. This distinguishes cone dystrophy from Stargardt disease and other macular dystrophies. At birth, no symptoms of cone dysfunction are present, unlike the disorders of cone or rod monochromatism.

The fundus appearance is variable. In the early stage, the fundus appears normal, or fine macular lesions and optic disc pallor may be the only signs. Pigmentary deposits resembling bony spicules can be found frequently in the macular area. Macular atrophy or a bull's-eye maculopathy, peripheral retinal pigment epithelium atrophy, intra-retinal pigmentation migration and arteriolar attenuation are shown as the disease progresses. It may be difficult to establish the correct diagnosis in the early stage of the disease because of the lack of observable retinal changes.

Electrophysiologic test confirms a marked generalized abnormality of cone function with comparatively little change in rod function in the early stage. The ERG shows a substantial loss of single-flash and 30-Hz flicker response, whereas rod and mixed responses are relatively spared. Older patients may show some loss of rod sensitivity also [2]. A subset of patients has been described in whom the full-field ERG appears normal, and involvement of only the foveal or central cones has been documented [3]. Macular focal cone ERG is useful to detect cone dystrophy as most of the patients show smaller responses than normal individuals and also to anticipate the progression of cone-rod dystrophy [4].

Peripheral visual fields remain normal, whereas the central visual field and visual acuity are decreased in young patients. Patchy losses of peripheral vision follow in the later phase of the disease.

10.3 Genetics of Cone/Cone-Rod Dystrophy

Cone dystrophies are most frequently nonsyndromic, however, they may also be part of several syndromes, such as Alström syndrome, Bardet-Biedl syndrome and Spinocerebellar Ataxia Type 7.

Nonsyndromic cone dystrophies are genetically heterogeneous (28 genes have been identified). The four most commonly mutated genes are ABCA4 (1p22.1), responsible for 30–60% of autosomal recessive CRDs, CRX (19q13.33) and GUCY2D (17p13.1), responsible for many reported cases of autosomal dominant CRDs, and RPGR (Xp11.4), responsible for X-linked CRDs [5–8].

Most of the sporadic cases of cone dystrophies are considered to be autosomal recessive genetic abnormality. The AR genes causing cone dystrophy include ABCA4, ADAM9, CACNA2D4, CDHR1, CNGB3, KCNV2, PDE6C, RAX2, RDH5, RPGRIP1. Biallelic variants of POC1B were recently reported to cause autosomal recessive nonsyndromic cone dystrophy [9]; POC1 B has been shown to play important roles in centriole assembly and/or stability and ciliogenesis [10].

Clinical features and progression patterns vary, even in the same family members with autosomal dominant cone dystrophy [11]. The genes inherited AD are PRPH2, AIPL1, HRG4, RIMS1, PITPNM3, PROM1, CRX, GUCA1A and GUCY2D. The GUCA1A and GUCY2D are associated with the cGMP pathway. CRX is a transcription factor of photoreceptor homeobox.

X-linked recessive cone dystrophies are associated with the genes such as RPGR, CACNA1F, or COD2 [12]. The female carrier may show subtle symptoms with various clinical presentations.

Taken together, it seems that most genes responsible for cone dystrophies or cone-rod dystrophies are involved in other types of retinal dystrophies, including RPs and other macular dystrophies. Any gene causing retinal dystrophy may potentially be involved in the pathogenesis of cone dystrophies, and the challenge is to understand the underlying mechanisms. Likewise, the question of why some mutations in a gene lead to CRD whereas others cause RP remains unresolved for several genes.

10.4 Differential Diagnosis

Differential diagnosis of cone dystrophy includes other hereditary cone disorders (including achromatopsia and allied cone dysfunction syndromes, cone dystrophy and Stargardt disease) and the rod-cone dystrophy, also known as retinitis pigmentosa, which is distinguished by the sequence of photoreceptor involvement (rod photoreceptors followed by cone photoreceptors).

Patients with retinitis pigmentosa typically present with night blindness in the early stage of the disease. In the fundus, pigment deposits are located in the periphery. In some cases, retinitis pigmentosa has a typical slow progression, but macular involvement occurs quite early, with some loss of central visual acuity. A disease history characterized by predominant night blindness and prominent rod involvement on ERG supports the diagnosis of retinitis pigmentosa. In the late-stage RP or cone dystrophy, the differential diagnosis may be difficult. At that time, the typical changes in ERG are undetectable.

Leber congenital amaurosis (LCA) is associated with a high degree of visual impairment, which is already present at birth, and appears either as a rod- or cone-predominant disease, or both. Nystagmus, poor light fixation and reactivity, visual acuity lower than 20/400 and flat ERG are cardinal signs of the disease. Differential diagnosis with early-onset CRD may be difficult because both diseases share the same clinical signs. The presence of a lapse time of several years before dramatic worsening of the visual disability will allow to classify the disease as CRD rather than LCA.

Stargardt disease is a maculopathy in which the peripheral retina usually remains free of lesions. The disease is easy to recognize with the presence of yellow flecks that may cover the entire fundus (fundus flavimaculatus), hyperfluorescent macular lesions (bull's eye) and dark choroid on the fluorescein angiography. However, there are extended lesions in some late-stage Stargardt cases, and in addition, a number of CRD are caused by the "Stargardt gene," ABCA4. In these cases, the early stage of the CRD may be similar to Stargardt disease, but in a decade, signs of peripheral involvement occur.

Achromatopsia is stationary cone dystrophy that appears at an earlier age and is inherited as an autosomal recessive trait. To date, three genes associated with achromatopsia have been characterized: CNGA3 and CNGB3, located at 2q11 and 8q21, which encode the α- and β-subunits of the cGMP-gated cation channel in cone cells, respectively, and GNAT2, located at 1p13, which encodes the cone α-transducin subunit [13–17]. Achromatopsia can be differentiated with progressive cone dystrophy based on the lack of disease evolution and the normal fundus.

10.5 Treatment

Currently, there is no therapy that stops the evolution of the disease or restores the vision, and the visual prognosis is variable, with early central vision loss and progressive visual dysfunction leading to legal blindness before 40 years of age in most cases.

Management aims at slowing down the degenerative process, treating the complications and visual rehabilitation.

Dark sunglasses or miotics may be helpful in reducing photophobia in some patients with cone dystrophies. Many patients also benefit from low vision aids such as magnifiers, closed-circuit television devices, and software for computer screen text enlargement.

Genetic counseling may be of benefit for patients and their families. A precise phenotypic diagnosis is always mandatory and is particularly useful in the absence of familial history or in sporadic cases (Fig. 10.1).

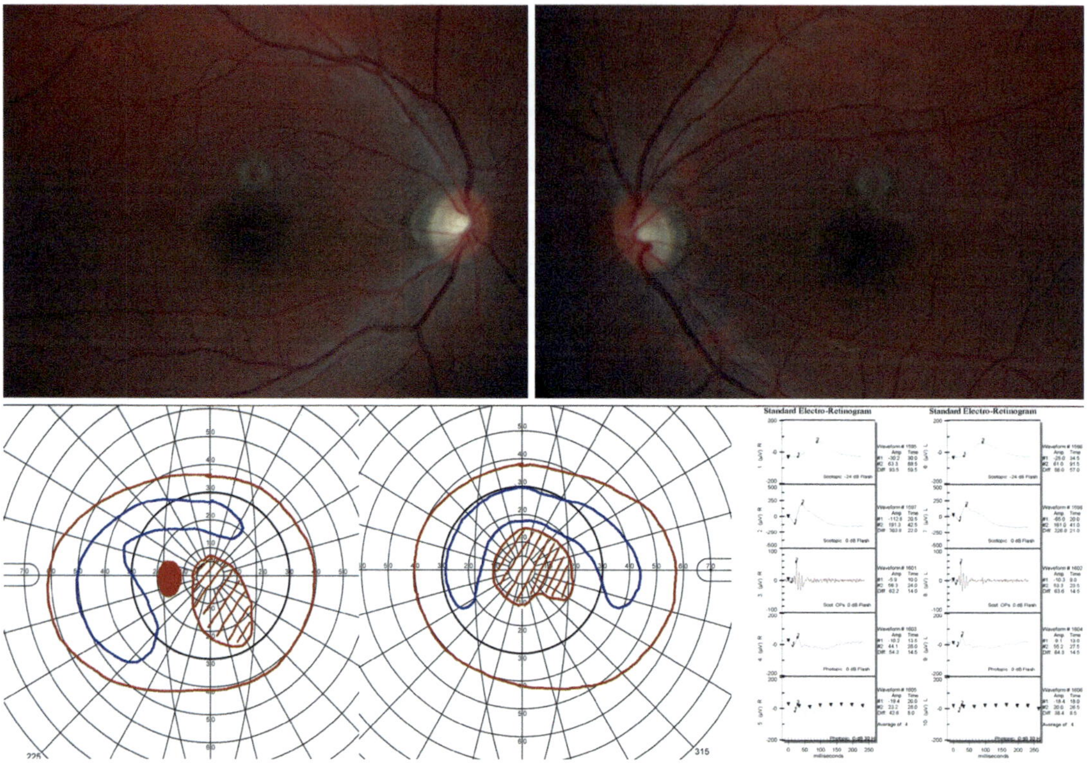

Fig. 10.1 A 19-year-old man has experienced a gradual decline of visual acuity for several years. The best-corrected visual acuities were 20/100 in OD and 20/200 in OS. Goldmann's visual field examination shows relative central scotoma. The fundus appears grossly normal; however, the electroretinography shows the decreased amplitude of cone responses (30 Hz flicker) which findings are compatible with cone dystrophy

References

1. Hamel CP, et al. Molecular genetics of pigmentary retinopathies: identification of mutations in CHM, RDS, RHO, RPE65, USH2A and XLRS1 genes. J Fr Ophtalmol. 2000;23(10):985–95.
2. Vincent A, et al. Phenotypic characteristics including in vivo cone photoreceptor mosaic in KCNV2-related “cone dystrophy with supernormal rod electroretinogram”. Invest Ophthalmol Vis Sci. 2013;54(1):898–908.
3. Gundogan FC, Tas A, Sobaci G. Electroretinogram in hereditary retinal disorders. Electroretinograms. 2011;95–132.
4. Galli-Resta L, et al. Early detection of central visual function decline in cone-rod dystrophy by the use of macular focal cone electroretinogram. Invest Ophthalmol Vis Sci. 2013;54(10):6560–9.
5. Xiao X, et al. A recurrent mutation in GUCY2D associated with autosomal dominant cone dystrophy in a Chinese family. Mol Vis. 2011;17:3271–8.
6. Thiadens AA, et al. Homozygosity mapping reveals PDE6C mutations in patients with early-onset cone photoreceptor disorders. Am J Hum Genet. 2009;85(2):240–7.
7. Chowers I, et al. Cone and rod dysfunction in the NARP syndrome. Br J Ophthalmol. 1999;83(2):190–3.
8. Kelsell RE, et al. Mutations in the retinal guanylate cyclase (RETGC-1) gene in dominant cone-rod dystrophy. Hum Mol Genet. 1998;7(7):1179–84.
9. Kominami A, et al. Case of cone dystrophy with normal fundus appearance associated with biallelic POC1B variants. Ophthalmic Genet. 2018;39(2):255–62.
10. Keller LC, et al. Molecular architecture of the centriole proteome: the conserved WD40 domain protein POC1 is required for centriole duplication and length control. Mol Biol Cell. 2009;20(4):1150–66.
11. Krill AE, Deutman AF. Dominant macular degenerations. The cone dystrophies. Am J Ophthalmol. 1972;73(3):352–69.
12. Jalkanen R, et al. X linked cone-rod dystrophy, CORDX3, is caused by a mutation in the CACNA1F gene. J Med Genet. 2006;43(8):699–704.
13. Wissinger B, et al. Human rod monochromacy: linkage analysis and mapping of a cone photoreceptor expressed candidate gene on chromosome 2q11. Genomics. 1998;51(3):325–31.

14. Kohl S, et al. Total colourblindness is caused by mutations in the gene encoding the alpha-subunit of the cone photoreceptor cGMP-gated cation channel. Nat Genet. 1998;19(3):257–9.
15. Kohl S, et al. Mutations in the CNGB3 gene encoding the beta-subunit of the cone photoreceptor cGMP-gated channel are responsible for achromatopsia (ACHM3) linked to chromosome 8q21. Hum Mol Genet. 2000;9(14):2107–16.
16. Aligianis IA, et al. Mapping of a novel locus for achromatopsia (ACHM4) to 1p and identification of a germline mutation in the alpha subunit of cone transducin (GNAT2). J Med Genet. 2002;39(9):656–60.
17. Kohl S, et al. Mutations in the cone photoreceptor G-protein alpha-subunit gene GNAT2 in patients with achromatopsia. Am J Hum Genet. 2002;71(2):422–5.

X-Linked Retinoschisis

11

Christopher Seungkyu Lee

11.1 Introduction

Since Josef Hass first described X-linked retinoschisis (XLRS, OMIM 312700) in two affected brothers in 1989 [1], XLRS has been shown to be one of the most common juvenile-onset retinal degeneration in males with an estimated prevalence of 1:5000–1:20,000 [2]. Haas believed that the disease was inflammatory in nature [1], but X-linked pattern of inheritance was demonstrated 15 years later [3], and the term "X-linked retinoschisis" was first coined in 1953 [4], which is widely accepted now.

11.2 Genetics

RS1, the causative gene for XLRS was identified in 1997 [5]. To date, over 200 different mutations in the *RS1* gene have been found (http://www.dmd.nl/rs/index.html). The *RS1* gene is organized in six exons and exclusively expressed in the photoreceptors and bipolar cells [6]. Its encoded protein, retinoschisin, however, is a secreted protein composed of 224-amino acids and can be found throughout the retinal layers [7, 8]. Retinoschisin is thought to be involved in cellular adhesion and cell–cell interaction through its discoidin domain, which is highly conserved across different species [5]. Most disease-causing *RS1* mutations are located within discoidin domain that is composed of approximately 150 amino acids, thus constituting the majority of the retinoschisin [9] (Fig. 11.1).

The penetrance of XLRS is nearly complete, but phenotype is highly variable; siblings, related individuals, and unrelated individuals with same mutation show significant phenotypic variability [10–15]. Unlike other X-linked retinal dystrophies such as choroideremia, female carriers rarely present with retinal abnormalities [14, 16, 17].

11.3 Clinical Features

Patients usually present with visual loss between the ages of 5 and 10 [18]. Visual acuity is highly variable, but usually better than 20/100, and asymmetry in visual acuity between two eyes in the individual patient is a frequent finding [18, 19]. The hallmark of XLRS is the presence of a spoke-wheel pattern of fold-like changes radiating from fovea in the fundus of young patients, typically younger than 30 years of age (Fig. 11.2). In patients older than 30 years, the foveal retinoschisis can present with nonspecific retinal abnormalities [2]. Peripheral retinoschisis mostly in the lower temporal quadrant is present in approximately 50% of patients [18]. The so-called

C. S. Lee (✉)
Retina and Uveitis Clinic, Department of Ophthalmology, Severance Hospital, Yonsei University College of Medicine, Seodaemun-gu, Seoul, Republic of Korea
e-mail: sklee219@yuhs.ac

H.-G. Yu (ed.), *Inherited Retinal Disease*, https://doi.org/10.1007/978-981-16-7337-5_11

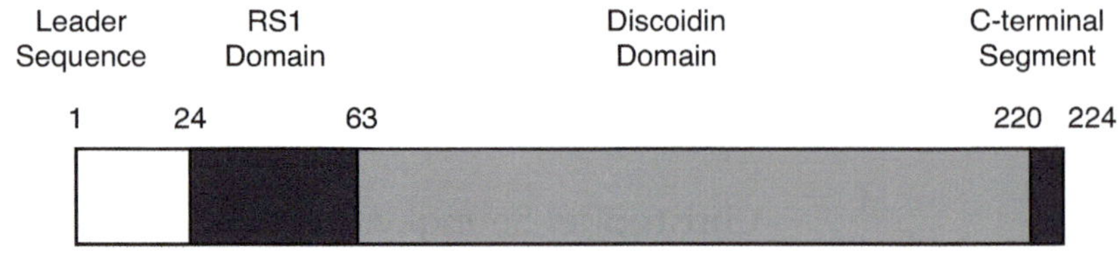

Fig. 11.1 Schematic diagram of retinoschisin. Most disease-causing mutations are located within discoidin domain

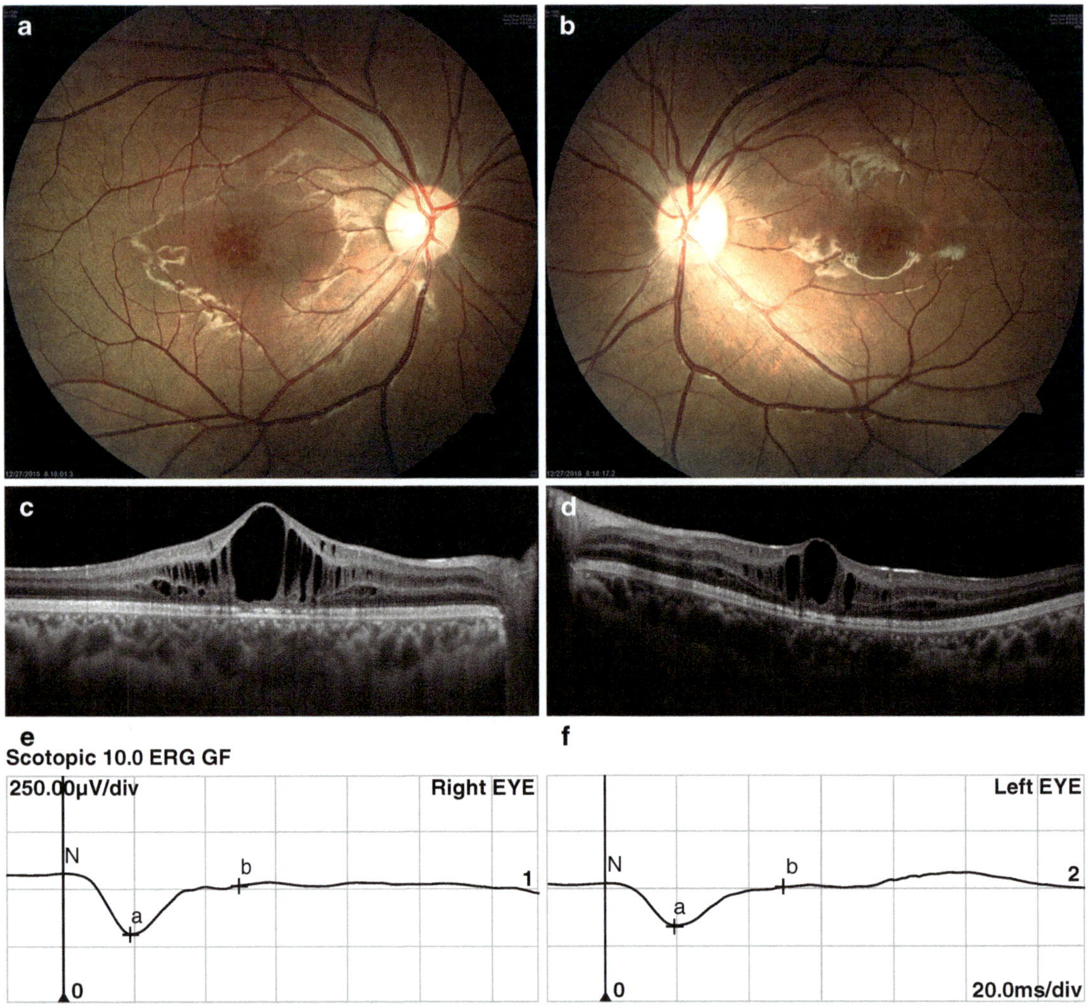

Fig. 11.2 Fundus images and electroretinogram (ERG) of an 18-year-old man clinically diagnosed with X-linked retinoschisis. His older brother showed similar retinal findings. Spoke-wheel pattern of folds radiating out from the fovea are seen in fundus photography of the right eye (**a**) and the left eye (**b**). Horizontal optical coherence tomography images through the fovea show schisis cavities in the ganglion cell layer, inner nuclear layer, and outer plexiform layer/outer nuclear layer in both the right eye (**c**) and the left eye (**d**). Dark-adapted 10.0 ERG shows 'negative' ERG with absent b-waves in both eyes (**e**, **f**). Note asymmetry in anatomical and functional findings between right and left eyes

vitreous veils may result if the thin inner wall of a peripheral schisis cavity is separated (Fig. 11.3). Bridging vessels can cross between two walls of schisis cavity and course directly into the vitreous, which can cause hemorrhage into the schisis cavity or vitreous cavity [18]. If additional break occurs in the outer wall of the schisis, retinal detachment may occur. Vitreous hemorrhage can

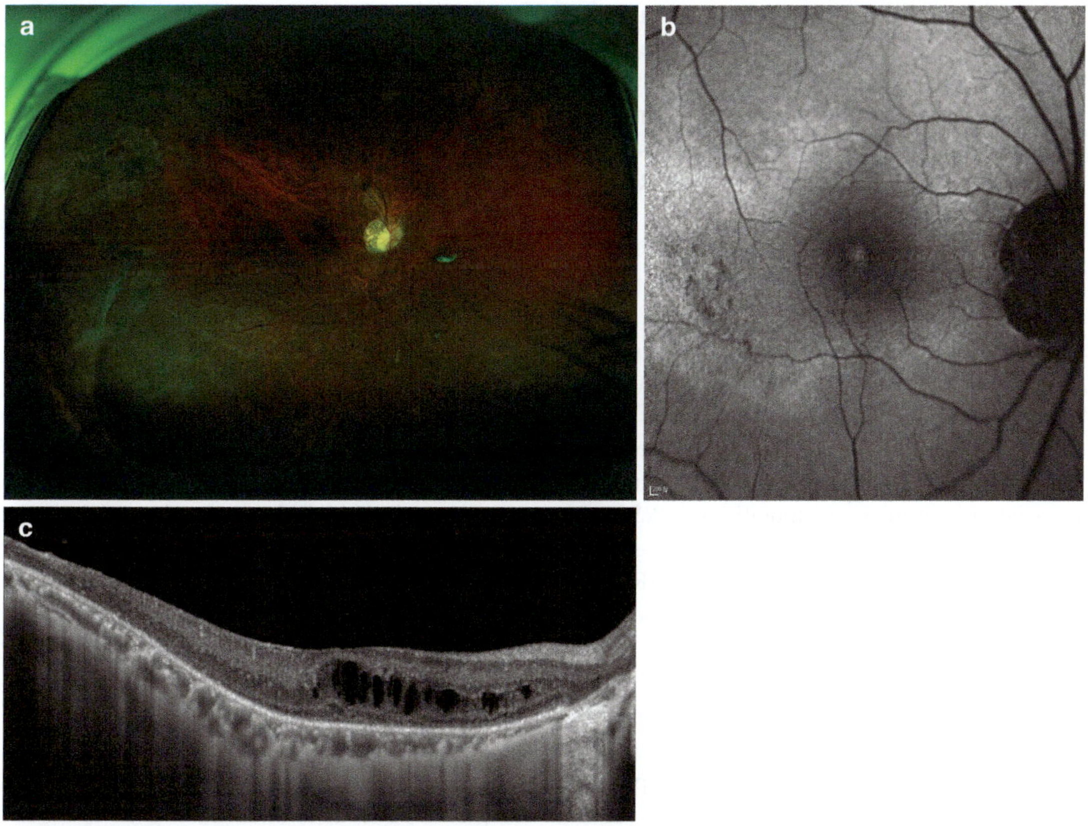

Fig. 11.3 Vitreous veil is seen in the inferotemporal quadrant of the peripheral retina in the right eye of a 53-year-old man with X-linked retinoschisis (XLRS) carrying an *RS1*-gene p.Arg102Trp mutation (**a**). Barrier laser photocoagulation scars are seen along the demarcation of peripheral retinoschisis. Autofluorescence imaging shows atrophic changes in the macula and irregular-shaped parafoveal autofluorescent ring (**b**). Splitting of the Spoke-wheel pattern abnormality in the fovea is not apparent in this adult XLRS patient. Horizontal optical coherence tomography image through the fovea shows that schisis is mostly located in the inner nuclear layer, more prominently on the nasal side of the macula (**c**)

occur in up to one third of patients [20] and retinal detachment can develop in about 5–20% of patients [12]. Development of full-thickness macular hole is a rare complication [21–23]. Additional retinal findings include Mizuo phenomenon [24], diffuse white retinal flecks [25], and Coats'-like exudative retinopathy [26] in few cases of XLRS.

Nowadays, spectral-domain optical coherence tomography (SD-OCT) is the major diagnostic tool for XLRS. The region of retinoschisis detected with SD-OCT often extends well beyond the area of ophthalmoscopically detected spoke-wheel pattern up to vascular arcades [16, 27]. Anatomical locations of schisis have long been a subject of interest. Histopathological study demonstrated the splitting of retinal nerve fiber layer (NFL) in enucleated eyes with advanced XLRS with retinal detachment, but schisis at foveomacular region was not described in these reports [28, 29]. OCT studies showed that the splitting of retina can involve any retinal layer, most frequently involving the inner nuclear layer (INL) and outer nuclear layer (ONL) in the foveomacular region [16, 27, 30–36]. More superficial splitting involving ganglion cell layer (GCL) and NFL appears to be present more frequently in extramacular region than foveomacular region [16, 27, 37]. These OCT findings are in agreement with the fact that retinoschisis protein is found in all retinal layers [7, 8] and suggest that different fundus locations and different retinal layers may have different levels of resistance to development of schisis, with INL at foveomacular region being the most vulnerable. In older patients, OCT may show the retinal thinning and epiretinal membrane without retinoschisis, which makes it difficult to differentiate XLRL with other macular diseases [38].

Electroretinogram (ERG) typically shows a so-called negative ERG, in which the a-wave is larger than the b-wave in contrast to the normal findings. But the a-wave can be normal or even reduced in XLRS patients due to aging and progressive atrophy of the retinal pigment epithelium (RPE) [39]. Negative ERG is present in about 50% of patients [2] and is less commonly associated with missense mutations in *RS1* gene than with nonsense, splice-site, or frame-shifting insertions/deletions [40]. The origin of ERG dysfunction is an abnormality in ON- and OFF-pathways on bipolar cells [41].

Fundus autofluorescence is often used for differential diagnosis of macular dystrophies. Spoke-wheel pattern of hyper-hypo autofluorescence can be seen in the fovea of XLRS patients. The parafoveal hyperautofluorescence is present in some older patients, which may represent an intermediate stage of increased metabolic load in photoreceptor and RPE [42] (Fig. 11.3b).

Fluorescein angiography is typically unremarkable and generally not required for diagnosis of XLRS, but it can be useful in differentiating foveomacular schisis in XLRS from other causes of cystoid macular edema showing angiographic leakage. Focal area of fluorescein leakage within peripheral schisis cavity or focal area of mottled hyperfluorescence due to RPE atrophy can be present in XLRS. Capillary nonperfusion area at the peripheral retina has been also described [43].

11.4 Differential Diagnosis

A foveal retinoschisis may by present in enhanced S-cone syndrome (Goldmann-Favre syndrome). Differential diagnosis of peripheral retinoschisis with early onset retinal detachments includes X-linked Norrie disease, familial exudative vitreoretinopathy (FEVR), and Stickler syndrome. Retinal detachments in Norrie disease are often present at birth and visual function is nearly absent. Avascular peripheral retina and dragged retinal vessels are typical features of FEVR. Stickler syndrome is often associated with hearing and facial abnormalities. Negative ERG in young males can be seen in congenital stationary night blindness.

11.5 Treatment Options

In general, treatment of XLRS is limited to low-vision aids at the moment. A few studies have shown some success with topical or oral carbonic anhydrase inhibitors in improving vision and decreasing retinal thickness [44–48]. Scatter laser photocoagulation performed to treat peripheral schisis and prevent retinal detachment may actually cause retinal detachment, possibly by making breaks of schisis outer wall [18, 49].

Surgical intervention is generally indicated in the context of severe complications including retinal detachment and vitreous hemorrhage. Surgical treatment of foveomacular schisis is not generally indicated. Because intercellular adhesion force in the retina could be 'weak' due to abnormal retinoschisin, only weak tractional force from the vitreous might be enough to aggravate the splitting of retina in foveomacular schisis. In this regard, vitrectomy with the intent of relieving vitreous traction has been advocated by some researchers, especially in cases of progressive XLRS, which in general resulted in greater degree of anatomical improvement, compared to visual improvement [50–52].

Gene therapy is a viable approach to treat patients with inherited retinal degeneration. There is no known naturally occurring animal model for XLRS, so retinoschisin knockout (*Rs1*-KO) mouse has been developed that displays features similar to human XLRS [53, 54], which were shown to be reversed by delivery of *RS1* gene [55–57]. In 2018, the result of phase I/IIa clinical trial with AAV8-*RS1* gene therapy for XLRS was published, which showed transient cavity closure in one of nine participants and dose-related intraocular inflammations [58].

11.6 Visual Prognosis

Visual prognosis of XLRS has been a controversial subject. Visual decline may be progressive in adulthood [59], but some studies reported relatively stable vision after teenage years in the absence of serious complications such as retinal detachment and vitreous hemorrhage [12, 19]. In older patients, macular atrophy may cause poor visual acuity [20]. These findings confirm the high degree of clinical variability in XLRS.

References

1. Hass J. Ueber das Zusammenvorkommen von Veraenderungen der Retina und Choroidea. Arch Augenheilkd. 1898;37:343–8.
2. Molday RS, Kellner U, Weber BH. X-linked juvenile retinoschisis: clinical diagnosis, genetic analysis, and molecular mechanisms. Prog Retin Eye Res. 2012;31(3):195–212. https://doi.org/10.1016/j.preteyeres.2011.12.002
3. Pagenstecher HE. Über eine unter dem Bilde der Netzhautablösung verlaufende, erbliche Erkrankung der Retina. Graefes Archiv Ophthalmol. 1913;86(3):457–62.
4. Jager G. A hereditary retinal disease. Trans Ophthalmol Soc U K. 1953;73:617–9.
5. Sauer CG, Gehrig A, Warneke-Wittstock R, et al. Positional cloning of the gene associated with X-linked juvenile retinoschisis. Nat Genet. 1997;17(2):164–70. https://doi.org/10.1038/ng1097-164
6. Molday LL, Hicks D, Sauer CG, et al. Expression of X-linked retinoschisis protein RS1 in photoreceptor and bipolar cells. Invest Ophthalmol Vis Sci. 2001;42(3):816–25. https://www.ncbi.nlm.nih.gov/pubmed/11222545
7. Grayson C, Reid SN, Ellis JA, et al. Retinoschisin, the X-linked retinoschisis protein, is a secreted photoreceptor protein, and is expressed and released by Weri-Rb1 cells. Hum Mol Genet. 2000;9(12):1873–9. https://doi.org/10.1093/hmg/9.12.1873
8. Prenner JL, Capone A Jr, Ciaccia S, et al. Congenital X-linked retinoschisis classification system. Retina. 2006;26(7 Suppl):S61–4. https://doi.org/10.1097/01.iae.0000244290.09499.c1
9. Curat CA, Eck M, Dervillez X, et al. Mapping of epitopes in discoidin domain receptor 1 critical for collagen binding. J Biol Chem. 2001;276(49):45952–8. https://doi.org/10.1074/jbc.M104360200
10. Eksandh LC, Ponjavic V, Ayyagari R, et al. Phenotypic expression of juvenile X-linked retinoschisis in Swedish families with different mutations in the XLRS1 gene. Arch Ophthalmol. 2000;118(8):1098–104. https://doi.org/10.1001/archopht.118.8.1098
11. Hewitt AW, FitzGerald LM, Scotter LW, et al. Genotypic and phenotypic spectrum of X-linked retinoschisis in Australia. Clin Exp Ophthalmol. 2005;33(3):233–9. https://doi.org/10.1111/j.1442-9071.2005.01018.x
12. Kellner U, Brummer S, Foerster MH, et al. X-linked congenital retinoschisis. Graefes Arch Clin Exp Ophthalmol. 1990;228(5):432–7. https://doi.org/10.1007/BF00927256
13. Kim SY, Ko HS, Yu YS, et al. Molecular genetic characteristics of X-linked retinoschisis in Koreans. Mol Vis. 2009;15:833–43. https://www.ncbi.nlm.nih.gov/pubmed/19390641
14. Renner AB, Kellner U, Fiebig B, et al. ERG variability in X-linked congenital retinoschisis patients with mutations in the RS1 gene and the diagnostic importance of fundus autofluorescence and OCT. Doc Ophthalmol. 2008;116(2):97–109. https://doi.org/10.1007/s10633-007-9094-5
15. Riveiro-Alvarez R, Trujillo-Tiebas MJ, Gimenez-Pardo A, et al. Correlation of genetic and clinical findings in Spanish patients with X-linked juvenile retinoschisis. Invest Ophthalmol Vis Sci. 2009;50(9):4342–50. https://doi.org/10.1167/iovs.09-3418
16. Gregori NZ, Lam BL, Gregori G, et al. Wide-field spectral-domain optical coherence tomography in patients and carriers of X-linked retinoschisis. Ophthalmology. 2013;120(1):169–74. https://doi.org/10.1016/j.ophtha.2012.07.051
17. Rodriguez FJ, Rodriguez A, Mendoza-Londono R, et al. X-linked retinoschisis in three females from the same family: a phenotype-genotype correlation. Retina. 2005;25(1):69–74. https://doi.org/10.1097/00006982-200501000-00010
18. Tantri A, Vrabec TR, Cu-Unjieng A, et al. X-linked retinoschisis: a clinical and molecular genetic review. Surv Ophthalmol. 2004;49(2):214–30. https://doi.org/10.1016/j.survophthal.2003.12.007
19. Roesch MT, Ewing CC, Gibson AE, et al. The natural history of X-linked retinoschisis. Can J Ophthalmol. 1998;33(3):149–58. https://www.ncbi.nlm.nih.gov/pubmed/9606571
20. George ND, Yates JR, Moore AT. Clinical features in affected males with X-linked retinoschisis. Arch Ophthalmol. 1996;114(3):274–80. https://doi.org/10.1001/archopht.1996.01100130270007
21. Brasil OF, da Cunha AL, de Castro MB, et al. Macular hole secondary to X-linked juvenile retinoschisis. Ophthalmic Surg Lasers Imaging. 2011;42(Online):e4–5. https://doi.org/10.3928/15428877-20110125-07
22. Shukla D, Naresh KB, Rajendran A, et al. Macular hole secondary to X-linked retinoschisis. Eye (Lond). 2006;20(12):1459–61. https://doi.org/10.1038/sj.eye.6702338
23. Stein GE, Lee SE, Chen RWS, et al. Surgical treatment of a macular hole in X-linked retinoschisis. Retin Cases Brief Rep. 2017;11(3):246–8. https://doi.org/10.1097/ICB.0000000000000332

24. Vincent A, Shetty R, Yadav NK, et al. Foveal schisis with Mizuo phenomenon: etio-pathogenesis of tapetal reflex in X-linked retinoschisis. Eye (Lond). 2009;23(5):1240–1. https://doi.org/10.1038/eye.2008.170
25. Hotta Y, Nakamura M, Okamoto Y, et al. Different mutation of the XLRS1 gene causes juvenile retinoschisis with retinal white flecks. Br J Ophthalmol. 2001;85(2):238–9. https://doi.org/10.1136/bjo.85.2.238
26. Fong DS, Frederick AR Jr, Blumenkranz MS, et al. Exudative retinal detachment in X-linked retinoschisis. Ophthalmic Surg Lasers. 1998;29(4):332–5. https://www.ncbi.nlm.nih.gov/pubmed/9571668
27. Yu J, Ni Y, Keane PA, et al. Foveomacular schisis in juvenile X-linked retinoschisis: an optical coherence tomography study. Am J Ophthalmol. 2010;149(6):973–8 e972. https://doi.org/10.1016/j.ajo.2010.01.031
28. Manschot WA. Pathology of hereditary juvenile retinoschisis. Arch Ophthalmol. 1972;88(2):131–8. https://doi.org/10.1001/archopht.1972.01000030133002
29. Yanoff M, Kertesz Rahn E, Zimmerman LE. Histopathology of juvenile retinoschisis. Arch Ophthalmol. 1968;79(1):49–53. https://doi.org/10.1001/archopht.1968.03850040051014
30. Apushkin MA, Fishman GA, Janowicz MJ. Correlation of optical coherence tomography findings with visual acuity and macular lesions in patients with X-linked retinoschisis. Ophthalmology. 2005;112(3):495–501. https://doi.org/10.1016/j.ophtha.2004.08.027
31. Brucker AJ, Spaide RF, Gross N, et al. Optical coherence tomography of X-linked retinoschisis. Retina. 2004;24(1):151–2. https://doi.org/10.1097/00006982-200402000-00021
32. Gao H, Kusumi R, Yung CW. Optical coherence tomographic findings in X-linked juvenile retinoschisis. Arch Ophthalmol. 2005;123(7):1006–8. https://doi.org/10.1001/archopht.123.7.1006
33. Gregori NZ, Berrocal AM, Gregori G, et al. Macular spectral-domain optical coherence tomography in patients with X linked retinoschisis. Br J Ophthalmol. 2009;93(3):373–8. https://doi.org/10.1136/bjo.2007.136127
34. Mastropasqua R, Toto L, Di Antonio L, et al. Optical coherence tomography angiography findings in X-linked retinoschisis. Ophthalmic Surg Lasers Imaging Retina. 2018;49(9):e20–31. https://doi.org/10.3928/23258160-20180907-03
35. Muscat S, Fahad B, Parks S, et al. Optical coherence tomography and multifocal electroretinography of X-linked juvenile retinoschisis. Eye (Lond). 2001;15(Pt 6):796–9. https://doi.org/10.1038/eye.2001.257
36. Stanga PE, Chong NH, Reck AC, et al. Optical coherence tomography and electrophysiology in X-linked juvenile retinoschisis associated with a novel mutation in the XLRS1 gene. Retina. 2001;21(1):78–80. https://doi.org/10.1097/00006982-200102000-00019
37. Urrets-Zavalia JA, Venturino JP, Mercado J, et al. Macular and extramacular optical coherence tomography findings in X-linked retinoschisis. Ophthalmic Surg Lasers Imaging. 2007;38(5):417–22. https://doi.org/10.3928/15428877-20070901-13
38. Menke MN, Feke GT, Hirose T. Effect of aging on macular features of X-linked retinoschisis assessed with optical coherence tomography. Retina. 2011;31(6):1186–92. https://doi.org/10.1097/IAE.0b013e3181ff0d2d
39. Miyake Y, Shiroyama N, Ota I, et al. Focal macular electroretinogram in X-linked congenital retinoschisis. Invest Ophthalmol Vis Sci. 1993;34(3):512–5. https://www.ncbi.nlm.nih.gov/pubmed/8449671
40. Vincent A, Robson AG, Neveu MM, et al. A phenotype-genotype correlation study of X-linked retinoschisis. Ophthalmology. 2013;120(7):1454–64. https://doi.org/10.1016/j.ophtha.2012.12.008
41. Khan NW, Jamison JA, Kemp JA, et al. Analysis of photoreceptor function and inner retinal activity in juvenile X-linked retinoschisis. Vision Res. 2001;41(28):3931–42. https://doi.org/10.1016/s0042-6989(01)00188-2
42. Tsang SH, Vaclavik V, Bird AC, et al. Novel phenotypic and genotypic findings in X-linked retinoschisis. Arch Ophthalmol. 2007;125(2):259–67. https://doi.org/10.1001/archopht.125.2.259
43. Green JL Jr, Jampol LM. Vascular opacification and leakage in X-linked (juvenile) retinoschisis. Br J Ophthalmol. 1979;63(5):368–73. https://doi.org/10.1136/bjo.63.5.368
44. Ali S, Seth R. X-linked juvenile retinoschisis in females and response to carbonic anhydrase inhibitors: case report and review of the literature. Semin Ophthalmol. 2013;28(1):50–4. https://doi.org/10.3109/08820538.2012.667496
45. Andreuzzi P, Fishman GA, Anderson RJ. Use of a carbonic anhydrase inhibitor in X-linked retinoschisis: effect on cystic-appearing macular lesions and visual acuity. Retina. 2017;37(8):1555–61. https://doi.org/10.1097/IAE.0000000000001379
46. Genead MA, Fishman GA, Walia S. Efficacy of sustained topical dorzolamide therapy for cystic macular lesions in patients with X-linked retinoschisis. Arch Ophthalmol. 2010;128(2):190–7. https://doi.org/10.1001/archophthalmol.2009.398
47. Testa F, Di Iorio V, Gallo B, et al. Carbonic anhydrase inhibitors in patients with X-linked retinoschisis: effects on macular morphology and function. Ophthalmic Genet. 2019;40(3):207–12. https://doi.org/10.1080/13816810.2019.1616303
48. Verbakel SK, van de Ven JP, Le Blanc LM, et al. Carbonic anhydrase inhibitors for the treatment of cystic macular lesions in children with X-linked juvenile retinoschisis. Invest Ophthalmol Vis Sci. 2016;57(13):5143–7. https://doi.org/10.1167/iovs.16-20078
49. Regillo CD, Custis PH. Surgical management of retinoschisis. Curr Opin Ophthalmol. 1997;8(3):80–6. https://doi.org/10.1097/00055735-199706000-00014

50. Byeon SH, Lee SC, Koh HJ, et al. Surgical removal of the internal limiting membrane in progressive macular change in x-linked juvenile retinoschisis. Retin Cases Brief Rep. 2007;1(3):156–9. https://doi.org/10.1097/01.ICB.0000279648.29819.4b
51. Ikeda F, Iida T, Kishi S. Resolution of retinoschisis after vitreous surgery in X-linked retinoschisis. Ophthalmology. 2008;115(4):718–22 e711. https://doi.org/10.1016/j.ophtha.2007.05.047
52. Yu H, Li T, Luo Y, et al. Long-term outcomes of vitrectomy for progressive X-linked retinoschisis. Am J Ophthalmol. 2012;154(2):394–402 e392. https://doi.org/10.1016/j.ajo.2012.02.005
53. Takada Y, Vijayasarathy C, Zeng Y, et al. Synaptic pathology in retinoschisis knockout (Rs1-/y) mouse retina and modification by rAAV-Rs1 gene delivery. Invest Ophthalmol Vis Sci. 2008;49(8):3677–86. https://doi.org/10.1167/iovs.07-1071
54. Weber BH, Schrewe H, Molday LL, et al. Inactivation of the murine X-linked juvenile retinoschisis gene, Rs1h, suggests a role of retinoschisin in retinal cell layer organization and synaptic structure. Proc Natl Acad Sci U S A. 2002;99(9):6222–7. https://doi.org/10.1073/pnas.092528599
55. Bush RA, Zeng Y, Colosi P, et al. Preclinical dose-escalation study of intravitreal AAV-RS1 gene therapy in a mouse model of X-linked retinoschisis: dose-dependent expression and improved retinal structure and function. Hum Gene Ther. 2016;27(5):376–89. https://doi.org/10.1089/hum.2015.142
56. Min SH, Molday LL, Seeliger MW, et al. Prolonged recovery of retinal structure/function after gene therapy in an Rs1h-deficient mouse model of x-linked juvenile retinoschisis. Mol Ther. 2005;12(4):644–51. https://doi.org/10.1016/j.ymthe.2005.06.002
57. Zeng Y, Takada Y, Kjellstrom S, et al. RS-1 gene delivery to an adult Rs1h knockout mouse model restores ERG b-wave with reversal of the electronegative waveform of X-linked retinoschisis. Invest Ophthalmol Vis Sci. 2004;45(9):3279–85. https://doi.org/10.1167/iovs.04-0576
58. Cukras C, Wiley HE, Jeffrey BG, et al. Retinal AAV8-RS1 gene therapy for X-linked retinoschisis: initial findings from a phase I/IIa trial by intravitreal delivery. Mol Ther. 2018;26(9):2282–94. https://doi.org/10.1016/j.ymthe.2018.05.025
59. Forsius H, Vainio-Mattila B, Eriksson A. X-linked hereditary retinoschisis. Br J Ophthalmol. 1962;46(11):678–81. https://doi.org/10.1136/bjo.46.11.678

Von Hippel Lindau Disease and Retinal Hemangioblastoma

12

Cheolmin Yun

12.1 Introduction

Von Hippel-Lindau Disease (VHL disease) is a syndrome characterized by a multiorgan neoplasm including retinal hemangioblastoma (RH), hemangioblastoma of brain and spinal cord, renal cell carcinoma, and pheochromocytoma [1, 2]. It is an autosomal dominant disorder caused by a mutation in the VHL gene located on chromosome 3 [1, 3]. The approximate incidence of VHL disease is 1 in 36,000 live births: one of the most common familial cancer syndrome [1, 4].

RH, also called as retinal capillary hemangioblastoma, retinal capillary hemangioma or retinal angioma, is a benign vascular neoplasm originating in the neurosensory retina or optic disc [1, 5]. The prevalence of VHL had been estimated to be 30–58% among the patients with RH, and sporadic RH can also arise in the absence of VHL disease [5, 6]. Because of the life-threatening manifestations and natures of the disease, proper ophthalmologic examination has a critical role in early diagnosis and treatment of VHL disease.

C. Yun (✉)
Department of Ophthalmology, Korea University College of Medicine, Korea University Ansan Hospital, Danwon-gu, Ansan-si, Gyeonggi-do, Korea
e-mail: yuncheolmin@korea.ac.kr

12.2 Genetics

VHL disease is caused by a germline alteration of VHL tumor suppressor gene located on chromosome 3 (3p25-26) [3, 7, 8]. The VHL protein (pVHL), product of the gene, participates in an adaptive response to hypoxic conditions [9]. The pVHL has a role in the ubiquitination and degradation of hypoxia-inducible factor-1 alpha (HIF-1 alpha), a transcription factor that induces vascular endothelial growth factor (VEGF) expression [10]. Deficiencies of pVHL can cause excessive accumulation of HIF, leading to the upregulation of genes associated with hypoxia [8, 11]. These can eventually induce the formation of various lesions including hemangioblastoma, cyst, and other types of tumors [8].

12.3 Clinical Features

12.3.1 Systemic Features

Various types of benign or malignant tumors or cysts can develop in multiple organs, including central nerve system (brainstem, cerebellum, endolymphatic sac, and spinal cord), eye (retina), visceral organs (adrenal glands, pancreas, and kidneys), and epididymis or broad ligament [1, 4, 5].

H.-G. Yu (ed.), *Inherited Retinal Disease*, https://doi.org/10.1007/978-981-16-7337-5_12

12.3.2 Ocular Features

RH is known as the most common presentation of VHL disease [5, 6, 12, 13]. The prevalence of ocular involvement in VHL disease is estimated to be from 38 to 60%, but because of the low prevalence of the disease, the accurate prevalence has not been clearly defined [12–14]. RH has been reported to be involved unilaterally in 42.1% and bilaterally in 57.9% in VHL patients [13].

RH can show different characteristics according to its type, location, and size [5]. During the early periods, RH can be seen as small and sessile lesions similar to microaneurysm. As the tumor grows, the features can be changed into a more nodular appearance [5]. It usually appears as a round, red, or grayish well-circumscribed lesion and can be accompanied by feeding arterioles and draining venules as the tumor aggravates. The course of the disease varies depending on its clinical characteristics, but most of RH grows over time and can cause lipid exudation, intraretinal edema, and exudative retinal detachment (Fig. 12.1) [15]. The tumor is exclusively found in peripheral retina (84.7%), less in juxtapapillary area only (8.0%), and both juxtapapillary area and peripheral retina (7.0%) [13].

Visual acuity of the patients with VHL disease and ocular involvement had been reported to be 20/20 or better in 84.6%, 20/25 to 20/40 in 9.5%, 20/50 to 20/160 in 3.0%, and 20/200 or worse in 3.0% [12]. Longitudinal analysis of RH in VHL disease revealed that most cases demon-

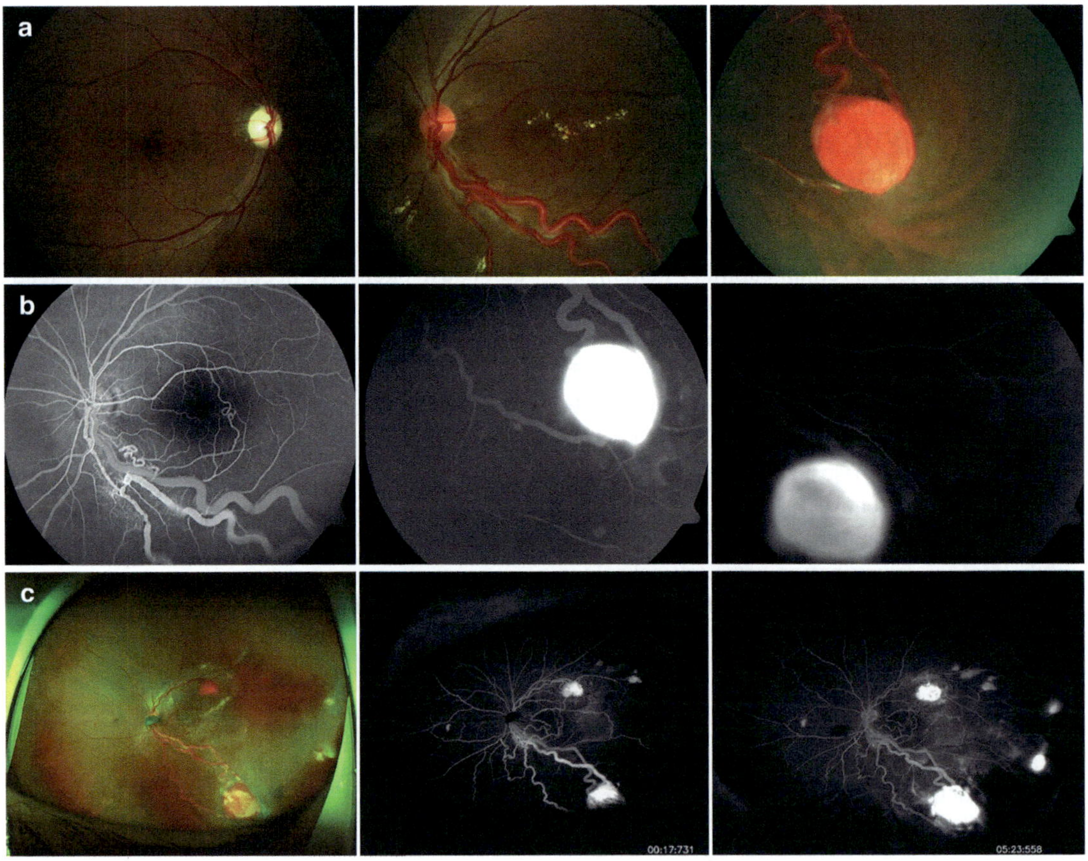

Fig. 12.1 A case of a 34-year-old male patient with von Hippel Lindau disease and retinal hemangioblastoma. (**a**) The tumor is located in inferotemporal retina on left eye. (**b**) The tumor shows hyperfluorescence and late leakage on a fluorescein angiography. (**c**) After 9 years, multiple new hemangioblastomas appeared on retina and the fluorescein angiography shows multiple hyperfluorescent lesions with leakage

strated relatively stable anatomy and visual function over 8 years, and 16.1% of the eyes experienced decreased vision more than ten letters [15]. Greater vision loss in ocular involvement was associated with the existence of juxtapapillary RH, additional development of RCH in new location, and increased number and extent of RH. Systemic factors associated with the poor prognosis were younger age at baseline and onset of ocular VHL disease, fellow eye involvement, and missense or protein-truncating germline mutations [15].

RH developed in juxtapapillary area or at disc may have different clinical characteristics and is perhaps difficult to discern with fundus examination [5, 12]. In some cases, the tumors appear as localized fullness at disc or disc margin, and these can be seen as distinct whitish-pink lesions with the growth. Feeder arterioles and draining venules are not typically visible (Fig. 12.2) [5, 12].

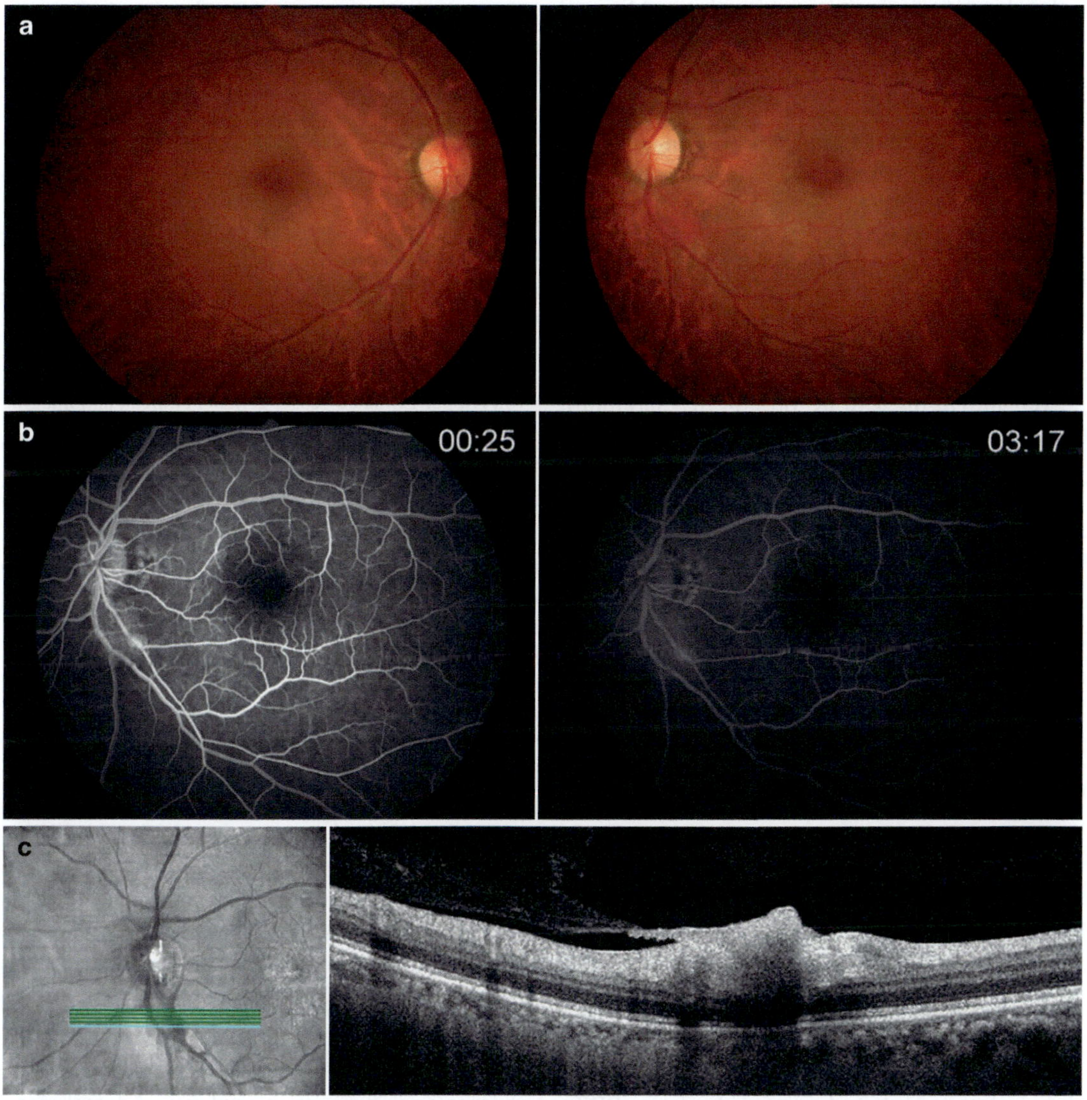

Fig. 12.2 A case of a 52-year-old male patient with von Hippel-Lindau disease and juxtapapillary hemangioblastoma. (**a**) A pinkish vascular lesion is noted inferior to the optic disc on left eye. (**b**) Fluorescein angiography shows early hyperfluorescence. (**c**) The tumor is located in inner retina with hyper-reflectivity (courtesy of Prof. Hyeong-Gon Yu, Seoul National University, Seoul, Korea)

12.4 Diagnosis of Retinal Hemangioblastoma and von Hippel-Lindau Disease

Based on the characteristic findings of the RH on fundus examination, the diagnosis can be made. Early RHs can show very small lesions and these may look similar to other microvascular abnormalities. Wide field fundus photography and fluorescein angiography are useful diagnostic tools. Wide field fundus photography may be helpful in monitoring tumor growth or additional development in new lesions. Fluorescein angiography shows early hyperfluorescence and late staining or leakage of the RH [5, 6, 13]. Optical coherence tomography may be useful in monitoring the macular edema, exudation, or traction caused by RH. Ultrasonography can be utilized to assess features, echogenicity, size, or diameter of the tumor. RH is seen as a solid mass with smooth margin and is usually not accompanied by posterior shadowing or choroidal properties [5, 12].

Because of the various, progressive and multifocal nature, comprehensive screening should be provided for patients. Recommended tests and intervals for screening for individuals at risk are summarized in Table 12.1 [1, 16].

Table 12.1 Recommended tests and time for screening of von Hippel-Lindau disease

Test	Start age and frequency
Ophthalmoscopic exam (Fundoscopy)	Infancy (every year)
Plasma, 24 h urinary catecholamines and metanephrines	At an age of 2 (every year or when blood pressure is elevated)
MRI (craniospinal axis)	At an age of 11 (every year)
CT and MRI (internal auditory canals)	Onset of auditory symptoms (hearing disturbance, tinnitus, vertigo, or difficulties of balance)
Ultrasound (abdomen)	At an age of 8 (every year, MRI if clinically indicated)
CT (abdomen)	At an age of 18 years or earlier if indicated clinically (every year)
Audiological assessment	If clinically indicated

CT, computed tomography; MRI, magnetic resonance imaging

Adapted from Lonser RR et al. von Hippel-Lindau disease. Lancet 2003; 361:2059–2067 and Choyke PL et al. von Hippel-Lindau disease: genetic, clinical, and imaging features. Radiology 1995; 194:629–642

12.5 Treatment of Ocular von Hippel-Lindau Disease

The main goal of treatment is a regression of a lesion without permanent adjacent retinal damage. Small extrapapillary RH can be ablated with focal laser treatment. However, as RH grows, ablation with laser can be difficult and may cause secondary adjacent retinal damage. Therefore, timely diagnosis and earlier treatment are essential. Several treatment modalities including laser photocoagulation, cryotherapy, radiotherapy (plaque radiotherapy, external beam radiation or proton beam radiation), trans-pupillary thermotherapy, photodynamic therapy (PDT), intravitreal injection of anti-VEGF drugs or steroid or vitreoretinal surgery can be considered (Fig. 12.3) [17–28].

Small extrapapillary RH smaller than 1.5 mm in diameter can be ablated with laser photocoagulation. Various types (argon green, diode, or krypton laser) can be used, and direct photocoagulation of the hemangioma and feeder vessel with a duration of 0.2–0.4 s may be helpful [18, 21, 22, 29, 30].

Extrapapillary RH with a diameter between 1.5 and 4.5 mm is difficult to be ablated with laser photocoagulation. Laser photocoagulation with a longer duration of more than 0.4 s may be needed to blanch the lesion. After the laser treatment, increase in retinal hemorrhage, exudative retinal detachment, or vitreous hemorrhage can rarely develop [31]. Trans-scleral cryotherapy or PDT can be applied in cases that do not respond to laser photocoagulation [17, 32–35].

In large extrapapillary RH or complicated by rhegmatogenous or tractional retinal detachment, surgical intervention may be helpful [36, 37]. The large tumor can be excised with en bloc resection and the retina can be attached with or

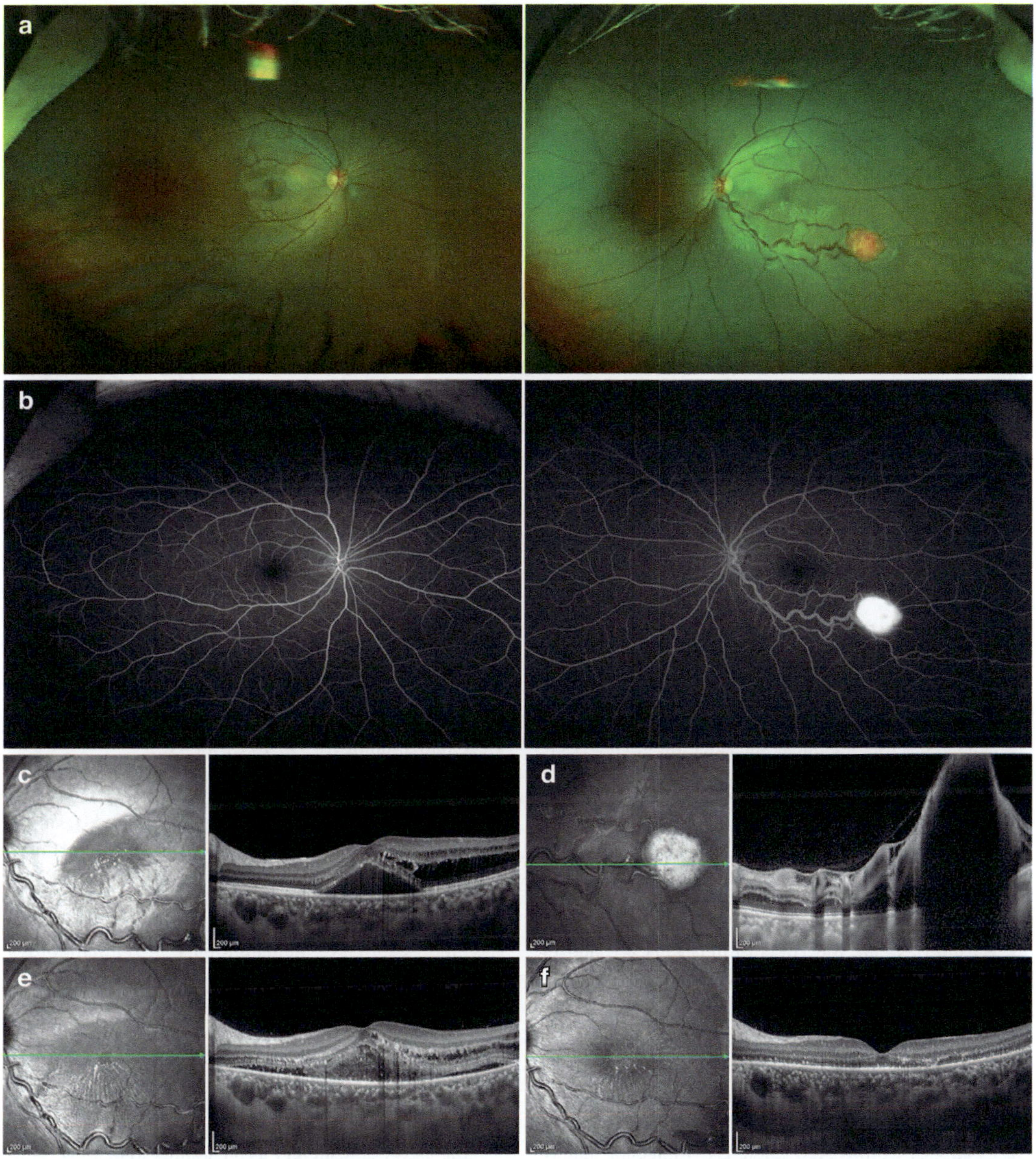

Fig. 12.3 A case of a 20-year-old female patient with von Hippel Lindau disease and retinal hemangioblastoma. The patient germline mutation was c.208G > A (p.Glu70Lys). (**a**) Retinal hemangioblastoma is located at inferotemporal quadrant with a dilated vessel of left eye. (**b**) Fluorescein angiography shows hyperfluorescence and staining of the lesion. (**c**, **d**) On optical coherence tomography, subretinal and intraretinal fluid with hyperreflective foci are shown and hemangioblastoma is found in retina. (**e**) After focal laser photocoagulation, macular edema was not resolved. (**f**) After intravitreal injection of bevacizumab, macular edema was diminished (courtesy of Prof. Hyeong-Gon Yu, Seoul National University, Seoul, Korea)

without retinectomy [36, 37]. Careful postoperative examination is needed due to the possible development of neovascular glaucoma or proliferative vitreoretinopathy [5, 36, 37].

In cases of juxtapapillary RH, direct photocoagulation can result in a decrease in visual field or visual acuity [38]. Therefore, asymptomatic lesions are usually observed with closed follow-up and examinations. In cases of RH affecting the central macula with exudation and visual acuity, PDT can decrease exudation in some cases [23, 35].

Based on the evidences implicating VEGF expression is involved in the pathogenesis of VHL disease, antiangiogenic pharmacotherapy had been tried in some trials [10, 39–41]. Dahr et al tried intravitreal pegaptanib sodium (3 mg) injection in patients with juxtapapillary or extra-paillary RH every 6 weeks for at least six times and two of five patients experienced a decrease in exudation, while other three patients did not respond to the treatment [39]. Wong et al. tried intravitreal ranibizumab (0.5 mg) injection every 4 weeks for 6–12 months, but the treatment showed limited beneficial effects [40].

References

1. Lonser RR, et al. von Hippel-Lindau disease. Lancet. 2003;361:2059–67.
2. Maher ER, Neumann HP, Richard S. von Hippel-Lindau disease: a clinical and scientific review. Eur J Hum Genet. 2011;19:617–23.
3. Latif F, et al. Identification of the von Hippel-Lindau disease tumor suppressor gene. Science. 1993;260:1317–20.
4. Neumann HP, Wiestler OD. Clustering of features and genetics of von Hippel-Lindau syndrome. Lancet. 1991;338:258.
5. Karimi S, et al. Von Hippel-Lindau disease and the eye. J Ophthalmic Vis Res. 2020;15:78–94.
6. Niemela M, et al. Hemangioblastomas of the retina: impact of von Hippel-Lindau disease. Invest Ophthalmol Vis Sci. 2000;41:1909–15.
7. Seizinger BR, et al. Von Hippel-Lindau disease maps to the region of chromosome 3 associated with renal cell carcinoma. Nature. 1988;332:268–9.
8. Chan CC, Collins AB, Chew EY. Molecular pathology of eyes with von Hippel-Lindau (VHL) disease: a review. Retina. 2007;27:1–7.
9. Nielsen SM, et al. Von Hippel-Lindau disease: genetics and role of genetic counseling in a multiple neoplasia syndrome. J Clin Oncol. 2016;34:2172–81.
10. Na X, et al. Overproduction of vascular endothelial growth factor related to von Hippel-Lindau tumor suppressor gene mutations and hypoxia-inducible factor-1 alpha expression in renal cell carcinomas. J Urol. 2003;170:588–92.
11. Iliopoulos O, et al. Negative regulation of hypoxia-inducible genes by the von Hippel-Lindau protein. Proc Natl Acad Sci U S A. 1996;93:10595–9.
12. Chew EY. Ocular manifestations of von Hippel-Lindau disease: clinical and genetic investigations. Trans Am Ophthalmol Soc. 2005;103:495–511.
13. Wong WT, et al. Clinical characterization of retinal capillary hemangioblastomas in a large population of patients with von Hippel-Lindau disease. Ophthalmology. 2008;115:181–8.
14. Maher ER, et al. Clinical features and natural history of von Hippel-Lindau disease. Q J Med. 1990;77:1151–63.
15. Toy BC, et al. Longitudinal analysis of retinal hemangioblastomatosis and visual function in ocular von Hippel-Lindau disease. Ophthalmology. 2012;119:2622–30.
16. Choyke PL, et al. von Hippel-Lindau disease: genetic, clinical, and imaging features. Radiology. 1995;194:629–42.
17. Amoils SP, Smith TR. Cryotherapy of angiomatosis retinae. Arch Ophthalmol. 1969;81:689–91.
18. Blodi CF, et al. Direct and feeder vessel photocoagulation of retinal angiomas with dye yellow laser. Ophthalmology. 1990;97:791–5. Discussion 796–7
19. Gorin MB. Von Hippel-Lindau disease: clinical considerations and the use of fluorescein-potentiated argon laser therapy for treatment of retinal angiomas. Semin Ophthalmol. 1992;7:182–91.
20. Kreusel KM, et al. Ruthenium-106 brachytherapy for peripheral retinal capillary hemangioma. Ophthalmology. 1998;105:1386–92.
21. Lane CM, et al. Laser treatment of retinal angiomatosis. Eye (Lond). 1989;3(Pt 1):33–8.
22. Schmidt D, Natt E, Neumann HP. Long-term results of laser treatment for retinal angiomatosis in von Hippel-Lindau disease. Eur J Med Res. 2000;5:47–58.
23. Schmidt-Erfurth UM, et al. Benefits and complications of photodynamic therapy of papillary capillary hemangiomas. Ophthalmology. 2002;109:1256–66.
24. Webster AR, Maher ER, Moore AT. Clinical characteristics of ocular angiomatosis in von Hippel-Lindau disease and correlation with germline mutation. Arch Ophthalmol. 1999;117:371–8.
25. Welch RB. Von Hippel-Lindau disease: the recognition and treatment of early angiomatosis retinae and the use of cryosurgery as an adjunct to therapy. Trans Am Ophthalmol Soc. 1970;68:367–424.
26. Agarwal A, Kumari N, Singh R. Intravitreal bevacizumab and feeder vessel laser treatment for a posteriorly located retinal capillary hemangioma. Int Ophthalmol. 2016;36:747–50.
27. Johnson MW, Flynn HW Jr, Gass JD. Pars plana vitrectomy and direct diathermy for complications of multiple retinal angiomas. Ophthalmic Surg. 1992;23:47–50.
28. Machemer R, Williams JM Sr. Pathogenesis and therapy of traction detachment in various retinal vascular diseases. Am J Ophthalmol. 1988;105:170–81.
29. Singh AD, et al. Treatment of retinal capillary hemangioma. Ophthalmology. 2002;109:1799–806.

30. Rosa RH Jr, Goldberg MF, Green WR. Clinicopathologic correlation of argon laser photocoagulation of retinal angiomas in a patient with von Hippel-Lindau disease followed for more than 20 years. Retina. 1996;16:145–56.
31. Huang C, et al. Long-Term therapeutic outcomes of photodynamic therapy-based or photocoagulation-based treatments on retinal capillary hemangioma. Photomed Laser Surg. 2018;36:10–7.
32. Shields JA. Response of retinal capillary hemangioma to cryotherapy. Arch Ophthalmol. 1993;111:551.
33. Watzke RC. Cryotherapy for retinal angiomatosis. A clinicopathologic report. Arch Ophthalmol. 1974;92:399–401.
34. Papastefanou VP, et al. Photodynamic therapy for retinal capillary hemangioma. Eye (Lond). 2013;27:438–42.
35. Sachdeva R, et al. Verteporfin photodynamic therapy of six eyes with retinal capillary haemangioma. Acta Ophthalmol. 2010;88:e334–40.
36. Gaudric A, et al. Vitreoretinal surgery for severe retinal capillary hemangiomas in von Hippel-Lindau disease. Ophthalmology. 2011;118:142–9.
37. Schlesinger T, et al. Internal en bloc resection and genetic analysis of retinal capillary hemangioblastoma. Arch Ophthalmol. 2007;125:1189–93.
38. Garcia-Arumi J, et al. Therapeutic options for capillary papillary hemangiomas. Ophthalmology. 2000;107:48–54.
39. Dahr SS, et al. Intravitreal anti-vascular endothelial growth factor therapy with pegaptanib for advanced von Hippel-Lindau disease of the retina. Retina. 2007;27:150–8.
40. Wong WT, et al. Intravitreal ranibizumab therapy for retinal capillary hemangioblastoma related to von Hippel-Lindau disease. Ophthalmology. 2008;115:1957–64.
41. George DJ, Kaelin WG Jr. The von Hippel-Lindau protein, vascular endothelial growth factor, and kidney cancer. N Engl J Med. 2003;349:419–21.

Other Macular Dystrophies 1

13

Joo Young Shin

Abstract

Various rare macular dystrophies have been reported with various prognoses, some with known causative genes with mutation. Diagnosis can be made clinically with typical cases, but many require genetic testing for confirmative diagnosis.

Keywords

Occult macular dystrophy · Butterfly-shaped pigment dystrophy · Pattern dystrophy · Sorsby fundus dystrophy · Bietti's crystalline retinopathy · Autosomal dominant radial drusen · Doyne honeycomb retinal dystrophy · North Carolina macular dystrophy · Dominant cystoid macular dystrophy

13.1 Occult Macular Dystrophy

In 1989, Miyake et al first reported three patients from a family that a hereditary macular dystrophy with no visible fundus abnormality [1].

Occult macular dystrophy shows bilateral progressive decrease in vision of 20/25–20/200 [2], with severe color vision impairment in most cases [3]. Onset of symptom varies, but disease severity seems to be worse with earlier onset of symptoms [4].

Typically, fundus appearance and fluorescein angiography show no abnormalities [5], but mild hyper-autofluorescence can be seen at the macula, which can aid in the diagnosis [6]. Cone function is decreased on electroretinography (ERG), and rod function is preserved especially in young age [7]. Macular waves are decreased or nearly absent on multifocal ERG [8]. Photoreceptor layer and outer nuclear layer defects can be found on optical coherence tomography [9–11]. Abnormal findings of multifocal ERG and optical coherence tomography were found to have significant correlation [12].

Most cases show autosomal dominant or sporadic inheritance patterns, and RP1L1 gene at 8p23 has been identified to be related with occult macular dystrophy [13]. Missense mutations in this gene are considered as the cause, but the exact pathophysiologic mechanism remains uncertain [14].

13.2 Butterfly-Shaped Pigment Dystrophy (Pattern Dystrophy)

Since its first reported in 1970 in a family of four siblings and their offspring with pigmentation in the macula in a butterfly-shaped pattern, many studies have been reported on butterfly-shaped pigment dystrophy, or pattern dystrophy [15].

Decreased visual function or metamorphopsia may be present, but many cases are identified on

J. Y. Shin (✉)
Department of Ophthalmology, Seoul National University College of Medicine, Seoul, Korea

H.-G. Yu (ed.), *Inherited Retinal Disease*, https://doi.org/10.1007/978-981-16-7337-5_13

routine eye exams because vision is preserved and progression is slow in many cases [16]. Bilateral symmetric pigmentation can be observed showing various shapes. Most cases show butterfly-shaped pigmentation in deep layers of the central retina, thus pigmentation can be poorly visualized with red-free light. The fovea and foveal reflex are normal, and the superficial layers of the retina including retinal vessels and optic nerve and choroid are normal. The butterfly-shaped pigmentation shows blocked fluorescence on fluorescein angiography with sharp margins. The photoreceptor layer and inner retinal layers are normal, and visual acuity, visual field, color vision, dark adaptation, and ERG are normal. Diffuse dysfunction of the retinal pigment epithelium causes abnormal electrooculography. On autopsy, photoreceptors and retinal pigment epithelium are lost in the areas of pigmentation, while choriocapillaris are normal. Lipofuscin accumulation can be observed outside the involved area.

Most cases are autosomal dominant [17]. Peripherin/RDS gene mutations are identified in many cases, but other genes associated with other macular dystrophies have also been found to be associated [18], and mutation in the CTNNA1 gene has also been identified [19]. Some cases show incomplete penetrance as in vitelliform macular dystrophy, and carriers can be identified with electrooculography.

The typical pigmentation makes it readily discriminative from other inherited macular dystrophies, but macular dystrophy in Steinert–Curschmann myotonic dystrophy shows similar appearance requiring differential diagnosis.

13.3 Sorsby Fundus Dystrophy

In 1949, Sorsby et al reported change in the fundus resembling inflammation in the posterior pole [20]. Bilateral change in the fundus was observed with abrupt decrease of vision, with autosomal dominant inheritance pattern. This lesion was similar with autosomal dominant central areolar choroidal dystrophy, and difficult to differentiate from disciform macular degeneration or true inflammatory reactions.

Visual loss and nyctalopia in the third to fourth decades of life are typical, with prominent presentation in the 40s. Fastly progressing central scotoma with abrupt increase in size and depth causing visual loss within several months accompanied with decreased color vision is the usual presentation.

The first signs on fundoscopy include bilateral macular edema with hemorrhage and exudation, progressing to pigmentation and scar formation. Atrophy of the retinal pigment epithelium becomes prominent with time, and underlying choroidal vessels are visible. This process progresses to the periphery through 3–4 years, and abnormal pigmentation and retinal pigment epithelium extend to the far periphery, resembling diffuse choroidal atrophy. Fluorescein angiography findings vary according to the stage of the disease, with filling defect of the choriocapillaris in early stages, progressing to atrophy of the choriocapillaris and prominent larger choroidal vessels in late stages. Choroidal neovascularization or polypoidal choroidal vasculopathy has also been reported [21]. Dark adaptation is usually not affected, but sometimes delayed with progressed disease. ERG is normal, but b wave is decreased with decreased rod function with progression.

The typical pathologic finding of Sorsby fundus dystrophy is lipid and protein accumulation between the Bruch's membrane and retinal pigment epithelium, up to 30 μm in some cases [22]. Subretinal hemorrhage and exudation can be present in some cases. Autosomal dominant inheritance is associated with mutation in 22q13, and tissue inhibitor of metalloproteinase-3 (TIMP3) gene mutation is considered as the causative mutation.

Other retinal and choroidal dystrophies should be differentiated, including vitelliform macular dystrophy, which may have a similar appearance due to exudation. Diffuse choroiditis and disciform macular degeneration should also be differentiated. Diffuse atrophy in the progressed stages can mimic diffuse atrophy due to high myopia, gyrate atrophy of the choroid, and choroideremia. Also, autosomal dominant central areolar choroidal dystrophy should also be considered. Treatment includes anti-vascular endothelial growth factor antibody injection for accompanied choroidal neovascularization or polypoidal choroidal vasculopathy [23–25].

13.4 Bietti's Crystalline Retinopathy

Crystalline retinopathy can be observed due to various causes, including toxic retinopathies, hereditary diseases, and chronic retinal detachment, but this rare form of crystalline retinopathy was first reported in 1937 by Bietti, described as yellow-white crystalline lipid deposits in the retina and sometimes cornea with tapetoretinal degeneration. The cause is unknown, but abnormality of the retinal pigment epithelium and disruption of the outer retinal blood barrier causing leak is the suspected pathophysiologic mechanism. Various degrees of retinal pigment epithelium and choriocapillaris loss are observed with crystalline deposits throughout all layers of the retina, also accompanied by superficial crystalline deposits in the corneal limbus [26, 27].

Typical crystalline deposits and choriocapillaris atrophy on fluorescein angiography usually lead to the diagnosis. Photoreceptor loss progresses with enlargement of this atrophy, and crystalline deposits disappear leaving choriocapillaris atrophy, which can be observed on optical coherence tomography [28, 29]. The size and location of the involved area determine the degree of involvement of visual acuity, dark adaptation, and ERG findings, with decrease of ERG and increased severity of nyctalopia with progression.

Differentiation with retinitis pigmentosa is needed, and up to 3–10% of cases of retinitis pigmentosa showing autosomal recessive pattern had been identified as crystalline retinopathy in a previous report. Less retinal vascular sclerosis is observed in crystalline retinopathy, and ERG is relatively preserved [27].

On biopsy of the cornea, complex lipid inclusions and cholesterol deposits were identified in fibroblasts and epithelial cells, also found in lymphocytes, leading to suspicion that abnormal systemic lipid metabolism is involved in the pathophysiology [30].

Autosomal recessive inheritance in suspected, but autosomal dominant cases has also been reported. Mutation in CYP4V2, one of the cytochrome p450 family, has been identified, which is involved in the metabolism of fatty acids. In a recent study on Korean and Japanese patients, over 50% of patients were found to have the c.802-8_810del17insGC mutation in both alleles, but was not associated with clinical severity [31].

13.5 Autosomal Dominant Radial Drusen (Doyne Honeycomb Retinal Dystrophy)

Autosomal dominant radial drusen are found inner to the Bruch's membrane and are thought to be secreted from the retinal pigment epithelial cells. Initially patients are asymptomatic and identified through routine funduscopic examinations, but eventually vision decreases accompanied by metamorphopsia. Usually patients present in their 20s and 30s [32], with a few round yellowish brown lesions in their posterior poles that turn white later. In their middle-ages, multiple white discrete dots cover the posterior pole, in a mosaic or honeycomb pattern. Usually bilateral and symmetric, the drusen are larger near the fovea, and are round and white and discrete compared to fundus flavimaculatus. As the disease progresses, the drusen near the center conglomerate, and retinal pigment epithelial atrophy appears in the retina. Pigmentation may increase and atrophy of the choriocapillaris and larger choroidal vessels occurs. Often drusen disappear leaving atrophic areas. Usually autosomal dominant radial drusen progress in radial fashion from the macula and optic disk area, leaving the optic disk and vessels and far periphery intact. On fluorescein angiography, multiple round hyperfluorescent dots are visible in the arterial phase, which partially correspond with the lesions visible on fundoscopy. Areas of retinal pigment epithelial atrophy not definitely visible on fundoscopy can be visualized with fluorescein angiography. Large drusen do not show hyperfluorescence due to blockage of choroidal fluorescence, while smaller ones allow visualization of the underlying background hyperfluorescence of the choroid. The lesions show no leakage, sparing the optic nerve, retinal vessels, and peripheral retina. Choroidal neovascularization may occur, which can be observed on optical coherence tomography [33, 34]. Vision remains normal in the early stages, progressively declining in further stages. As deposits are accumulated under the retinal pigment epithelium toward the choroid, photoreceptors remain intact longer than in fundus flavimaculatus, but after 10–20 years, photoreceptor damage may occur. Vision loss is rare before 40, but may progresses to central scotoma. Color vision remains normal while visual function is spared as in other macular diseases. Dark adaptation is normal, but may be slightly decreased in advanced cases. ERG is normal, but increased b wave latency may be observed in advanced cases. Electrooculography is normal, but becomes subnormal with increased area of involvement. Symptoms and findings are usually less severe than fundus flavimaculatus.

Round accumulation of hyaline bodies in retinal pigment epithelium is observed histologically. When compared to drusen in age-related macular degeneration, collagen type IV was found only in autosomal dominant radial drusen, but other components were similar [35].

Autosomal dominant inheritance with mutation of the fibulin gene (EFEMP1) on chromosome 2 is reported as the genetic cause [36, 37].

Differentiation with degenerative drusen of age-related macular degeneration is required. Degenerative drusen can also be observed in other diseases such as hyalinosis cutis et mucosae (Urbach–Wiethe syndrome). Fundus flavimaculatus, fundus albipunctatus, and fleck retina of Kandori should also be differentiated.

13.6 Others

13.6.1 North Carolina Macular Dystrophy

North Carolina macular dystrophy was first reported in 1971 by Lefler et al in an Iris family in North Carolina with retinopathy and aminoaciduria [38]. Symmetric bilateral large lesions are seen on the macula at birth, with no progression during lifetime. Mutation in the MCDR1 gene on 6q [39] involved in regulation of retinal transcription factor PRDM13 has been reported [40, 41].

13.6.2 Dominant Cystoid Macular Dystrophy

Initially cystoid macular edema occurs with progression to macular atrophy and surrounding pigmentation. Mild decrease in vision occurs in young patients, but progresses with age. The retinal vessels and optic nerve head are spared late into the disease. On fluorescein angiography, typical capillary leak around the macula can be found, which progresses to window defects in atrophic areas. ERG is usually normal, but electrooculography is subnormal, also progressing with age. Yellow-blue and red-green color vision are all decreased. Initially the retinal pigment epithelium is involved, but inner and outer blood retinal barrier seems to be broken down secondarily. Mutation at 7p15.3 is thought to be associated, but the exact gene has not been identified yet [42].

References

1. Miyake Y, Ichikawa K, Shiose Y, Kawase Y. Hereditary macular dystrophy without visible fundus abnormality. Am J Ophthalmol. 1989;108(3):292–9.
2. Ahn SJ, Cho SI, Ahn J, Park SS, Park KH, Woo SJ. Clinical and genetic characteristics of Korean occult macular dystrophy patients. Invest Ophthalmol Vis Sci. 2013;54(7):4856–63.
3. Kim YG, Baek SH, Moon SW, Lee HK, Kim US. Analysis of spectral domain optical coherence tomography findings in occult macular dystrophy. Acta Ophthalmol. 2011;89(1):e52–6.
4. Fujinami K, Yang L, Joo K, Tsunoda K, Kameya S, Hanazono G, et al. Clinical and genetic characteristics of east Asian patients with occult macular dystrophy (Miyake disease): East Asia occult macular dystrophy studies report number 1. Ophthalmology. 2019;126(10):1432–44.
5. Tsunoda K, Usui T, Hatase T, Yamai S, Fujinami K, Hanazono G, et al. Clinical characteristics of occult macular dystrophy in family with mutation of RP1l1 gene. Retina. 2012;32(6):1135–47.

6. Fujinami K, Tsunoda K, Hanazono G, Shinoda K, Ohde H, Miyake Y. Fundus autofluorescence in autosomal dominant occult macular dystrophy. Arch Ophthalmol. 2011;129(5):597–602.
7. Miyake Y, Horiguchi M, Tomita N, Kondo M, Tanikawa A, Takahashi H, et al. Occult macular dystrophy. Am J Ophthalmol. 1996;122(5):644–53.
8. Piao CH, Kondo M, Tanikawa A, Terasaki H, Miyake Y. Multifocal electroretinogram in occult macular dystrophy. Invest Ophthalmol Vis Sci. 2000;41(2):513–7.
9. Park SJ, Woo SJ, Park KH, Hwang JM, Chung H. Morphologic photoreceptor abnormality in occult macular dystrophy on spectral-domain optical coherence tomography. Invest Ophthalmol Vis Sci. 2010;51(7):3673–9.
10. Ahn SJ, Ahn J, Park KH, Woo SJ. Multimodal imaging of occult macular dystrophy. JAMA Ophthalmol. 2013;131(7):880–90.
11. Kitaguchi Y, Kusaka S, Yamaguchi T, Mihashi T, Fujikado T. Detection of photoreceptor disruption by adaptive optics fundus imaging and Fourier-domain optical coherence tomography in eyes with occult macular dystrophy. Clin Ophthalmol. 2011;5:345–51.
12. Yang L, Joo K, Tsunoda K, Kondo M, Fujinami-Yokokawa Y, Arno G, et al. Spatial functional characteristics of east Asian patients with occult macular dystrophy (Miyake disease); EAOMD report no. 2. Am J Ophthalmol. 2021;221:169–80.
13. Akahori M, Tsunoda K, Miyake Y, Fukuda Y, Ishiura H, Tsuji S, et al. Dominant mutations in RP1L1 are responsible for occult macular dystrophy. Am J Hum Genet. 2010;87(3):424–9.
14. Chen CJ, Scholl HP, Birch DG, Iwata T, Miller NR, Goldberg MF. Characterizing the phenotype and genotype of a family with occult macular dystrophy. Arch Ophthalmol. 2012;130(12):1554–9.
15. Deutman AF, van Blommestein JD, Henkes HE, Waardenburg PJ, Solleveld-van DE. Butterfly-shaped pigment dystrophy of the fovea. Arch Ophthalmol. 1970;83(5):558–69.
16. Zhang K, Garibaldi DC, Li Y, Green WR, Zack DJ. Butterfly-shaped pattern dystrophy: a genetic, clinical, and histopathological report. Arch Ophthalmol. 2002;120(4):485–90.
17. Khoubian FJ, Shakin EP, Tantri A, Kim DY, Edwards AO, Donoso LA. Autosomal dominant pattern dystrophy: identification of a novel splice site mutation in the peripherin/RDS gene. Retina. 2005;25(8):999–1004.
18. Boon CJ, den Hollander AI, Hoyng CB, Cremers FP, Klevering BJ, Keunen JE. The spectrum of retinal dystrophies caused by mutations in the peripherin/RDS gene. Prog Retin Eye Res. 2008;27(2):213–35.
19. Saksens NT, Krebs MP, Schoenmaker-Koller FE, Hicks W, Yu M, Shi L, et al. Mutations in CTNNA1 cause butterfly-shaped pigment dystrophy and perturbed retinal pigment epithelium integrity. Nat Genet. 2016;48(2):144–51.
20. Sorsby A, Mason ME. A fundus dystrophy with unusual features. Br J Ophthalmol. 1949;33(2):67–97.
21. Koutresi D, Clarke B, Lotery AJ, De Salvo G. Sorsby fundus dystrophy with polypoidal choroidal vasculopathy: Extending TIMP3 phenotypes. Clin Exp Ophthalmol. 2019;47(9):1214–8.
22. Capon MR, Marshall J, Krafft JI, Alexander RA, Hiscott PS, Bird AC. Sorsby's fundus dystrophy. A light and electron microscopic study. Ophthalmology. 1989;96(12):1769–77.
23. Gliem M, Muller PL, Mangold E, Holz FG, Bolz HJ, Stohr H, et al. Sorsby fundus dystrophy: novel mutations, novel phenotypic characteristics, and treatment outcomes. Invest Ophthalmol Vis Sci. 2015;56(4):2664–76.
24. Spaide RF. Long-term visual acuity preservation in Sorsby fundus dystrophy with corticosteroid treatment. Retin Cases Brief Rep. 2019; https://doi.org/10.1097/ICB.0000000000000946.
25. Gemenetzi MK, Luff AJ, Lotery AJ. Successful treatment of choroidal neovascularization secondary to sorsby fundus dystrophy with intravitreal bevacizumab. Retin Cases Brief Rep. 2011;5(2):132–5.
26. Ahmed I, McDonald HR, Schatz H, Johnson RN, Ai E, Cruess AF, et al. Crystalline retinopathy associated with chronic retinal detachment. Arch Ophthalmol. 1998;116(11):1449–53.
27. Bernauer W, Daicker B. Bietti's corneal-retinal dystrophy. A 16-year progression. Retina. 1992;12(1):18–20.
28. Miyata M, Oishi A, Hasegawa T, Ishihara K, Oishi M, Ogino K, et al. Choriocapillaris flow deficit in Bietti crystalline dystrophy detected using optical coherence tomography angiography. Br J Ophthalmol. 2018;102(9):1208–12.
29. Hirashima T, Miyata M, Ishihara K, Hasegawa T, Sugahara M, Ogino K, et al. Choroidal vasculature in Bietti crystalline dystrophy with CYP4V2 mutations and in retinitis pigmentosa with EYS mutations. Invest Ophthalmol Vis Sci. 2017;58(10):3871–8.
30. Wilson DJ, Weleber RG, Klein ML, Welch RB, Green WR. Bietti's crystalline dystrophy. A clinicopathologic correlative study. Arch Ophthalmol. 1989;107(2):213–21.
31. Murakami Y, Koyanagi Y, Fukushima M, Yoshimura M, Fujiwara K, Akiyama M, et al. Genotype and long-term clinical course of Bietti crystalline dystrophy in Korean and Japanese patients. Ophthalmol Retina. 2021; https://doi.org/10.1016/j.oret.2021.02.009.
32. Tsang SH, Sharma T. Doyne honeycomb retinal dystrophy (malattia leventinese, autosomal dominant drusen). Adv Exp Med Biol. 2018;1085:97–102.
33. Serra R, Coscas F, Messaoudi N, Srour M, Souied E. Choroidal neovascularization in malattia leventinese diagnosed using optical coherence tomography angiography. Am J Ophthalmol. 2017;176:108–17.
34. Corbelli E, Corvi F, Carnevali A, Querques L, Zucchiatti I, Bandello F, et al. Optical coherence tomography angiography demonstration of choroidal neovascularization in malattia leventinese. Ophthalmic Surg Lasers Imaging Retina. 2016;47(6):602–4.

35. Sohn EH, Wang K, Thompson S, Riker MJ, Hoffmann JM, Stone EM, et al. Comparison of drusen and modifying genes in autosomal dominant radial drusen and age-related macular degeneration. Retina. 2015;35(1):48–57.
36. Stone EM, Lotery AJ, Munier FL, Heon E, Piguet B, Guymer RH, et al. A single EFEMP1 mutation associated with both Malattia Leventinese and Doyne honeycomb retinal dystrophy. Nat Genet. 1999;22(2):199–202.
37. Zhang K, Sun X, Chen Y, Zhong Q, Lin L, Gao Y, et al. Doyne honeycomb retinal dystrophy/malattia leventinese induced by EFEMP1 mutation in a Chinese family. BMC Ophthalmol. 2018;18(1):318.
38. Lefler WH, Wadsworth JA, Sidbury JB Jr. Hereditary macular degeneration and amino-aciduria. Am J Ophthalmol. 1971;71(1 Pt 2):224–30.
39. Small KW, Weber JL, Roses A, Lennon F, Vance JM, Pericak-Vance MA. North Carolina macular dystrophy is assigned to chromosome 6. Genomics. 1992;13(3):681–5.
40. Weleber RG. Dysregulation of retinal transcription factor PRDM13 and North Carolina macular dystrophy. Ophthalmology. 2016;123(1):2–4.
41. Small KW, DeLuca AP, Whitmore SS, Rosenberg T, Silva-Garcia R, Udar N, et al. North Carolina macular dystrophy is caused by dysregulation of the retinal transcription factor PRDM13. Ophthalmology. 2016;123(1):9–18.
42. Saksens NT, van Huet RA, van Lith-Verhoeven JJ, den Hollander AI, Hoyng CB, Boon CJ. Dominant cystoid macular dystrophy. Ophthalmology. 2015;122(1):180–91.

Other Macular Dystrophies 2

14

In Hwan Cho

Abstract

The differential diagnosis of macular dystrophies may be challenging because of their overlapping clinical phenotypes. Genetic testing may contribute to define and diagnose these diseases accurately. This chapter deals with several macular dystrophies, including Sorsby fundus dystrophy, North Carolina macular dystrophy, Doyne honeycomb retinal dystrophy, and Bietti's crystalline dystrophy, in which gene variants have been identified as a cause of the disease. The purpose of this chapter is to provide an overview of these disorders.

Keywords

Sorsby fundus dystrophy · North Carolina macular dystrophy · Doyne honeycomb retinal dystrophy · Bietti's crystalline dystrophy

The original version of this chapter has been revised. The correction to this chapter can be found at https://doi.org/10.1007/978-981-16-7337-5_18

I. H. Cho (✉)
Department of Ophthalmology, College of Medicine, Soonchunhyang University,
Dongnam-gu, Cheonan, Korea

14.1 Sorsby Fundus Dystrophy

Sorsby fundus dystrophy (SFD) is a fully penetrant autosomal dominant degenerative disease of the macula, which was first described by Sorsby and Mason in 1949 [1].

14.1.1 Molecular Genetics

SFD is caused by variants in the gene encoding the tissue inhibitor of metalloproteinases-3 (TIMP3), located on chromosome 22q12.3 [2]. Most of the known variants of TIMP3 are Ser181Cys [2], Ser156Cys [3], and Tyr172Cys [4]. These SFD-associated TIMP3 variants promote the formation of higher molecular weight protein complexes, which is a product of dimerization/multimerization of the variant TIMP3 molecules [5]. This may alter TIMP3-mediated extracellular matrix turnover and result in the accumulation of TIMP3 variants in the Bruch's membrane (BM) of patients with SFD [6]. The formation of drusen-like deposits in the BM could contribute to the thickening of this membrane with pathological outcomes, including impaired transport of nutrients and growth factors, leading to retinal pigment epithelium (RPE)/photoreceptor dysfunction [7]. In addition, Majid et al. demonstrated that a TIMP3 variant can induce apoptosis of RPE cells, suggesting that this apoptosis may be the final pathway of SFD [8]. Furthermore, TIMP3 has been recently

H.-G. Yu (ed.), *Inherited Retinal Disease*, https://doi.org/10.1007/978-981-16-7337-5_14

shown to be a potent inhibitor of angiogenesis, which may, in part, account for the complication of choroidal neovascularization (CNV) found in SFD [9].

14.1.2 Clinical Manifestation

Patients with SFD are usually asymptomatic during the first decades of life. Some patients may be aware of the difficulties in dark adaptation and color vision for a decade or more prior to losing their central vision. Central visual loss typically occurs in the fourth to sixth decades because of CNV and subretinal hemorrhage. According to a previous study, the median age of severe visual loss in the first and second eye was 45 and 59 years, respectively [10]. Preneovascular fundus examination shows normal to diffuse or focal subretinal yellow-white deposits at the level of the BM [11]. Later in the course of the SFD, retinal degeneration progresses to involve the retina anterior to the macula. The peripheral retina is usually spared from degeneration.

14.1.3 Differential Diagnosis

The differential diagnosis includes retinal diseases-associated macular atrophy and/or CNV, including age-related macular degeneration (AMD), Doyne honeycomb retinal dystrophy, pattern dystrophy, and late-stage Best disease. SFD has considerable phenotypic overlap with AMD; however, earlier onset, strong inheritance pattern, and late involvement of peripheral chorioretinal atrophy are important distinguishing characteristics of SFD.

14.1.4 Management

Jacobson et al. [12] suggested that night blindness from SFD was caused by the chronic deprivation of vitamin A from the photoreceptors due to the thickened BM separating the RPE from the choriocapillaris. A short-term reversal of night blindness at the early stage of SFD after oral administration of vitamin A at a dose of 50,000 IU/day has been reported [12]. However, vitamin A is not a widely used treatment because of the potential toxicity associated with its long-term use at high doses [13]. Treatment for CNV in SFD includes laser treatment, photodynamic therapy, and intravitreal steroid injection; however, their efficacy is limited. Intravitreal anti-vascular endothelial growth factor (VEGF) injections, such as bevacizumab and ranibizumab have shown promise in delaying visual loss due to CNV [10, 13].

14.2 North Carolina Macula Dystrophy

North Carolina macular dystrophy (NCDM) is an autosomal dominant macular dystrophy with a variable phenotype. NCDM is a congenital developmental abnormality of the macula that does not progress in severity [14]. However, some progression and vision loss can occur because of the development of CNV [15].

Small et al. [15] described the grading system of NCDM as follows:

- Grade 1: good visual acuity (20/20–20/30) with bilateral multiple small drusen-like deposits in the central macula.
- Grade 2: good to moderate visual acuity (20/25–20/200) with bilateral confluent drusen-like deposits in the central macula.
- Grade 3: moderate to poor visual acuity (20/20–count fingers) with bilateral excavated lesions of the macula. The macular atrophic lesion commonly has a ring of pigmentation and fibrous tissue at its peripheral edge.

Even in the case of grade 3 NCDM, the visual acuity is better than that could be predicted from the fundus appearance. Grade 3 macular atrophic lesions could be confused with congenital toxoplasmosis, but visual acuity is generally worse in the latter. Notably, approximately half of the patients with NCDM are asymptomatic; therefore, the absence of a history of other affected family members may not be useful in correctly diagnosing NCDM.

Full-field electroretinogram (ERG) shows normal findings, indicating that retinal dysfunction is confined to the macular area. The ERG pattern is usually normal in grades 1 and 2 but abnormal in grade 3. The electrooculogram (EOG) is either normal or shows a mildly reduced Arden ratio. Interestingly, dark adaptation and color vision are normal in patients with NCDM [14].

Through linkage analysis, Small et al. [16] mapped NCDM to chromosome 6q. Although most families show linkage to the 6q locus, two families with identical phenotypes (MCDR3) have been mapped to chromosome 5q, indicating genetic heterogeneity in this disorder [17, 18].

14.3 Doyne Honeycomb Retinal Dystrophy/Malattia Leventinese/Autosomal Dominant Drusen

In 1899, Doyne honeycomb retinal dystrophy (DHRD) was first described phenotypically by Doyne [19]. He found early-onset retinal dystrophy with white deposits in a honeycomb pattern at the macula and nasal to the disk in the eyes of four sisters. In 1925, Vogt reported similar phenotypic fundus findings in a cluster of likely related individuals in the Leventine Valley of Switzerland [20]. He named it Malattia Leventinese (ML). Until 1999, DHRD and ML were considered separate entities because of their phenotypic variability and histopathological findings [21]. However, Stone et al. [22] identified a missense mutation (Arg345Trp) in the EGF-containing fibrillin-like extracellular matrix protein 1 (*EFEMP1*) gene on chromosome 2 in both families with DHRD and MLVT, confirming that the two represented slight phenotypic variants of the same disease.

14.3.1 Molecular Genetics

DHRD is characterized by an autosomal dominant mutation (Arg345Trp) in the *EFEMP1* gene encoding fibulin-3 [22]. *EFEMP1* is located on chromosome 2p16. Fibulin-3 is widely expressed in the extracellular matrix throughout the body; however, its exact function is unknown [23]. Arg345Trp mutation may induce resistance to the degradation of fibulin-3 rather than impairment of function [23]. Fue et al. [24] found that *EFEMP1*-Arg345Trp knockin mice developed deposits between the BM and the RPE. Such deposits may contain an increased amount of fibulin-3. In a recent study, Stanton et al. [25] suggested that fibulin-3 plays a central role in the development of basal laminar deposits, and deletion of *EFEMP1* in mice protects against the development of basal laminar deposits. These deposits could contribute to RPE/photoreceptor dysfunction and may induce sequelae, including geographic atrophy and CNV.

14.3.2 Clinical Manifestation

The disease severity of DHRD varies widely with the evidence of interocular, intrafamilial, and interfamilial variability in visual loss and natural history [20]. Patients with DHRD may be asymptomatic early in the course of the disease, and the onset of symptoms is usually at the age of 30–50 years. Patients may describe an initial insidious onset of visual symptoms, such as reduced central vision, photophobia, slow dark adaptation, paracentral scotoma, and metamorphopsia [26–28]. Loss of color vision occurs at a later stage [28]. In the advanced stage of the disease, which usually occurs in the seventh or eighth decade of life, central vision is involved, and visual acuity is severely impaired, predominantly because of RPE atrophy and scarring [29, 30]. CNV can develop but it is a rare complication [28, 31–33]; however, it can sometimes be associated with subretinal hemorrhage [34].

Fundus findings are typically characterized by early-onset drusenoid deposits involving the posterior pole and peripapillary area. These small drusen at the early stage can become large and more confluent at later stages [35, 36] (Fig. 14.1). Optical coherence tomography (OCT) imaging can reveal focal dome-shaped, saw-tooth, or diffuse hyperreflective deposits with elevation between the BM and RPE, usually becoming more confluent over time [37]. The outer retinal

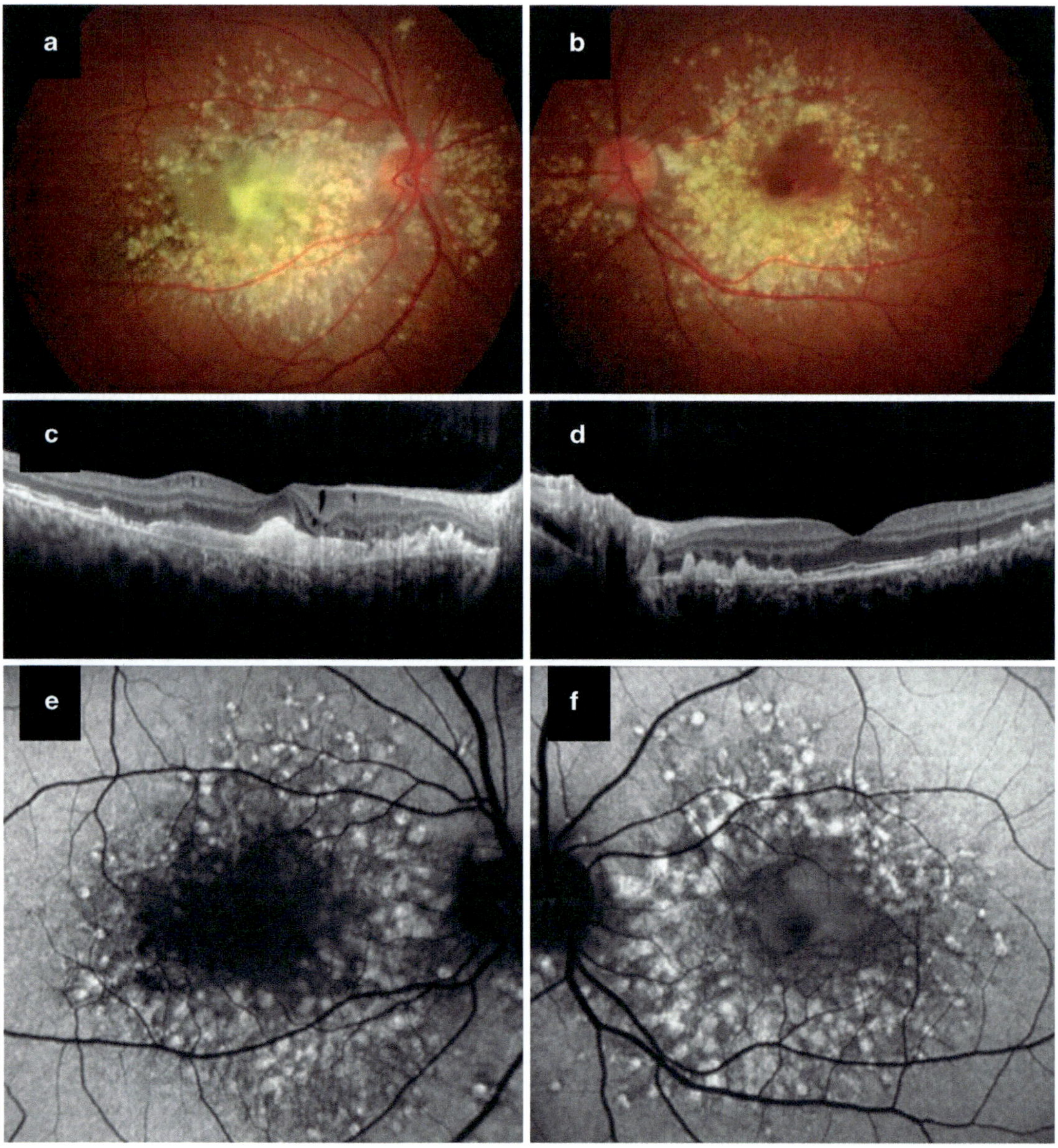

Fig. 14.1 Fundus photography, optical coherence tomography, and fundus autofluorescence of a 32-year-old man with Doyne honeycomb retinal dystrophy. (**a**, **b**) Fundus photographs show diffuse and confluent drusen with variable size, widely distributed in the posterior pole and peripapillary area. (**c**, **d**) Optical coherence tomography reveals bilateral extensive hyperreflective thickening beneath the retinal pigment epithelium accompanied by wavy uplift and intraretinal fluid accumulation in the right eye. (**e**, **f**) Fundus autofluorescence shows hyperautofluorescent spots corresponding to large drusen (Courtesy of Prof. Eun Kyoung Lee, Seoul National University, Seoul, Korea)

layer may be preserved early in the disease, but later stages can show variable or diffuse inner segment/outer segment junction (IS/OS junction) loss and outer retinal disruption. OCT is also useful for detecting CNV and geographic atrophy (Fig. 14.1). Fundus autofluorescence (FAF) [36] allows visualization of the health of the RPE/photoreceptor complex. Drusen of DHRD can be hypo-or hyper-autofluorescent, but one study showed that larger drusen are typically more hyper-autofluorescent [37]. Central areas of the posterior pole may be hypo-autofluorescent because of central geographic atrophy and loss or dysfunction of the RPE. On fluorescein angiography (FA) and indocyanine green angiography (ICG), large round drusen are hypofluorescent at the early phase and become hyperfluorescent at the late phase. However, small drusen are hyperfluorescent at the early phase and decrease their fluorescence toward the late phase [36–38] (Fig. 14.2).

14.3.3 Differential Diagnosis

Differential diagnosis for patients with early-onset drusen include Stargardt disease, North Carolina macular dystrophy, Sorsby fundus dystrophy, Best disease, Pattern dystrophy, and age-related macular degeneration.

14.3.4 Treatment

Currently, there is no proven treatment for DHRD. Typically, patients with DHRD are managed conservatively by observation. A series of anti-VEGF agents can be used for CNV development.

14.4 Bietti's Crystalline Dystrophy

Bietti's crystalline dystrophy (BCD) is an autosomal recessive retinal degeneration that was first described by Bietti in 1937 [39]. He reported three patients with crystalline deposits in the retina, scattered retinal pigment, chorioretinal atrophy, and yellow-white spots in the limbal cornea. In 1968, Bagolini and Ioli-Spada presented a 30-year follow-up data on these three patients and an additional six patients and designated this condition as Bietti's tapetoretinal degeneration with marginal corneal dystrophy [39]. They confirmed that BCD is a progressive and degenerative condition. Welch [40] identified the presence of lipid inclusion in the fibroblasts and corneal epithelium by analyzing a corneal limbus biopsy obtained from a patient with BCD, and described the condition as "crystalline retinopathy." Li et al. [41] identified the *CYP4V2* gene as a causative gene variant of BCD, which is involved in fatty acid metabolism. Lockhart et al. [42] developed an animal model that showed retinal crystalline deposits and metabolic lipid disturbances in *Cyp4v3*$^{-/-}$ knockout mice, corresponding with BCD findings in humans.

14.4.1 Molecular Genetics

The *CYP4V2* variant is related to the pathogenesis of BCD, which is expressed in a vast majority of body tissues, especially the RPE and retina, with a lesser degree of expression in the cornea [41, 43]. The *CYP4V2* gene belongs to the cytochrome p450 gene family. It is an 11-exon sequence that encodes a 525-amino acid protein, and plays an important role in lipid metabolism [43]. Functional alteration of *CYP4V2* may lead to impaired binding, elongation, or desaturation of fatty acids [44]. Lee et al. [44] found that the conversion of fatty acid precursors into n-3 polyunsaturated fatty acids is lower than normal in patients with BCD. This may be caused by a dysfunction of microsomal omega hydroxylase, which degrades lipids with mitochondrial and peroxisomal beta-oxidation enzymes, and the protein is encoded by *CYP4V2* [45]. Histopathologic studies have found panchorioretinal atrophy with complex lipid inclusion in choroidal fibroblasts [46], which may be a cause of progressive atrophy of the choriocapillaris and RPE layer in patients with BCD [47].

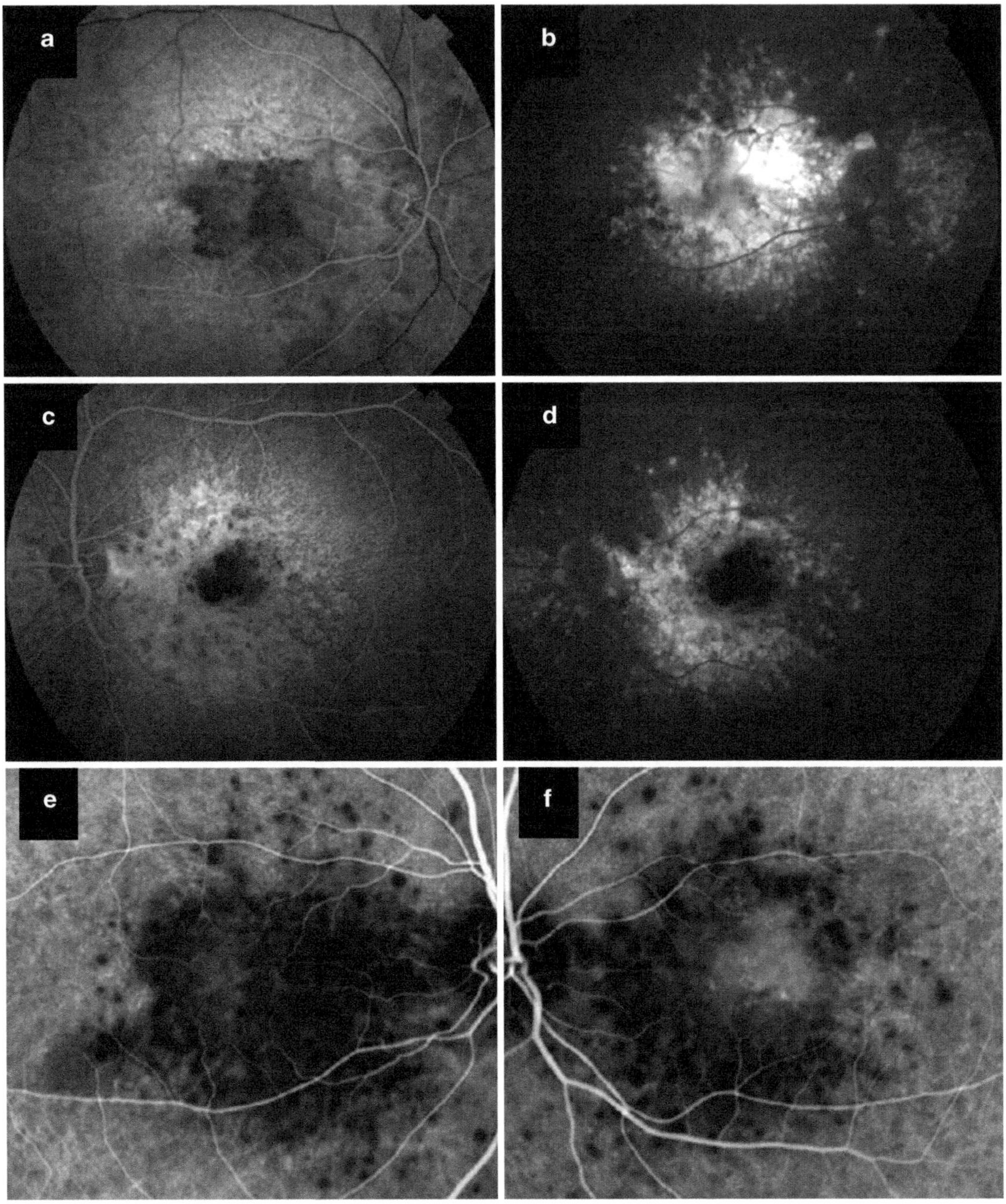

Fig. 14.2 Fluorescein angiography and indocyanine green angiography of the same patient as in Fig. 14.1. (**a**, **c**) In the early phase of fluorescein angiography, indistinct hypofluorescence corresponding to large drusen and diffuse pinpoint hyperfluorescence corresponding to small drusen are noticed. (**b**, **d**) In the late phase of fluorescein angiography, ill-defined zone of hyperfluorescence corresponding to large drusen and less intense hyperfluorescence of the small drusen are visible. (**e**, **f**) Indocyanine green angiography reveals multiple hypofluorescent dots corresponding to large drusen with small hyperfluorescent spots of the small drusen (Courtesy of Prof. Eun Kyoung Lee, Seoul National University, Seoul, Korea)

14.4.2 Clinical Manifestation

The hallmark sign of BCD is white spots or crystals in the retina and corneal stroma. Initially, patients with BCD are often asymptomatic, and the first clinical manifestation most commonly appears between the second and third decade of life. As BCD progresses, symptoms appear gradually and painlessly and include night blindness, visual field constriction, color vision impairment, floaters, and photopsias. At the advanced stage of BCD, patients experience profound visual impairment and become legally blind.

In 1986, Yugawa et al. [48] classified BCD into the following three stages:

- Stage 1: RPE atrophy with uniform fine white crystalline deposits is observed in the macular area.
- Stage 2: RPE atrophy extends beyond the posterior pole. Choriocapillaris atrophy, in addition to RPE atrophy, appears markedly at the posterior pole. Crystalline deposits in the lesion vary in shape and size and tend to become confluent. The number of crystalline deposits is lower in the advanced atrophic areas of the RPE-choriocapillaris complex.
- Stage 3: RPE-choriocapillaris complex atrophy is observed throughout the fundus. The total number of crystalline deposits decreases.

Corneal involvement of crystalline deposits can be observed by slit lamp examination. The crystalline deposits are of variable size and are situated throughout the corneal stroma. They are more numerous near the corneal limbus and do not disturb the visual acuity. In contrast to retinal crystalline deposits, they persist in the advanced stages of BCD (Fig. 14.3).

OCT imaging shows global thinning in the posterior pole and the presence of crystalline deposits (Fig. 14.4). The crystalline deposits appear as hyperreflective spots. These spots can be observed not only in the RPE and BM but also throughout the neurosensory retina and choroid [41, 49, 50]. OCT also shows the loss of the IS/OS junction and external limiting membrane, as well as the formation of tubulations in the outer retina [47]. CNV is not common in patients with BCD; however, if present, careful evaluation and management are required.

FAF can be used to detect the progression of BCD. Hypoautofluorescence is representative of RPE cell loss, and it corresponds to atrophic lesions on OCT. Notably, crystalline deposits in BCD cannot be found in FAF because these deposits are a collection of cholesterol esters [51]. In the early stages of BCD, FA shows hyperfluorescent window defects. Hypofluorescent areas can be seen in the FA in the late stage of the BCD. FA is also useful for the detection of CNVs. ICG shows a lobular

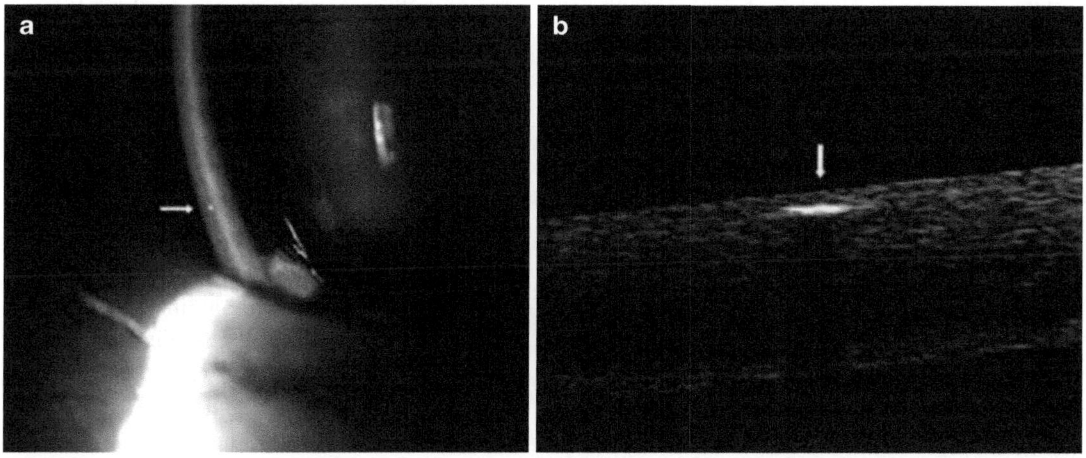

Fig. 14.3 (**a**) Slit-lamp biomicroscopic images showing glistening white crystal-like deposits (arrow) in the cornea. (**b**) Anterior segment OCT shows hyperreflective plaques (arrow) located beneath the corneal epithelium in the corresponding area of **a**

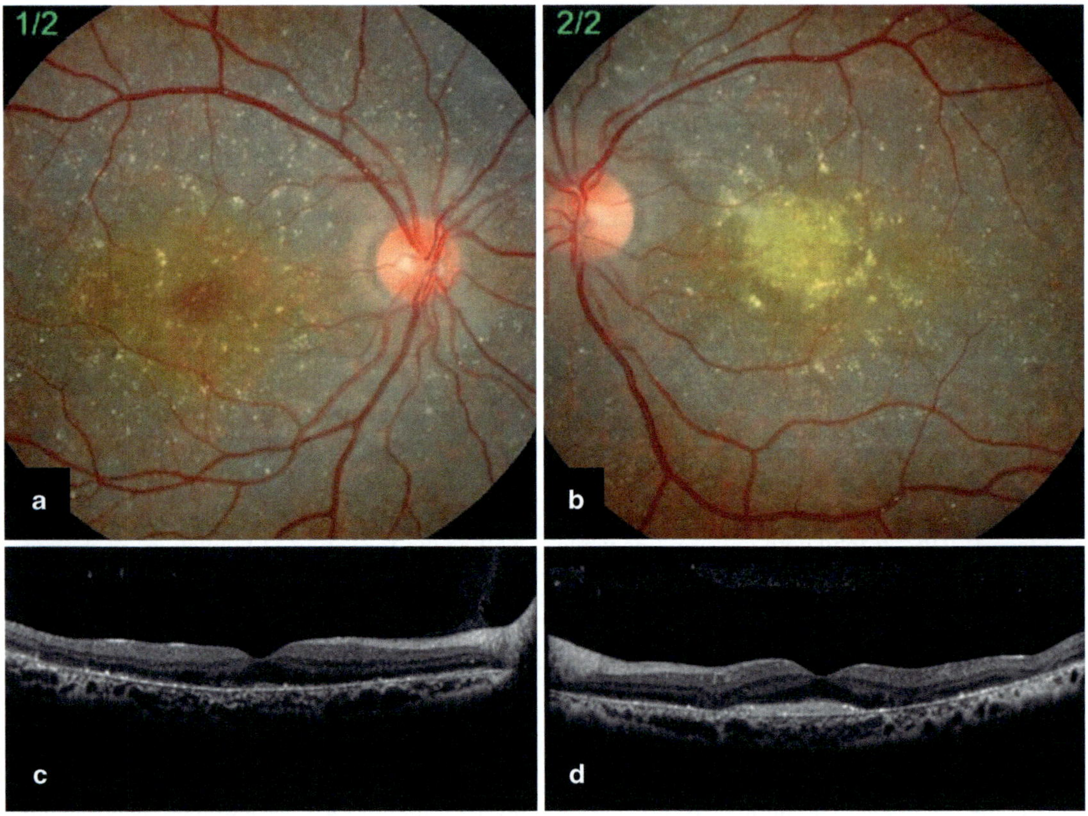

Fig. 14.4 Fundus photography (**a**, **b**) and OCT findings (**c**, **d**) of a patient with BCD. (**a**, **b**) Fundus examination shows mild retinal atrophy and multiple crystalline deposits. CNV membrane is observed in the left eye. (**c**, **d**) OCT shows crystalline deposits as hyperreflective spots. CNV membrane can also be found between the outer retina and RPE

pattern of hypofluorescent lesions in the late phase, and these lesions are thought to be areas of choriocapillaris nonperfusion [52]. The ERG pattern is related to the severity of BCD. Various features of ERG have been described, such as reduced amplitude of scotopic response, photopic response, and non-recordable ERG [53].

14.4.3 Differential Diagnosis

Retinal diseases that present with crystalline deposits in the retina need to be differentiated from BCD. Nadim et al. classified these diseases into systemic disorders, drug-induced disorders, primary ocular disorders, and embolic diseases [54]. Since diffuse RPE dystrophy without obvious crystalline deposits occurs in the advanced stage of BCD, it is difficult to differentiate it from retinal degenerative diseases, such as retinitis pigmentosa and choroideremia.

- Systemic disorders: oxalosis, cystinosis, hyperornithinemia, and Sjögren–Larsson syndrome.
- Drug-induced disorders: tamoxifen, canthaxanthin, talc, and nitrofurantoin.
- Primary ocular disorders: calcified macular drusen, idiopathic parafoveal telangiectasis, and long-standing retinal detachment.
- Embolic diseases: calcium emboli and cholesterol emboli.

14.4.4 Treatment

Currently, there is no proven medical or surgical treatment for BCD. In cases of coexisting CNV, ophthalmologists should be aware that they can be treated with intravitreal anti-VEGF injections [55].

References

1. Sorsby A, Mason MEJ, Gardener N. A fundus dystrophy with unusual features (late onset and dominant inheritance of a central retinal lesion showing oedema, haemorrhage and exudates developing into generalised choroidal atrophy with massive pigment proliferation). Br J Ophthalmol. 1949;33(2):67.
2. Weber BH, Vogt G, Pruett RC, Stöhr H, Felbor U. Mutations in the tissue inhibitor of metalloproteinases-3 (TIMP3) in patients with Sorsby's fundus dystrophy. Nat Genet. 1994;8(4):352–6.
3. Felbor U, Stohr H, Amann T, Schonherr U, Weber BH. A novel Ser156Cys mutation in the tissue inhibitor of metalloproteinases-3 (TIMP3) in Sorsby's fundus dystrophy with unusual clinical features. Hum Mol Genet. 1995;4(12):2415–6. https://doi.org/10.1093/hmg/4.12.2415.
4. Jacobson SG, Cideciyan AV, Bennett J, Kingsley RM, Sheffield VC, Stone EM. Novel mutation in the TIMP3 gene causes Sorsby fundus dystrophy. Arch Ophthalmol. 2002;120(3):376–9. https://doi.org/10.1001/archopht.120.3.376.
5. Langton KP, Barker MD, McKie N. Localization of the functional domains of human tissue inhibitor of metalloproteinases-3 and the effects of a Sorsby's fundus dystrophy mutation. J Biol Chem. 1998;273(27):16778–81. https://doi.org/10.1074/jbc.273.27.16778.
6. Langton KP, McKie N, Curtis A, Goodship JA, Bond PM, Barker MD, et al. A novel tissue inhibitor of metalloproteinases-3 mutation reveals a common molecular phenotype in Sorsby's fundus dystrophy. J Biol Chem. 2000;275(35):27027–31. https://doi.org/10.1074/jbc.M909677199.
7. Langton KP, McKie N, Smith BM, Brown NJ, Barker MD. Sorsby's fundus dystrophy mutations impair turnover of TIMP-3 by retinal pigment epithelial cells. Hum Mol Genet. 2005;14(23):3579–86. https://doi.org/10.1093/hmg/ddi385.
8. Majid MA, Smith VA, Easty DL, Baker AH, Newby AC. Sorsby's fundus dystrophy mutant tissue inhibitors of metalloproteinase-3 induce apoptosis of retinal pigment epithelial and MCF-7 cells. FEBS Lett. 2002;529(2–3):281–5.
9. Qi JH, Ebrahem Q, Moore N, Murphy G, Claesson-Welsh L, Bond M, et al. A novel function for tissue inhibitor of metalloproteinases-3 (TIMP3): inhibition of angiogenesis by blockage of VEGF binding to VEGF receptor-2. Nat Med. 2003;9(4):407–15. https://doi.org/10.1038/nm846.
10. Sivaprasad S, Webster AR, Egan CA, Bird AC, Tufail A. Clinical course and treatment outcomes of Sorsby fundus dystrophy. Am J Ophthalmol. 2008;146(2):228–34. https://doi.org/10.1016/j.ajo.2008.03.024.
11. Hamilton WK, Ewing CC, Ives EJ, Carruthers JD. Sorsby's fundus dystrophy. Ophthalmology. 1989;96(12):1755–62. https://doi.org/10.1016/s0161-6420(89)32647-9.
12. Jacobson SG, Cideciyan AV, Regunath G, Rodriguez FJ, Vandenburgh K, Sheffield VC, et al. Night blindness in Sorsby's fundus dystrophy reversed by vitamin A. Nat Genet. 1995;11(1):27–32.
13. Gliem M, Muller PL, Mangold E, Holz FG, Bolz HJ, Stohr H, et al. Sorsby fundus dystrophy: novel mutations, novel phenotypic characteristics, and treatment outcomes. Invest Ophthalmol Vis Sci. 2015;56(4):2664–76. https://doi.org/10.1167/iovs.14-15733.
14. Small KW. North Carolina macular dystrophy, revisited. Ophthalmology. 1989;96(12):1747–54. https://doi.org/10.1016/s0161-6420(89)32655-8.
15. Small KW, Killian J, McLean WC. North Carolina's dominant progressive foveal dystrophy: how progressive is it? Br J Ophthalmol. 1991;75(7):401–6. https://doi.org/10.1136/bjo.75.7.401.
16. Small KW, Weber JL, Hung WY, Vance J, Roses A, Pericak-Vance M. North Carolina macular dystrophy: exclusion map using RFLPs and microsatellites. Genomics. 1991;11(3):763–6. https://doi.org/10.1016/0888-7543(91)90087-u.
17. Michaelides M, Johnson S, Tekriwal AK, Holder GE, Bellmann C, Kinning E, et al. An early-onset autosomal dominant macular dystrophy (MCDR3) resembling North Carolina macular dystrophy maps to chromosome 5. Invest Ophthalmol Vis Sci. 2003;44(5):2178–83. https://doi.org/10.1167/iovs.02-1094.
18. Rosenberg T, Roos B, Johnsen T, Bech N, Scheetz TE, Larsen M, et al. Clinical and genetic characterization of a Danish family with North Carolina macular dystrophy. Mol Vis. 2010;16:2659–68.
19. Doyne RW. Peculiar condition of choroiditis occurring in several members of the same family. Trans Ophthalmol Soc UK. 1899;19:71.
20. Vaclavik V, Munier FL. Malattia Leventinese (autosomal dominant drusen). In: Querques G, Souied E, editors. Macular dystrophies. Cham: Springer; 2016. p. 39–51.
21. Forni S, Babel J. Etude clinique et histologique de la malattia leventinese. Ophthalmologica. 1962;143(5):313–22.
22. Stone EM, Lotery AJ, Munier FL, Heon E, Piguet B, Guymer RH, et al. A single EFEMP1 mutation associated with both Malattia Leventinese and Doyne honeycomb retinal dystrophy. Nat Genet. 1999;22(2):199–202. https://doi.org/10.1038/9722.

23. Marmorstein LY, Munier FL, Arsenijevic Y, Schorderet DF, McLaughlin PJ, Chung D, et al. Aberrant accumulation of EFEMP1 underlies drusen formation in Malattia Leventinese and age-related macular degeneration. Proc Natl Acad Sci U S A. 2002;99(20):13067–72. https://doi.org/10.1073/pnas.202491599.
24. Fu L, Garland D, Yang Z, Shukla D, Rajendran A, Pearson E, et al. The R345W mutation in EFEMP1 is pathogenic and causes AMD-like deposits in mice. Hum Mol Genet. 2007;16(20):2411–22. https://doi.org/10.1093/hmg/ddm198.
25. Stanton JB, Marmorstein AD, Zhang Y, Marmorstein LY. Deletion of Efemp1 is protective against the development of sub-RPE deposits in mouse eyes. Invest Ophthalmol Vis Sci. 2017;58(3):1455–61. https://doi.org/10.1167/iovs.16-20955.
26. Gerber DM, Munier FL, Niemeyer G. Cross-sectional study of visual acuity and electroretinogram in two types of dominant drusen. Invest Ophthalmol Vis Sci. 2003;44(2):493–6. https://doi.org/10.1167/iovs.01-0787.
27. Haimovici R, Wroblewski J, Piguet B, Fitzke FW, Holder GE, Arden GB, et al. Symptomatic abnormalities of dark adaptation in patients with EFEMP1 retinal dystrophy (Malattia Leventinese/Doyne honeycomb retinal dystrophy). Eye (Lond). 2002;16(1):7–15. https://doi.org/10.1038/sj.eye.6700018.
28. Michaelides M, Jenkins SA, Brantley MA, Andrews RM, Waseem N, Luong V, et al. Maculopathy due to the R345W substitution in fibulin-3: distinct clinical features, disease variability, and extent of retinal dysfunction. Invest Ophthalmol Vis Sci. 2006;47(7):3085–97.
29. Evans K, Gregory CY, Wijesuriya SD, Kermani S, Jay MR, Plant C, et al. Assessment of the phenotypic range seen in Doyne honeycomb retinal dystrophy. Arch Ophthalmol. 1997;115(7):904–10. https://doi.org/10.1001/archopht.1997.01100160074012.
30. Heon E, Piguet B, Munier F, Sneed SR, Morgan CM, Forni S, et al. Linkage of autosomal dominant radial drusen (malattia leventinese) to chromosome 2p16-21. Arch Ophthalmol. 1996;114(2):193–8. https://doi.org/10.1001/archopht.1996.01100130187014.
31. Sohn EH, Patel PJ, MacLaren RE, Adatia FA, Pal B, Webster AR, et al. Responsiveness of choroidal neovascular membranes in patients with R345W mutation in fibulin 3 (Doyne honeycomb retinal dystrophy) to anti-vascular endothelial growth factor therapy. Arch Ophthalmol. 2011;129(12):1626–8. https://doi.org/10.1001/archophthalmol.2011.338.
32. Takeuchi T, Hayashi T, Bedell M, Zhang K, Yamada H, Tsuneoka H. A novel haplotype with the R345W mutation in the EFEMP1 gene associated with autosomal dominant drusen in a Japanese family. Invest Ophthalmol Vis Sci. 2010;51(3):1643–50. https://doi.org/10.1167/iovs.09-4497.
33. Zhang T, Xie X, Cao G, Jiang H, Wu S, Su Z, et al. Malattia leventinese/Doyne honeycomb retinal dystrophy in a Chinese family with mutation of the EFEMP1 gene. Retina. 2014;34(12):2462–71. https://doi.org/10.1097/IAE.0000000000000259.
34. Pager CK, Sarin LK, Federman JL, Eagle R, Hageman G, Rosenow J, et al. Malattia leventinese presenting with subretinal neovascular membrane and hemorrhage. Am J Ophthalmol. 2001;131(4):517–8. https://doi.org/10.1016/s0002-9394(00)00821-7.
35. Gregory CY, Evans K, Wijesuriya SD, Kermani S, Jay MR, Plant C, et al. The gene responsible for autosomal dominant Doyne's honeycomb retinal dystrophy (DHRD) maps to chromosome 2p16. Hum Mol Genet. 1996;5(7):1055–9. https://doi.org/10.1093/hmg/5.7.1055.
36. Song JS, Oh BL, Park UC, Yu HG, Lee EK. Autosomal dominant drusen confirmed by molecular genetics. J Korean Ophthalmol Soc. 2021;62(1):120–126.
37. Querques G, Guigui B, Leveziel N, Querques L, Bandello F, Souied EH. Multimodal morphological and functional characterization of Malattia Leventinese. Graefes Arch Clin Exp Ophthalmol. 2013;251(3):705–14. https://doi.org/10.1007/s00417-012-2106-5.
38. Guigui B, Leveziel N, Martinet V, Massamba N, Sterkers M, Coscas G, et al. Angiography features of early onset drusen. Br J Ophthalmol. 2011;95(2):238–44. https://doi.org/10.1136/bjo.2009.178400.
39. Kang EY-C, Wang N-K. Bietti's crystalline dystrophy. In: Cheung G, editor. Hereditary chorioretinal disorders. Singapore: Springer; 2020. p. 119–38.
40. Welch RB. Bietti's tapetoretinal degeneration with marginal corneal dystrophy crystalline retinopathy. Trans Am Ophthalmol Soc. 1977;75:164–79.
41. Li A, Jiao X, Munier FL, Schorderet DF, Yao W, Iwata F, et al. Bietti crystalline corneoretinal dystrophy is caused by mutations in the novel gene CYP4V2. Am J Hum Genet. 2004;74(5):817–26. https://doi.org/10.1086/383228.
42. Lockhart CM, Nakano M, Rettie AE, Kelly EJ. Generation and characterization of a murine model of Bietti crystalline dystrophy. Invest Ophthalmol Vis Sci. 2014;55(9):5572–81. https://doi.org/10.1167/iovs.13-13717.
43. Lee J, Jiao X, Hejtmancik JF, Kaiser-Kupfer M, Chader GJ. Identification, isolation, and characterization of a 32-kDa fatty acid-binding protein missing from lymphocytes in humans with Bietti crystalline dystrophy (BCD). Mol Genet Metab. 1998;65(2):143–54. https://doi.org/10.1006/mgme.1998.2723.
44. Lee J, Jiao X, Hejtmancik JF, Kaiser-Kupfer M, Gahl WA, Markello TC, et al. The metabolism of fatty acids in human Bietti crystalline dystrophy. Invest Ophthalmol Vis Sci. 2001;42(8):1707–14.
45. Kelly EJ, Nakano M, Rohatgi P, Yarov-Yarovoy V, Rettie AE. Finding homes for orphan cytochrome P450s. CYP4V2 and CYP4F22 in disease states. Mol Interv. 2011;11(2):124–32. https://doi.org/10.1124/mi.11.2.10.
46. Kaiser-Kupfer MI, Chan C-C, Markello TC, Crawford MA, Caruso RC, Csaky KG, et al. Clinical biochemical and pathologic correlations in Bietti's crystalline dystrophy. Am J Ophthalmol. 1994;118(5):569–82.

47. Halford S, Liew G, Mackay DS, Sergouniotis PI, Holt R, Broadgate S, et al. Detailed phenotypic and genotypic characterization of Bietti crystalline dystrophy. Ophthalmology. 2014;121(6):1174–84. https://doi.org/10.1016/j.ophtha.2013.11.042.
48. Yuzawa M, Mae Y, Matsui M. Bietti's crystalline retinopathy. Ophthalmic Paediatr Genet. 1986;7(1):9–20.
49. Rossi S, Testa F, Li A, Yaylacioglu F, Gesualdo C, Hejtmancik JF, et al. Clinical and genetic features in Italian Bietti crystalline dystrophy patients. Br J Ophthalmol. 2013;97(2):174–9. https://doi.org/10.1136/bjophthalmol-2012-302469.
50. Toto L, Carpineto P, Parodi MB, Di Antonio L, Mastropasqua A, Mastropasqua L. Spectral domain optical coherence tomography and in vivo confocal microscopy imaging of a case of Bietti's crystalline dystrophy. Clin Exp Optom. 2013;96(1):39–45. https://doi.org/10.1111/j.1444-0938.2012.00784.x.
51. Wilson DJ, Weleber RG, Klein ML, Welch RB, Green WR. Bietti's crystalline dystrophy: a clinicopathologic correlative study. Arch Ophthalmol. 1989;107(2):213–21.
52. Fong AM, Koh A, Lee K, Ang CL. Bietti's crystalline dystrophy in Asians: clinical, angiographic and electrophysiological characteristics. Int Ophthalmol. 2009;29(6):459–70. https://doi.org/10.1007/s10792-008-9266-7.
53. Yanagi Y, Tamaki Y, Takahashi H, Sekine H, Mori M, Hirato T, et al. Clinical and functional findings in crystalline retinopathy. Retina. 2004;24(2):267–74.
54. Nadim F, Walid H, Adib J. The differential diagnosis of crystals in the retina. Int Ophthalmol. 2001;24(3):113–21.
55. Fuerst NM, Serrano L, Han G, Morgan JI, Maguire AM, Leroy BP, et al. Detailed functional and structural phenotype of Bietti crystalline dystrophy associated with mutations in CYP4V2 complicated by choroidal neovascularization. Ophthalmic Genet. 2016;37(4):445–52. https://doi.org/10.3109/13816810.2015.1126616.

Hereditary Vitreoretinal Degenerations

15

So Hyun Bae

Abstract

The hereditary vitreoretinal degenerations contain a heterogenous group of disease entities with a wide variability of phenotypes. Clinical diagnosis of these conditions would be difficult due to overlapping clinical features among them. Now, the advances in clinical and molecular genetic studies have contributed to the assessment to define and diagnose these conditions properly. This chapter deals with several types of disorders covering chondrodysplasias with vitreoretinal degeneration including Stickler syndrome, Wagner syndrome, snowflake vitreoretinal degeneration, retinal nuclear receptor-related diseases including enhanced S-cone syndrome and autosomal dominant vitreoretinochoroidopathy. The purpose of this chapter is to provide an overview of these disorders.

Keywords

Snowflake vitreoretinal degeneration
Stickler syndrome · Wagner syndrome
Enhanced S-cone syndrome
Goldmann–Favre syndrome

S. H. Bae (✉)
Department of Ophthalmology, Kangnam Sacred Heart Hospital, Hallym University School of Medicine, Yeongdeungpo-gu, Seoul, South Korea

15.1 Chondrodysplasias Associated with Vitreoretinal Degeneration

In 1965, Stickler et al. [1] published their report on hereditary progressive arthro-ophthalmopathy. Now it is known to contain five subgroups that belong to the family of chondrodysplasias associated with vitreoretinal degeneration as follows; Stickler syndrome, Marshall syndrome, Knobloch syndrome, Kniest dysplasia, and Weissenbacher–Zweymüller syndrome.

15.1.1 Stickler Syndrome

15.1.1.1 Molecular Genetics

Stickler syndrome is a connective disorder that affects the systemic formation of collagen resulting in ocular, orofacial, auditory, and musculoskeletal abnormalities. In the human vitreous, collagen forms a network of heterotypic fibrils which consists of type II, V/XI, and IX. Collagen consists of a trimer of three α chains (peptide) which are folded into a helical structure. Collagen type II is the most abundant collagen in the vitreous. It consists of three identical α chains (homotrimer) encoded in a single gene of *COL2A1* (COL=collagen, 2=type II, A1=α1 peptide). Whereas collagen type IX and XI are formed by different peptide chains (heterotrimers). Type IX collagen is encoded in three different genes called *COL9A1, COL9A2,* and

H.-G. Yu (ed.), *Inherited Retinal Disease*, https://doi.org/10.1007/978-981-16-7337-5_15

COL9A3. Type XI collagen is encoded in genes called *COL11A1, COL11A2,* and *COL2A1*. Type XI collagen is found in distinct forms in cartilage and vitreous; the α1(IX) chain is expressed in both cartilage and vitreous while the α2(XI) chain is chiefly in non-ocular tissue. Thus, mutations in the *COL11A2* gene do not affect ocular tissue resulting in non-ocular Stickler syndrome (type 3).

Stickler syndrome is subclassified into several types based on genetic heterogeneity. The majority of patients have type 1 Stickler syndrome, which is caused by mutations in the *COL2A1* gene on chromosome 12q13, encoding type II collagen [2]. The families with premature stop codon mutations in exon 2 of the *COL2A1* gene exhibited predominant ocular features with no or minimal extraocular abnormalities, known as ocular only Stickler syndrome [3]. Other types of mutations in the *COL2A1* gene cause a wide range of severity in skeletal dysplasia as follows: severe dysplasia in achondrogenesis type II and hypochondrogenesis and intermediate severity in spondyloepiphyseal dysplasia congenita and Kniest dysplasia. Type 1 Stickler syndrome is the most common type II collagenopathy with a mild phenotype.

Types 2 and 3 Stickler syndromes are caused by mutations in the *COL11A1* gene on chromosome 1p21 [4] and in the *COL11A2* gene on chromosome 6p21 encoding type XI collagen [5], respectively. Type 3 Stickler syndrome is known as non-ocular Stickler syndrome which has only extraocular findings as stated above. Stickler syndrome, types 1, 2, and 3 are inherited in autosomal dominant patterns with high penetrance. In addition, several studies described autosomal recessive Stickler syndrome caused by mutations in collagen IX genes, such as *COL9A1* (type 4), *COL9A2* (type 5), and *COL9A3*, which locate on chromosome 6q13, 1p34, and 20q13 [6–8]. Recently, small families in the autosomal recessive pattern were found to have mutations in *LRP2* (lipoprotein receptor-related protein-2) and *LOXL3* (encoding lysyl oxidase-like 3) [9, 10].

15.1.1.2 Clinical Phenotypes

Ocular Findings

Patients with Stickler syndrome can present a wide range of ocular phenotypes including congenital high myopia, cataract, glaucoma, and vitreoretinal abnormalities such as congenital vitreous anomaly, radial perivascular retinal degeneration, and rhegmatogenous retinal detachment.

Most of the patients are myopic, which is typically congenital, non-progressive, and of a high degree. Patients may present congenital and non-progressive cataracts, shown as a distinctive wedge or fleck-shaped cataract such as quadrantic lamellar feature (Fig. 15.1). Drainage angle abnormalities may predispose patients to glaucoma. The optic nerve is normal.

Congenital vitreous anomaly is the pathognomonic feature of Stickler syndrome. Type 1 Stickler syndrome usually has a membranous vitreous anomaly presenting as retrolental folded membrane behind which it is empty vitreous space [11]. While an irregular and beaded vitreous is presented in type 2 Stickler syndrome [12]. Ocular only Stickler syndrome presents hypoplastic vitreous which may be optically empty [13]. In Stickler syndrome, radial perivascular

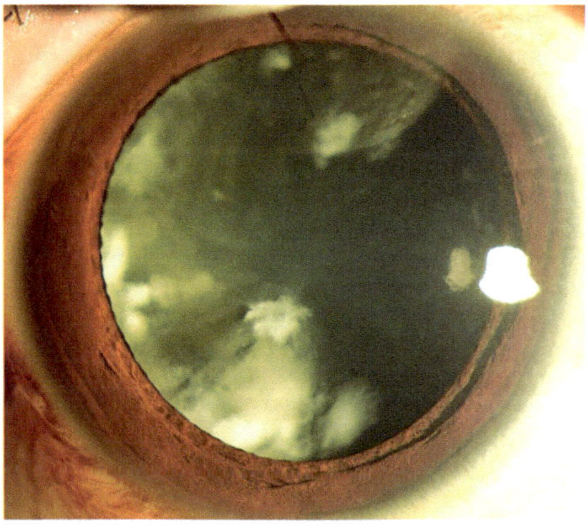

Fig. 15.1 Quadrantic lamellar cataract in Stickler syndrome

retinal degeneration [14] may develop in childhood which becomes worse with age resulting in perivascular pigment accumulation (Fig. 15.2). In addition, circumferential lattice degeneration is frequently observed.

Stickler syndrome is the most common inherited cause of non-traumatic rhegmatogenous retinal detachment in childhood (Fig. 15.3). The patients with Stickler syndrome have life-long risks of retinal detachment with the age of onset mostly ranging from 10 to 30 years [15, 16]. The incidence of retinal detachment has been reported up to 60% [17]. In addition, Ang et al. [18] has reported even higher risk over 70% in type 1 Stickler syndrome with almost half of them having bilateral giant retinal tears in childhood. Multiple or posteriorly located retinal tears are also often detected. Abnormalities of vitreous and vitreoretinal interface have been regarded as a predisposing factor to retinal detachment.

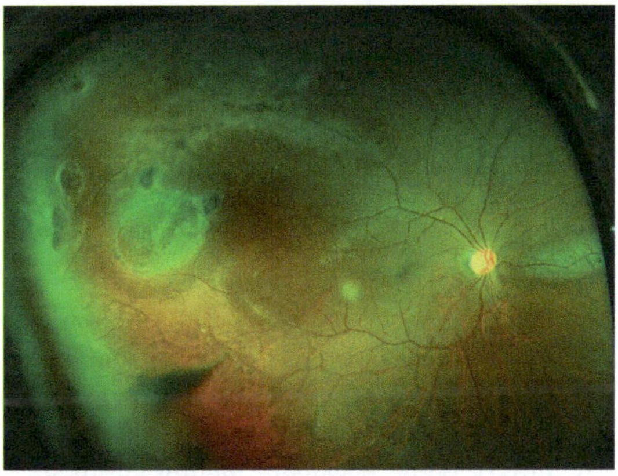

Fig. 15.2 Radial perivascular retinal degeneration with clumps of pigmentation in Stickler syndrome

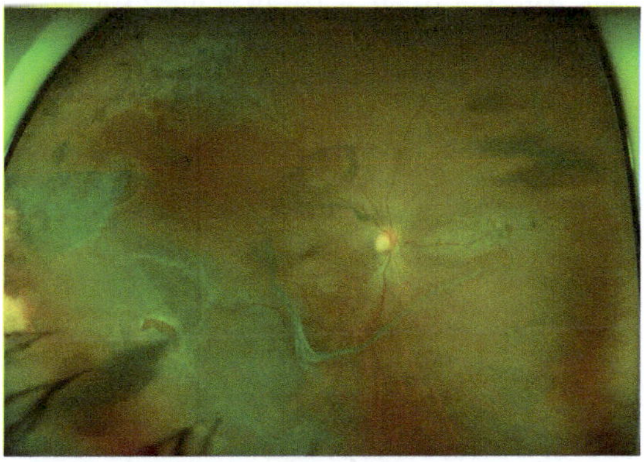

Fig. 15.3 Rhegmatogenous retinal detachment in Stickler syndrome. All images are provided by Sang Jin Kim in Sungkyunkwan university

Extraocular Findings

Orofacial abnormalities in Stickler syndrome include mid-face hypoplasia, micrognathia, as well as midline cleft ranging from cleft palate to bifid uvula. Hearing difficulties are well-known in Stickler syndrome. Although its pathogenesis is not clear, the causes of hearing loss would be a conductive or sensorineural loss. Conductive hearing deficits may result from recurrent otitis media secondary to palate abnormalities or ossicle defects [19]. Sensorineural hearing loss may be associated with abnormal structure of the cochlear. In addition, patients with non-ocular Stickler syndrome have been reported to experience worse hearing loss. Patients with Stickler syndrome have a wide range of musculoskeletal manifestations. Joint hypermobility may be common in younger patients; however, it reduces with age resulting in early-onset degenerative osteoarthritis by the third or fourth decade [20]. Spine abnormalities are frequently found such as flattened vertebral bodies, endplate abnormalities, and scoliosis. Mild spondyloepiphyseal dysplasia is also common. Slender extremities and long fingers have been reported. Height is normal. Liberfarb and Goldblatt [21] reported mitral valve prolapse in 45.6% of Stickler syndrome patients; however, a more recent study by Snead [22] did not detect any valvular disease in Stickler syndrome.

15.1.1.3 Management

Management of retinal detachment in Stickler syndrome is challenging, often needs multiple surgeries due to re-detachment. Therefore, prophylactic treatments have been tried to reduce the risk of retinal detachment. Several retrospective studies have reported the favorable efficacy and safety of prophylactic treatments including cryotherapy or laser photocoagulation [18, 23, 24]. In 2008, a retrospective study by Ang et al. [18] demonstrated the benefits of 360° cryotherapy against retinal detachment from giant retinal tears in type 1 Stickler syndrome [18]. In this study, 73% of patients untreated with cryotherapy experienced retinal detachment with 48% of them bilateral. In contrast, only 8% of patients who underwent cryotherapy developed retinal detachment without a case of bilateral detachment. In 2014, they have reported extended results of prophylactic cryotherapy in 487 type 1 patients referred as the Cambridge prophylactic cryotherapy protocol [23]. They demonstrated a 7.4-fold increased risk of retinal detachment in the controls compared to the bilateral prophylaxis group. In addition, the risk of development of a second eye retinal detachment without cryotherapy was 10.3-fold compared to those who underwent cryotherapy after retinal detachment in the fellow eyes. However, these studies would be biased due to their study design. In addition, circumferential interventions could not prevent retinal detachment secondary to posterior retinal tears. To determine the guidelines for prophylactic interventions, more well-designed clinical trials are needed.

15.1.2 Marshall Syndrome

Marshall syndrome is characterized by myopia, congenital cataract, liquefied vitreous, midfacial hypoplasia, and congenital hearing loss [25]. It shows a round face with a very flat nasal bridge, while Stickler syndrome has a long face with a normal nasal bridge. Ectodermal abnormalities have been reported in Marshall syndrome. It is inherited in autosomal dominant pattern. It is caused by a mutation of the *COL11A1* gene, like type 2 Stickler syndrome. The splicing mutations of 54-bp exons in the C-terminal region of the *COL11A1* gene have been reported in Marshall syndrome [26]. There has been a debate whether Marshall syndrome belongs to a different disease entity from Stickler syndrome. Ayme and Preus [27] concluded that Marshall syndrome is a distinct disorder based on their cluster analysis.

15.1.3 Knobloch Syndrome

Knobloch syndrome is an autosomal recessive developmental disorder characterized by distinct ocular and occipital abnormalities. The ocular abnormalities include high myopia, absence of iris crypt, cataract, lens subluxation, vitreoretinal degeneration, and retinal detachment. Khan et al. described typical features of vitreoretinal degeneration including severe chorioretinal atrophy with prominent choroidal vessel show, macular atrophy, and white fibrillar vitreous condensations [28]. The occipital anomalies have variable phenotypes ranging from occult cutis aplasia to occipital skull defect with or without encephalocele [28]. In 2000, Sertie et al. [29] identified homozygous acceptor splice mutation in the *COL18A1* gene on chromosome 21q22 in a Brazilian family with Knobloch syndrome. *COL18A1* encodes a basement membrane proteoglycan, collagen XVIII, which is widely expressed in multiple organs, especially in ocular tissue including iris, ciliary body, basement membrane of RPE and Bruch's membrane. It has an important role in ocular and neurologic development. Until now, numerous mutations in *COL18A1* have been detected in other families with Knobloch syndrome such as homozygous frameshift mutation [30]. Whereas, Aldahmesh et al. [31] has proposed the *ADAMTS18* gene as a causal gene for Knobloch syndrome in one Saudi patient. However, they later found aberrant splicing in the *COL18A1* gene in the same patient, concluding that *ADAMTS18* did not cause this condition [32].

15.1.4 Kniest Dysplasia

Kniest dysplasia is an autosomal dominant disorder that is caused by heterozygous mutations in the *COL2A1* gene like type 1 Stickler syndrome. Kniest dysplasia has distinguishable skeletal and craniofacial abnormalities including dwarfism with a short trunk and limbs, kyphoscoliosis, enlargement and contracture of joints and cleft palate. It has abnormal ocular features such as congenital myopia, vitreous degeneration, and retinal detachment [33]. In addition, hearing loss often occurs. Skeletal deformity becomes worse with age, resulting in severe dwarfism.

15.1.5 Weissenbacher–Zweymüller Syndrome

Weissenbacher–Zweymüller syndrome (WZS) is characterized by the Pierre-Robin sequence, midfacial hypoplasia, snub nose, short proximal limb with dumbbell-shaped femora, and humeri without any ocular abnormalities [34]. In contrast to Kniest dysplasia, the bone changes subsequently resolved resulting in normal growth in adulthood. Sensorineural hearing loss was reported. It is caused by a mutation in the *COL11A2* gene on chromosome 6p21 like non-ocular Stickler syndrome. Giedion et al. [35] proposed WZS to be named as otospondylomegaepiphyseal dysplasia. While, Pihlajamaa et al. [36] suggested that WZS and non-ocular Stickler syndrome are the same disorder.

15.2 Wagner Syndrome

Wagner syndrome was firstly described in a Swiss family in 1938 [37]. Historically, it was considered as the same entity with Stickler syndrome, referred to Wagner–Stickler syndrome due to overlapping clinical features. However, now, Wagner syndrome is considered as a distinct entity from Stickler syndrome with the advance of genetic analysis. Whereas, previously, erosive vitreoretinopathy and Jansen syndrome have been described to share similar clinical features with Wagner syndrome. Subsequent linkage studies revealed that these diseases were also linked to regions of chromosome 5, where is also critical for Wagner syndrome [38, 39]. Now they are considered allelic disorders, named as the chromosome 5q retinopathies.

15.2.1 Molecular Genetics

Wagner syndrome is inherited in an autosomal dominant pattern with complete penetrance. Wagner syndrome was first identified to be linked to chromosome 5q13-14 in 1995 [16]. In 2005, Miyamoto et al. [40] found abnormal splicing in the chondroitin sulfate proteoglycan 2 gene (*CSPG2*), now named *VCAN*, encoding for the versican. In human vitreous, versican is known to bind to hyaluronate and link protein, resulting in the formation of large aggregates which support the structural integrity, as well as maintain and regulate the retinal cells [40]. The altered versican might lead to abnormal interaction with vitreous and subsequent severe syneresis of vitreous; however, the mechanism is not certain yet.

15.2.2 Clinical Phenotypes

The phenotypes of Wagner syndrome have a wide range of spectrum and show a progressive course age-dependently. The hallmark of Wagner syndrome is congenitally optically empty vitreous with fibrillary condensations or preretinal avascular membrane, described as strands, veils, or sheets [41–43]. Vitreous abnormalities are usually shown in childhood. Recent study revealed a thick multilayered membrane detached from the fovea with persistent attachment to peri fovea on optical coherence tomography (OCT), which is different from age-related posterior vitreous detachment [44]. Wagner syndrome often presents early-onset cataracts and mild myopia. Pseudostrabismus with a large positive angle kappa was reported due to ectopic fovea in some pedigrees with Wagner syndrome [40, 42, 43].

Chorioretinal degeneration has a progressive course with variable expression. It includes loss of RPE, perivascular or peripheral pigmentation, and chorioretinal atrophy starting from the periphery, eventually involving the posterior pole in advanced cases. Rhegmatogenous retinal detachment is less complicated, late-onset, and occurs infrequently compared to Stickler syndrome. Whereas, the incidence of peripheral tractional retinal detachment has been reported as

25% and even over 50% in patients over age 45 in a follow-up study with the original pedigree [42]. Peripheral vascular sheathing, inverted papilla, and glaucoma may be detected. In contrast to Stickler syndrome, the patients with Wagner syndrome do not have any systemic manifestations such as midfacial hypoplasia, arthropathy, or hearing loss.

In early ages, nyctalopia can be present, but vision is usually normal. With advancing age, progressive chorioretinal atrophy or cataract leads to gradual loss of vision even in absence of retinal detachment. Visual field can show variable findings including diffuse peripheral loss or ring scotoma with progressive chorioretinal atrophy [42]. Electrophysiological tests are also usually nearly normal in young patients but become progressively abnormal including impaired dark adaptation, progressive reduction in a- and b-wave amplitudes with better preservation of the b-wave on ERG [41, 42].

In summary, Wagner syndrome has differentiating features from Stickler syndrome such as nyctalopia, progressive chorioretinal atrophy, lower risk of retinal detachment, abnormal retinal function, and absence of systemic findings.

15.2.3 Management

There is no established guideline to treat this condition. The patients should be examined regularly to detect the development of cataracts and retinal detachment. Refractive error, cataract, and retinal detachment should be managed properly.

15.3 Snowflake Vitreoretinal Degeneration

Snowflake vitreoretinal degeneration (SVD) was firstly described in a family, an American family of European ancestry by Hirose et al. in 1974 [45]. The original family of this condition is characterized by cataract, fibrillar vitreous degeneration, and peripheral minute crystallin-like retinal deposits.

15.3.1 Molecular Genetics

SVD shows autosomal dominant inheritance. The mutations in the *KCNJ13* gene on chromosome 2q36, encoding Kir7.1 was reported to cause SVD [46]. Inwardly rectifying potassium channel Kir7.1 is highly expressed in internal limiting membrane and retinal pigment epithelium (RPE). Impaired potassium transport might lead to vitreoretinal degeneration by Müller cell dysfunction [46].

15.3.2 Clinical Phenotypes

Hirose's original family [45] exhibited several distinguishing features including early-onset cataracts, fibrillar vitreous degeneration, and peripheral crystalline-like deposits resembling a snowflake. Although several studies referred to snowflake-like lesions in other families, only one family by Pollack et al. [47] showed clinically identical conditions with Hirose's original family until now. In 2003, Lee et al. [48] reported follow-up results of this original family and described additional distinct features including corneal guttae similar to Fuchs' corneal endothelial dystrophy. In their report, the patients exhibit optic nerve head abnormalities including waxy pallor, peripapillary atrophy, flat-appearing or dysmorphic nerve head [48]. They showed moderate myopia with a mean spherical equivalent of -2.9 diopters [48]. Peripheral retinal deposits are characteristic features represented as minute, yellow-white crystalline-like deposits called snowflakes. Corneal guttae and peripheral retinal degeneration might be progressive resulting in increased retinal pigmentation and sheathing of retinal vessels. Rhegmatogenous retinal detachment was reported in 21% of this family members [48], a relatively lower rate compared to those with Stickler syndrome. In contrast to Stickler syndrome, there are no radial or circumferential lattice degeneration and systemic manifestations such as midfacial maldevelopment, hearing loss, or arthropathy [48]. Hirose et al. [49] demonstrated impaired retinal function with elevated rod thresholds in dark-adaptation tests and reduced scotopic b-wave in dim white light on electroretinogram(ERG); however, the vision is relatively good.

15.3.3 Management

There is no specific management until now. The patients should be educated and examined regularly to detect cataract and retinal detachment.

15.4 Retinal Nuclear Receptor (*NR2E3*)-Related Diseases

15.4.1 Molecular Genetics

The *NR2E3* gene (nuclear receptor subfamily 2, Group E, member 3), also known as photoreceptor-specific nuclear receptor (PNR), encodes a nuclear hormone receptor of ligand-dependent transcription factor which is expressed in photoreceptors [50]. The *NR2E3* gene is located on chromosome 15q23. The NR2E3 protein has a critical role in the regulation of embryogenic development and maintenance of photoreceptors. It enhances the expression of rod-specific genes but represses the cone-specific genes synergistically with other transcription factors such as cone-rod homeobox (CRX) and neural retinal leucine zipper (NRL) [51]. CRX is essential for the expression of photoreceptor-specific genes, such as opsins. NRL promotes rhodopsin expression and represses cone cell fate in photoreceptor progenitor cells. In human retina, there are three cone types referred to long-, middle-, and short-wavelength-sensitive (L, M, and S) cones. The *NR2E3* mutations result in an abnormal ratio of S- to L-/M-cones, suggesting abnormal switching between S- and other cones [52]. Put together, dysfunction of *NR2E3* leads to abnormal differentiation and degeneration of photoreceptors, specifically rod cell differentiation, resulting in excess S-cones at the expense of M- and L-cones and absence of rod [53].

Mutations in the *NR2E3* gene are associated with autosomal recessive vitreoretinal degeneration including Goldmann–Favre syndrome (GFS), enhanced S-cone syndrome (ESCS), and clumped pigmentary retinal degeneration (CPRD). In addition to these recessive retinal degenerations, dominant mutations in *NR2E3* are linked to some autosomal dominant retinitis pigmentosa. Now, GFS, ESCS, and CPRD are considered as the same disease entity in a wide spectrum of manifestations based on electrophysiological, psychophysical, and molecular genetic findings [54].

15.4.2 Clinical Phenotypes

The clinical features in patients with *NR2E3*-related recessive retinal degenerations have great variability in the phenotypes and onset even with the high intrafamilial variability [55]. Those were characterized by early-onset nyctalopia, pigmentary retinal degeneration, retinoschisis, vitreous degeneration, posterior subcapsular cataract, and markedly abnormal ERG findings. Pigmentary retinal degeneration is typically presented as mid-peripheral nummular pigment deposits in the area of the vascular arcades rather than the bone spicule seen in retinitis pigmentosa. While, only subtle pigmentary changes would be also detected shown as white spots, yellow flecks, or focal hyperpigmentation [55–57]. However, clumped pigment retinopathy is not a pathognomic finding for *NR2E3*-related degeneration, since similar fundus findings have been reported in Bardet-Biedl syndrome [58] or some retinitis pigmentosa such as non-syndromic form [59]. Previous OCT study revealed disorganized retinal lamination and the rosette formation in the outer nuclear layer at an advanced stage [57]. Some patients would have cystoid maculopathy or retinoschisis in either macula or peripheral retina similar to X-linked retinoschisis. Vitreous is usually severely liquefied resulting in an optically empty cavity containing vitreous strands or membranes. Visual acuity loss is a variable ranging from normal to marked reduction regardless of age. Poor visual acuity is often related to macular retinoschisis, cataract, and pigmentary retinal degeneration. Visual field tests show defects similar to retinitis pigmentosa corresponding to the areas of retinoschisis and retinal degeneration.

15.4.3 Electrophysiology

There is a high variability of severity in ERG abnormalities, even reported cases with mild impairment and preserved rod function. However, the traditional full-field ERG results include the following findings: (1) undetectable rod response; (2) similar waveforms to a standard single flash under photopic and scotopic; and (3) abnormally reduced amplitude of photopic 30-Hz flicker ERG rather than that of a-wave in single flash photopic ERG [56]. Spectral ERG testing revealed a hypersensitivity of the S-cones and reduced sensitivity of M- or L-cones [60]. The ERG testing shows great amplitude to a blue light flash on an orange background and severely reduced response to an intensity-matched, orange light flash on a green background. While Audo et al. [56] reported the progressively reduced amplitudes of b-wave without a change of a-wave as the stimulus duration of blue flash increased, suggesting OFF-related ERG activity in some patients with ESCS. However, in normal retina, S-cones are connected to ON-bipolar cells, while M- and L-cones connected to both ON- and OFF-bipolar cells. This may reflect an abnormal development of second-order neural network indicating S-cones connected to ON- and OFF-bipolar cells or secondary replacement of M- and L-cone opsins by S-cone opsin, although there is no established consensus yet [56, 61].

15.4.4 Management

There is no specific treatment for this condition.

15.5 Autosomal Dominant Vitreoretinochoroidopathy

Autosomal dominant vitreoretinochoroidopathy (ADVIRC) was firstly described in 1982 by Kaufman et al. [62] This condition is characterized by peripheral circumferential hyperpigmentation which is sharply demarcated from the normal central retina, midperipheral chorioretinal atrophy, fibrillar vitreous condensation, intraretinal white opacities, preretinal neovascularization, and macular edema [62]. It is also associated with abnormal ocular development including nanophthalmos, microcornea, iris dysgenesis, angle-closure glaucoma, optic nerve dysplasia, and cataract [63]. In 2004, Yardley et al. [64] found the missense mutations in the *BEST1* gene in the patients with ADVIRC, which was originally known to cause Best vitelliform macular dystrophy. The *Best1* gene encodes the transmembrane bestrophin-1 protein which is expressed in the basolateral membrane of RPE [65]. The electrooculogram is usually severely reduced in *BEST1*-related ADVIRC patients [63], supporting the abnormalities at the level of RPE. However, in some cases with mild phenotypes, it may be nearly normal. The ERG findings vary between the patients from normal to reduced rod and cone responses in advanced cases. Nyctalopia is absent.

References

1. Stickler GB, Belau PG, Farrell FJ, Jones JD, Pugh DG, Steinberg AG, et al. Hereditary progressive arthro-ophthalmopathy. Mayo Clin Proc. 1965;40:433–55.
2. Snead MP, Payne SJ, Barton DE, Yates JR, al-Imara L, Pope FM, et al. Stickler syndrome: correlation between vitreoretinal phenotypes and linkage to COL 2A1. Eye (Lond). 1994;8(Pt 6):609–14. https://doi.org/10.1038/eye.1994.153.
3. Richards AJ, Martin S, Yates JR, Scott JD, Baguley DM, Pope FM, et al. COL2A1 exon 2 mutations: relevance to the Stickler and Wagner syndromes. Br J Ophthalmol. 2000;84(4):364–71. https://doi.org/10.1136/bjo.84.4.364.
4. Richards AJ, Yates JR, Williams R, Payne SJ, Pope FM, Scott JD, et al. A family with Stickler syndrome type 2 has a mutation in the COL11A1 gene resulting in the substitution of glycine 97 by valine in alpha 1 (XI) collagen. Hum Mol Genet. 1996;5(9):1339–43. https://doi.org/10.1093/hmg/5.9.1339.
5. Sirko-Osadsa DA, Murray MA, Scott JA, Lavery MA, Warman ML, Robin NH. Stickler syndrome without eye involvement is caused by mutations in COL11A2, the gene encoding the alpha2(XI) chain of type XI collagen. J Pediatr. 1998;132(2):368–71. https://doi.org/10.1016/s0022-3476(98)70466-4.
6. Nikopoulos K, Schrauwen I, Simon M, Collin RW, Veckeneer M, Keymolen K, et al. Autosomal recessive Stickler syndrome in two families is caused by mutations in the COL9A1 gene. Invest Ophthalmol Vis Sci. 2011;52(7):4774–9. https://doi.org/10.1167/iovs.10-7128.

7. Baker S, Booth C, Fillman C, Shapiro M, Blair MP, Hyland JC, et al. A loss of function mutation in the COL9A2 gene causes autosomal recessive Stickler syndrome. Am J Med Genet A. 2011;155A(7):1668–72. https://doi.org/10.1002/ajmg.a.34071.
8. Faletra F, D'Adamo AP, Bruno I, Athanasakis E, Biskup S, Esposito L, et al. Autosomal recessive Stickler syndrome due to a loss of function mutation in the COL9A3 gene. Am J Med Genet A. 2014;164A(1):42–7. https://doi.org/10.1002/ajmg.a.36165.
9. Schrauwen I, Sommen M, Claes C, Pinner J, Flaherty M, Collins F, et al. Broadening the phenotype of LRP2 mutations: a new mutation in LRP2 causes a predominantly ocular phenotype suggestive of Stickler syndrome. Clin Genet. 2014;86(3):282–6. https://doi.org/10.1111/cge.12265.
10. Alzahrani F, Al Hazzaa SA, Tayeb H, Alkuraya FS. LOXL3, encoding lysyl oxidase-like 3, is mutated in a family with autosomal recessive Stickler syndrome. Hum Genet. 2015;134(4):451–3. https://doi.org/10.1007/s00439-015-1531-z.
11. Vu CD, Brown J Jr, Korkko J, Ritter R 3rd, Edwards AO. Posterior chorioretinal atrophy and vitreous phenotype in a family with Stickler syndrome from a mutation in the COL2A1 gene. Ophthalmology. 2003;110(1):70–7. https://doi.org/10.1016/s0161-6420(02)01446-x.
12. Donoso LA, Edwards AO, Frost AT. Ritter R, 3rd, Ahmad N, Vrabec T et al. Clinical variability of Stickler syndrome: role of exon 2 of the collagen COL2A1 gene. Surv Ophthalmol. 2003;48(2):191–203. https://doi.org/10.1016/s0039-6257(02)00460-5.
13. Richards AJ, McNinch A, Martin H, Oakhill K, Rai H, Waller S, et al. Stickler syndrome and the vitreous phenotype: mutations in COL2A1 and COL11A1. Hum Mutat. 2010;31(6):E1461–71. https://doi.org/10.1002/humu.21257.
14. Hagler WS, Crosswell HH Jr. Radial perivascular chorioretinal degeneration and retinal detachment. Trans Am Acad Ophthalmol Otolaryngol. 1968;72(2):203–16.
15. Stickler GB, Hughes W, Houchin P. Clinical features of hereditary progressive arthro-ophthalmopathy (Stickler syndrome): a survey. Genet Med. 2001;3(3):192–6. https://doi.org/10.1097/00125817-200105000-00008.
16. Abeysiri P, Bunce C, da Cruz L. Outcomes of surgery for retinal detachment in patients with Stickler syndrome: a comparison of two sequential 20-year cohorts. Graefes Arch Clin Exp Ophthalmol. 2007;245(11):1633–8. https://doi.org/10.1007/s00417-007-0609-2.
17. Carroll C, Papaioannou D, Rees A, Kaltenthaler E. The clinical effectiveness and safety of prophylactic retinal interventions to reduce the risk of retinal detachment and subsequent vision loss in adults and children with Stickler syndrome: a systematic review. Health Technol Assess. 2011;15(16):iii–xiv, 1–62. https://doi.org/10.3310/hta15160.
18. Ang A, Poulson AV, Goodburn SF, Richards AJ, Scott JD, Snead MP. Retinal detachment and prophylaxis in type 1 Stickler syndrome. Ophthalmology. 2008;115(1):164–8. https://doi.org/10.1016/j.ophtha.2007.03.059.
19. Szymko-Bennett YM, Mastroianni MA, Shotland LI, Davis J, Ondrey FG, Balog JZ, et al. Auditory dysfunction in Stickler syndrome. Arch Otolaryngol Head Neck Surg. 2001;127(9):1061–8. https://doi.org/10.1001/archotol.127.9.1061.
20. Acke FR, Malfait F, Vanakker OM, Steyaert W, De Leeneer K, Mortier G, et al. Novel pathogenic COL11A1/COL11A2 variants in Stickler syndrome detected by targeted NGS and exome sequencing. Mol Genet Metab. 2014;113(3):230–5. https://doi.org/10.1016/j.ymgme.2014.09.001.
21. Liberfarb RM, Goldblatt A. Prevalence of mitral-valve prolapse in the Stickler syndrome. Am J Med Genet. 1986;24(3):387–92. https://doi.org/10.1002/ajmg.1320240302.
22. Snead MP. Hereditary vitreopathy. Eye (Lond). 1996;10(Pt 6):653–63. https://doi.org/10.1038/eye.1996.158.
23. Fincham GS, Pasea L, Carroll C, McNinch AM, Poulson AV, Richards AJ, et al. Prevention of retinal detachment in Stickler syndrome: the Cambridge prophylactic cryotherapy protocol. Ophthalmology. 2014;121(8):1588–97. https://doi.org/10.1016/j.ophtha.2014.02.022.
24. Leiba H, Oliver M, Pollack A. Prophylactic laser photocoagulation in Stickler syndrome. Eye (Lond). 1996;10(Pt 6):701–8. https://doi.org/10.1038/eye.1996.164.
25. Marshall D. Ectodermal dysplasia; report of kindred with ocular abnormalities and hearing defect. Am J Ophthalmol. 1958;45(4 Pt 2):143–56.
26. Annunen S, Korkko J, Czarny M, Warman ML, Brunner HG, Kaariainen H, et al. Splicing mutations of 54-bp exons in the COL11A1 gene cause Marshall syndrome, but other mutations cause overlapping Marshall/Stickler phenotypes. Am J Hum Genet. 1999;65(4):974–83. https://doi.org/10.1086/302585.
27. Ayme S, Preus M. The Marshall and Stickler syndromes: objective rejection of lumping. J Med Genet. 1984;21(1):34–8. https://doi.org/10.1136/jmg.21.1.34.
28. Khan AO, Aldahmesh MA, Mohamed JY, Al-Mesfer S, Alkuraya FS. The distinct ophthalmic phenotype of Knobloch syndrome in children. Br J Ophthalmol. 2012;96(6):890–5. https://doi.org/10.1136/bjophthalmol-2011-301396.
29. Sertie AL, Sossi V, Camargo AA, Zatz M, Brahe C, Passos-Bueno MR. Collagen XVIII, containing an endogenous inhibitor of angiogenesis and tumor growth, plays a critical role in the maintenance of retinal structure and in neural tube closure (Knobloch syndrome). Hum Mol Genet. 2000;9(13):2051–8. https://doi.org/10.1093/hmg/9.13.2051.
30. Najmabadi H, Hu H, Garshasbi M, Zemojtel T, Abedini SS, Chen W, et al. Deep sequencing

reveals 50 novel genes for recessive cognitive disorders. Nature. 2011;478(7367):57–63. https://doi.org/10.1038/nature10423.
31. Aldahmesh MA, Khan AO, Mohamed JY, Alkuraya H, Ahmed H, Bobis S, et al. Identification of ADAMTS18 as a gene mutated in Knobloch syndrome. J Med Genet. 2011;48(9):597–601. https://doi.org/10.1136/jmedgenet-2011-100306.
32. Aldahmesh MA, Khan AO, Mohamed JY, Levin AV, Wuthisiri W, Lynch S, et al. No evidence for locus heterogeneity in Knobloch syndrome. J Med Genet. 2013;50(8):565–6. https://doi.org/10.1136/jmedgenet-2013-101755.
33. Maumenee IH, Traboulsi EI. The ocular findings in Kniest dysplasia. Am J Ophthalmol. 1985;100(1):155–60. https://doi.org/10.1016/s0002-9394(14)74998-0.
34. Weissenbacher G, Zweymueller E. [Simultaneous occurrence of the Pierre Robin syndrome and fetal chondrodysplasia]. Monatsschr Kinderheilkd. 1964;112:315–7.
35. Giedion A, Brandner M, Lecannellier J, Muhar U, Prader A, Sulzer J, et al. Oto-spondylo-megaepiphyseal dysplasia (OSMED). Helv Paediatr Acta. 1982;37(4):361–80.
36. Pihlajamaa T, Prockop DJ, Faber J, Winterpacht A, Zabel B, Giedion A, et al. Heterozygous glycine substitution in the COL11A2 gene in the original patient with the Weissenbacher-Zweymuller syndrome demonstrates its identity with heterozygous OSMED (nonocular Stickler syndrome). Am J Med Genet. 1998;80(2):115–20. https://doi.org/10.1002/(sici)1096-8628(19981102)80:2<115::aid-ajmg5>3.0.co;2-o.
37. Wagner H. Ein bisher unbekanntes Erbleiden des Auges (Degeneratio hyaloideo-retinalis hereditaria), beobachtet im Kanton Zurich. Klin Monatsbl Augenheilkd. 1938;100:840–57.
38. Perveen R, Hart-Holden N, Dixon MJ, Wiszniewski W, Fryer AE, Brunner HG, et al. Refined genetic and physical localization of the Wagner disease (WGN1) locus and the genes CRTL1 and CSPG2 to a 2- to 2.5-cM region of chromosome 5q14.3. Genomics. 1999;57(2):219–26. https://doi.org/10.1006/geno.1999.5766.
39. Mukhopadhyay A, Nikopoulos K, Maugeri A, de Brouwer AP, van Nouhuys CE, Boon CJ, et al. Erosive vitreoretinopathy and Wagner disease are caused by intronic mutations in CSPG2/Versican that result in an imbalance of splice variants. Invest Ophthalmol Vis Sci. 2006;47(8):3565–72. https://doi.org/10.1167/iovs.06-0141.
40. Miyamoto T, Inoue H, Sakamoto Y, Kudo E, Naito T, Mikawa T, et al. Identification of a novel splice site mutation of the CSPG2 gene in a Japanese family with Wagner syndrome. Invest Ophthalmol Vis Sci. 2005;46(8):2726–35. https://doi.org/10.1167/iovs.05-0057.
41. Brown DM, Graemiger RA, Hergersberg M, Schinzel A, Messmer EP, Niemeyer G, et al. Genetic linkage of Wagner disease and erosive vitreoretinopathy to chromosome 5q13-14. Arch Ophthalmol. 1995;113(5):671–5. https://doi.org/10.1001/archopht.1995.01100050139045.
42. Graemiger RA, Niemeyer G, Schneeberger SA, Messmer EP. Wagner vitreoretinal degeneration. Follow-up of the original pedigree. Ophthalmology. 1995;102(12):1830–9. https://doi.org/10.1016/s0161-6420(95)30787-7.
43. Meredith SP, Richards AJ, Flanagan DW, Scott JD, Poulson AV, Snead MP. Clinical characterisation and molecular analysis of Wagner syndrome. Br J Ophthalmol. 2007;91(5):655–9. https://doi.org/10.1136/bjo.2006.104406.
44. Rothschild PR, Burin-des-Roziers C, Audo I, Nedelec B, Valleix S, Brezin AP. Spectral-domain optical coherence tomography in Wagner syndrome: characterization of vitreoretinal interface and foveal changes. Am J Ophthalmol. 2015;160(5):1065–72.e1. https://doi.org/10.1016/j.ajo.2015.08.012.
45. Hirose T, Lee KY, Schepens CL. Snowflake degeneration in hereditary vitreoretinal degeneration. Am J Ophthalmol. 1974;77(2):143–53. https://doi.org/10.1016/0002-9394(74)90665-5.
46. Hejtmancik JF, Jiao X, Li A, Sergeev YV, Ding X, Sharma AK, et al. Mutations in KCNJ13 cause autosomal-dominant snowflake vitreoretinal degeneration. Am J Hum Genet. 2008;82(1):174–80. https://doi.org/10.1016/j.ajhg.2007.08.002.
47. Pollack A, Uchenik D, Chemke J, Oliver M. Prophylactic laser photocoagulation in hereditary snowflake vitreoretinal degeneration. A family report. Arch Ophthalmol. 1983;101(10):1536–9. https://doi.org/10.1001/archopht.1983.01040020538005.
48. Lee MM, Ritter R 3rd, Hirose T, Vu CD, Edwards AO. Snowflake vitreoretinal degeneration: follow-up of the original family. Ophthalmology. 2003;110(12):2418–26. https://doi.org/10.1016/S0161-6420(03)00828-5.
49. Hirose T, Wolf E, Schepens CL. Retinal functions in snowflake degeneration. Ann Ophthalmol. 1980;12(10):1135–46.
50. Kobayashi M, Takezawa S, Hara K, Yu RT, Umesono Y, Agata K, et al. Identification of a photoreceptor cell-specific nuclear receptor. Proc Natl Acad Sci U S A. 1999;96(9):4814–9. https://doi.org/10.1073/pnas.96.9.4814.
51. Cheng H, Khanna H, Oh EC, Hicks D, Mitton KP, Swaroop A. Photoreceptor-specific nuclear receptor NR2E3 functions as a transcriptional activator in rod photoreceptors. Hum Mol Genet. 2004;13(15):1563–75. https://doi.org/10.1093/hmg/ddh173.
52. Milam AH, Rose L, Cideciyan AV, Barakat MR, Tang WX, Gupta N, et al. The nuclear receptor NR2E3 plays a role in human retinal photoreceptor differentiation and degeneration. Proc Natl Acad Sci U S A. 2002;99(1):473–8. https://doi.org/10.1073/pnas.022533099.
53. Peng GH, Ahmad O, Ahmad F, Liu J, Chen S. The photoreceptor-specific nuclear receptor Nr2e3 interacts with Crx and exerts opposing effects on the tran-

scription of rod versus cone genes. Hum Mol Genet. 2005;14(6):747–64. https://doi.org/10.1093/hmg/ddi070.

54. Jacobson SG, Roman AJ, Roman MI, Gass JD, Parker JA. Relatively enhanced S cone function in the Goldmann-Favre syndrome. Am J Ophthalmol. 1991;111(4):446–53. https://doi.org/10.1016/s0002-9394(14)72379-7.
55. Jurklies B, Weismann M, Kellner U, Zrenner E, Bornfeld N. Clinical findings in autosomal recessive syndrome of blue cone hypersensitivity. Ophthalmologe. 2001;98(3):285–93. https://doi.org/10.1007/s003470170164.
56. Audo I, Michaelides M, Robson AG, Hawlina M, Vaclavik V, Sandbach JM, et al. Phenotypic variation in enhanced S-cone syndrome. Invest Ophthalmol Vis Sci. 2008;49(5):2082–93. https://doi.org/10.1167/iovs.05-1629.
57. Jacobson SG, Sumaroka A, Aleman TS, Cideciyan AV, Schwartz SB, Roman AJ, et al. Nuclear receptor NR2E3 gene mutations distort human retinal laminar architecture and cause an unusual degeneration. Hum Mol Genet. 2004;13(17):1893–902. https://doi.org/10.1093/hmg/ddh198.
58. Franceschetti A, Francois J, Babel J. Chorioretinal heredodegenerations. Springfield, IL: Charles C. Thomas; 1974.
59. Sharon D, Sandberg MA, Caruso RC, Berson EL, Dryja TP. Shared mutations in NR2E3 in enhanced S-cone syndrome, Goldmann-Favre syndrome, and many cases of clumped pigmentary retinal degeneration. Arch Ophthalmol. 2003;121(9):1316–23. https://doi.org/10.1001/archopht.121.9.1316.
60. Jacobson SG, Marmor MF, Kemp CM, Knighton RW. SWS (blue) cone hypersensitivity in a newly identified retinal degeneration. Invest Ophthalmol Vis Sci. 1990;31(5):827–38.
61. Roman AJ, Jacobson SG. S cone-driven but not S cone-type electroretinograms in the enhanced S cone syndrome. Exp Eye Res. 1991;53(5):685–90. https://doi.org/10.1016/0014-4835(91)90230-c.
62. Kaufman SJ, Goldberg MF, Orth DH, Fishman GA, Tessler H, Mizuno K. Autosomal dominant vitreoretinochoroidopathy. Arch Ophthalmol. 1982;100(2):272–8. https://doi.org/10.1001/archopht.1982.01030030274008.
63. Vincent A, McAlister C, Vandenhoven C, Heon E. BEST1-related autosomal dominant vitreoretinochoroidopathy: a degenerative disease with a range of developmental ocular anomalies. Eye (Lond). 2011;25(1):113–8. https://doi.org/10.1038/eye.2010.165.
64. Yardley J, Leroy BP, Hart-Holden N, Lafaut BA, Loeys B, Messiaen LM, et al. Mutations of VMD2 splicing regulators cause nanophthalmos and autosomal dominant vitreoretinochoroidopathy (ADVIRC). Invest Ophthalmol Vis Sci. 2004;45(10):3683–9. https://doi.org/10.1167/iovs.04-0550.
65. Marmorstein AD, Marmorstein LY, Rayborn M, Wang X, Hollyfield JG, Petrukhin K. Bestrophin, the product of the Best vitelliform macular dystrophy gene (VMD2), localizes to the basolateral plasma membrane of the retinal pigment epithelium. Proc Natl Acad Sci U S A. 2000;97(23):12758–63. https://doi.org/10.1073/pnas.220402097.

Hereditary Choroidal Dystrophy 16

Sang Jin Kim

Abstract

Hereditary choroidal dystrophies include central areolar choroidal dystrophy, gyrate atrophy of the choroid and retina, choroideremia, etc. Although traditionally these conditions have been classified as choroidal dystrophies, the primary pathogenic process is thought to occur in the retinal pigment epithelium, not in the choroid. The underlying genetic causes result in the degeneration of both the RPE and choroid. In gyrate atrophy, dietary modifications to lower ornithine levels may slow the progression of chorioretinal atrophy and improve cystoid macular edema. For the treatment of choroideremia, clinical trial of gene therapy using adeno-associated viral vector encoding REP1 is currently underway.

Keywords

Central areolar choroidal dystrophy
Choroideremia · Gyrate atrophy

S. J. Kim (✉)
Department of Ophthalmology, Samsung Medical Center, Sungkyunkwan University School of Medicine, Gangnam-gu, Seoul, Korea
e-mail: sangjinkim@skku.edu

16.1 Choroideremia

Choroideremia is an X-linked, recessive inherited chorioretinal disorder causing progressive degeneration of the retina, retinal pigment epithelium (RPE), and choroid [1–3]. Affected male patients develop night blindness with progressive peripheral vision loss and eventual central vision loss. Female carriers may be asymptomatic but may show patchy chorioretinal atrophy. *CHM* gene, which encodes Rab escort protein 1 (REP1) is a gene responsible for choroideremia.

16.1.1 Clinical Features

In patients with choroideremia, visual field constriction and vision loss is progressive leading to blindness. Typically, choroideremia patients show night blindness in their first or second decade of life, and in their third decade of life, patients report peripheral field constriction [4]. Central vision is preserved until later in life (usually until their 40s), resulting in tunnel vision [4]. Jolly et al. [5] reported that the median age for retaining 20/20 BCVA (best-corrected visual acuity) was 39 years. Around 60–70 years of age, patients show severe vision loss and often complete blindness.

Full-field ERG shows abnormal scotopic responses in choroideremia, which correlate symptomatically with a reduction in night vision. Later in life, cone cell dysfunction also occurs,

H.-G. Yu (ed.), *Inherited Retinal Disease*, https://doi.org/10.1007/978-981-16-7337-5_16

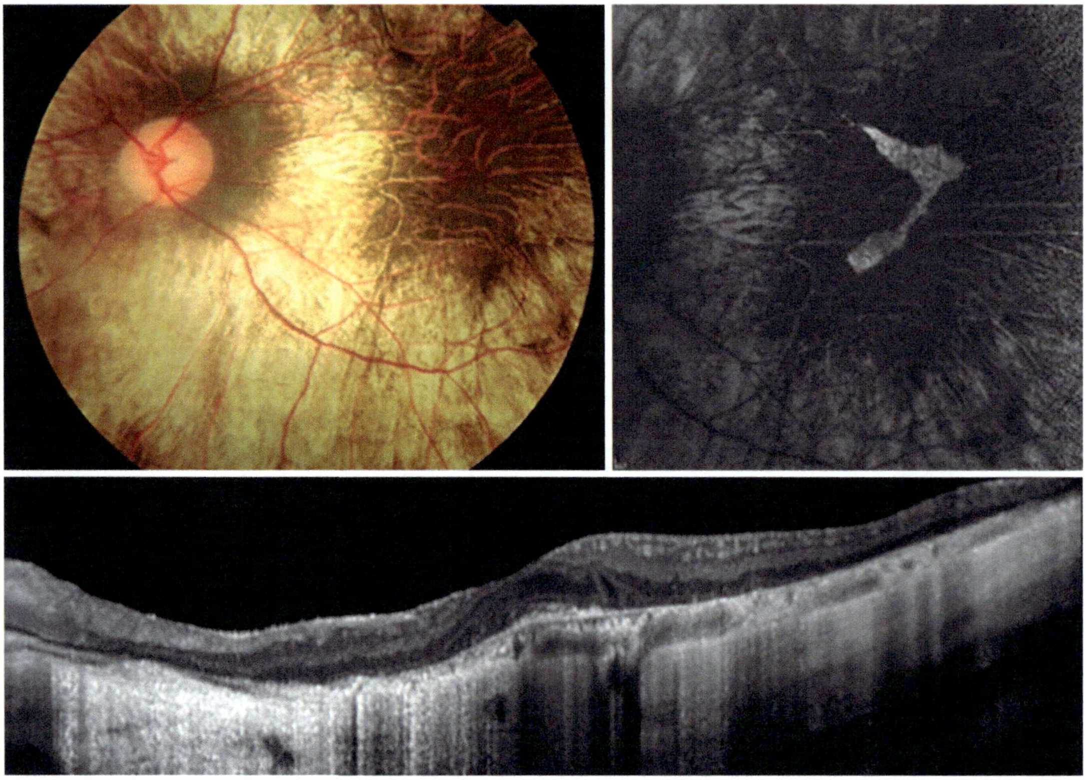

Fig. 16.1 (Top left) Color fundus photograph shows extensive chorioretinal atrophy in a 50-year-old male patient with choroideremia; (top right). Fundus autofluorescence reveals loss of RPE with sparing of the small macular area; (bottom) OCT shows thinning of choroid layer and outer retinal layers

resulting in abnormal photopic responses. Fundus autofluorescence (FAF) reveals areas of chorioretinal atrophy (Figs. 16.1 and 16.2) and is useful for evaluating disease progression. OCT shows decreased RPE reflectance and thinning of the outer retinal layers and further loss of RPE reflectivity (Figs. 16.1 and 16.2). Outer retinal tubulation on OCT is a common finding in choroideremia. Some patients develop cystoid macular edema, mostly located in the outer retinal layers. By combining FAF and OCT, the loss of both RPE and photoreceptors can be followed over time [4].

16.1.2 Molecular Genetics and Pathophysiology

CHM encodes Rab Escort Protein-1 (REP-1) which facilitates posttranslational modification of Rab proteins regulating intracellular trafficking. Various types of variants of the *CHM* gene have been identified in patients with choroideremia. These include small deletions, nonsense mutations, missense mutations, frameshift mutations, splice site defects, deletion of an exon, and deletion of the entire gene, causing truncation, loss of functional domain, or absence of REP-1 [6]. Subsequently, prenylation deficiency due to the absence of REP1 was identified as the cause of retinal degeneration in choroideremia.

Because choroideremia is often caused by large deletion of *CHM*, next-generation sequencing-based gene testing alone may not reveal *CHM* mutations. Therefore, for the molecular diagnosis of choroideremia, combined molecular genetic techniques including direct *CHM* sequencing and RNA (cDNA) sequencing as well as NGS-based approach should be considered [6].

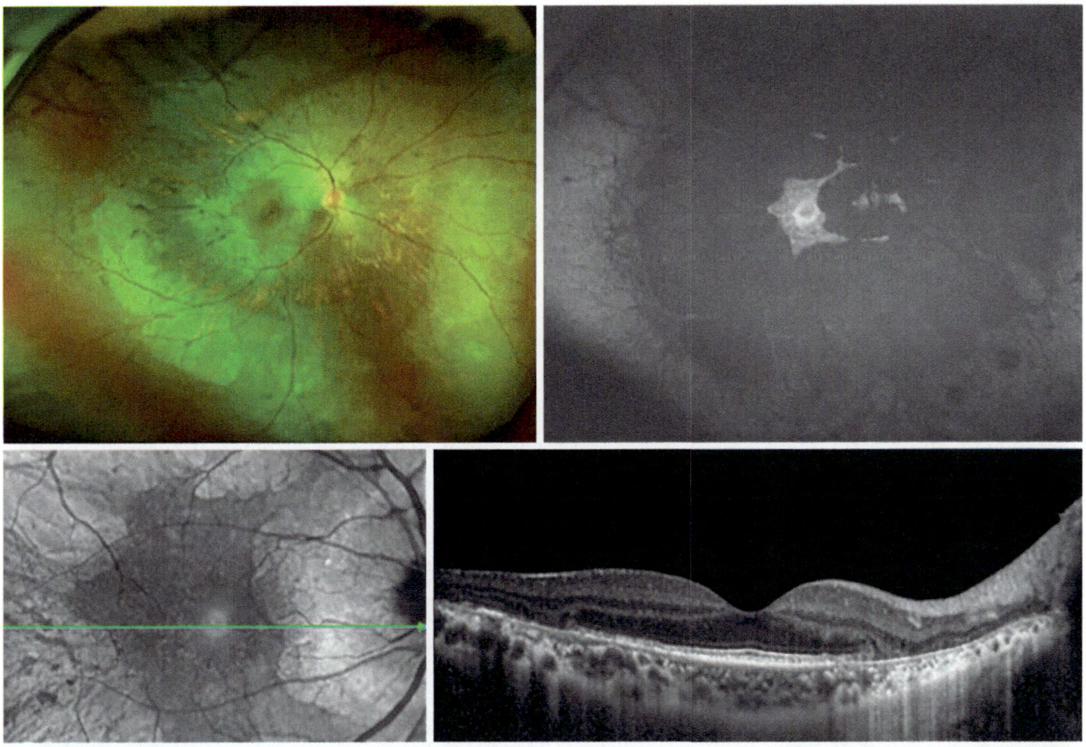

Fig. 16.2 (Top left) Ultra-wide-field fundus photograph shows extensive chorioretinal atrophy in a 30-year-old male patient with choroideremia; (top right). Ultra-wide-field Fundus autofluorescence reveals loss of RPE with sparing of the macular area; (bottom) OCT shows thinning of choroid layer and outer retinal layers. Compared to Fig. 16.1, this 30-year-old patient reveals more preserved area of retina and RPE on fundus photographs and OCT

16.1.3 Gene Therapy

Preclinical studies using animal models and human cells showed restoration of REP1 expression and function following AAV2-mediated gene delivery [7]. Clinical trials of gene therapy using adeno-associated viral vector encoding REP1 is currently underway. In 2014, the initial findings of phase 1/2 clinical trial of subfoveal administration of AAV-REP1 showed that gene delivery was successful that overcome any negative effects of temporary retinal detachment involving fovea [8]. In 2019, Fischer et al. [9] reported the results of phase 2 clinical trial to assess the safety and efficacy of retinal gene therapy with an AAV2 designed to deliver a functional version of the CHM gene (AAV2-REP1) for treatment of patients with choroideremia. In this study, among six participants, gene therapy with AAV2-REP1 was associated with maintenance or improvement of visual acuity, although no significant difference was found from control eyes. In another phase 2 trial using AAV2-REP1, Lam et al. [10] reported sustained improvement or maintenance of BCVA is achievable in choroideremia with high-dose AAV2-REP1. The safety profile of these clinical trials was fair. Further clinical trials are underway.

16.2 Gyrate Atrophy

Gyrate atrophy of the choroid and retina is an extremely rare autosomal recessive chorioretinal dystrophy. Mutation in the OAT gene causes deficiency of the enzyme ornithine aminotransferase with subsequent hyperornithinemia, which is toxic to choroid and RPE cells [11]. Patients with gyrate atrophy show night blindness and progressive visual field constriction with eventual blindness [11].

16.2.1 Clinical Features

Patients with gyrate atrophy present with night blindness and progressive visual field constriction in their first or second decade of life. Loss of central vision may occur in the fourth to fifth decades. The fundus findings of gyrate atrophy are quite characteristic: fundus showed well-demarcated chorioretinal atrophy that progressively coalesces together (Fig. 16.3). In most cases, the fundus finding of scalloped chorioretinal atrophy in the midperiphery with visible large choroidal vessels is sufficient to suspect gyrate atrophy. Patients with GA may also have (high) myopia and posterior subcapsular cataract. A gradual decrease in central vision occurs when the macula is involved or posterior subcapsular cataract develops. Macular abnormalities include cystoid macular edema (Fig. 16.4), foveoschisis, epiretinal membrane, and atrophy. According to the natural history study by Takki and Milton [12], visual acuities in phakic eyes tended to decrease from 20/30 to 20/200 in 10 years or less. Without the benefit of cataract surgery, the percentage of eyes with acuity 20/200 or worse

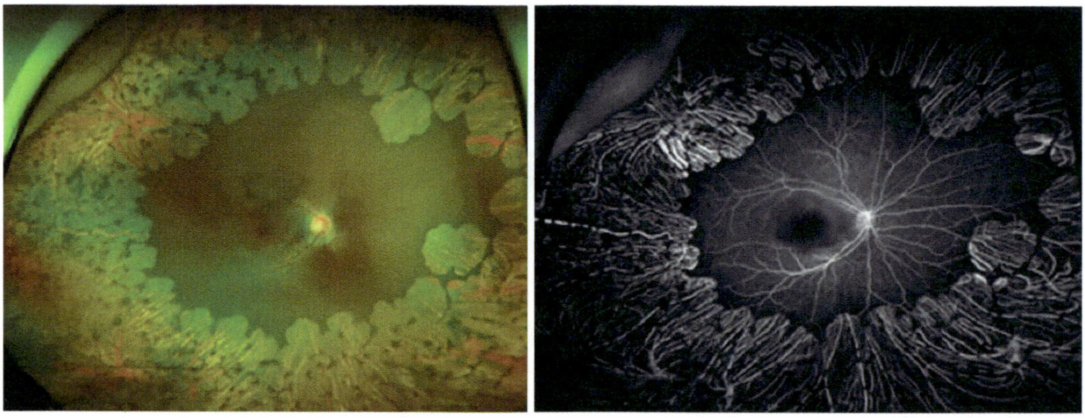

Fig. 16.3 Scalloped chorioretinal atrophy in the midperiphery with visible large choroidal vessels in a patient with gyrate atrophy

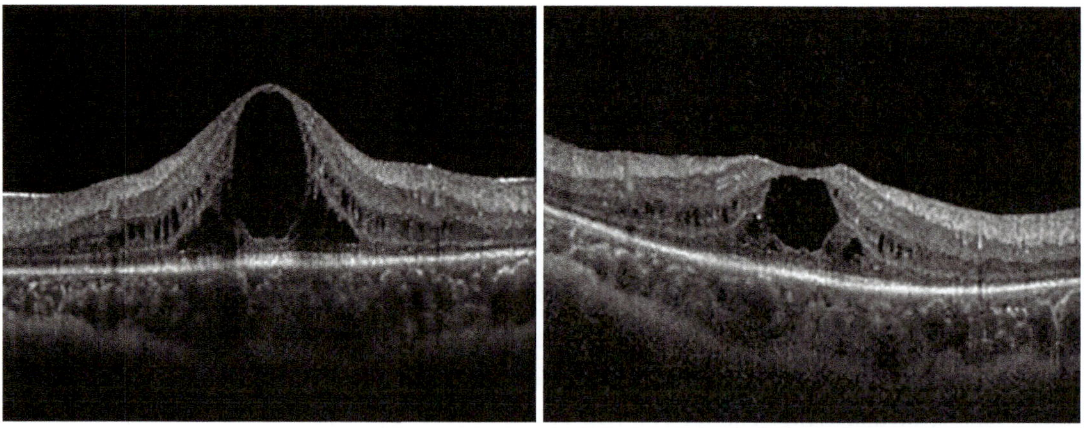

Fig. 16.4 (Left) Cystoid macular before dietary modifications in a patient with gyrate atrophy; (right) After arginine restriction, macular edema improved

would have been 37% at age 30 and 64% at age 40. Most patients usually show vision of less than 20/200 between 40 and 55 years of age due to chorioretinal atrophy [12].

16.2.2 Molecular Genetics and Pathophysiology

Gyrate atrophy of the choroid and retina results from mutations of the *OAT* gene on chromosome 10q26, leading to deficiency of the ornithine aminotransferase, a vitamin B6-dependent mitochondrial matrix enzyme, which normally metabolizes the amino acid ornithine into pyrroline-5-carboxylic acid. A deficiency of OAT leads to ornithine accumulation, with levels 10- to 20-fold above normal. There are more than 50 reported variants in the OAT gene that lead to gyrate atrophy. These mutations result in truncation of the enzyme, causing protein degradation. Accumulation of excessive ornithine occurs in the plasma, urine, cerebrospinal fluid, and aqueous humor. The toxic effects of hyperornithinemia on the RPEs may lead to progressive choriocapillaris atrophy which can be seen as characteristic chorioretinal degenerative patches on fundus examination [13].

Histopathologic studies revealed focal areas of atrophy of the photoreceptors with hyperplasia of the adjacent RPE [14]. The retina had focal areas of photoreceptor atrophy with adjacent RPE hyperplasia. An abrupt transition from the near-normal retina to a zone of near-total atrophy of the retina, RPE, and choroid was present.

16.2.3 Management of Gyrate Atrophy

Dietary modifications to lower ornithine levels can be helpful. Food rich in arginine includes nuts, seeds, dairy products, seafood, meat, chocolate, etc. The restriction of arginine in the diet, the precursor amino acid for ornithine, can effectively lower plasma ornithine levels and slow the progression of chorioretinal atrophy. Kaiser-Kupfer et al. [15, 16] reported that long-term reduction of ornithine with an arginine-restricted diet dramatically slowed the progression of gyrate atrophy and that If started at an early age, long-term substantial reduction of plasma ornithine levels might slow the progression of the chorioretinal lesions.

However, lowering plasma ornithine is not always successful in slowing the progression of chorioretinal degeneration. Vannas-Sulonen et al. [17] reported that despite the lowered plasma ornithine levels, electroretinographic changes progressed in two patients, and the chorioretinal atrophy progressed steadily in all the patients throughout the diet. This could be due to the genetic heterogeneity associated with gyrate atrophy.

Some patients with gyrate atrophy showed a significant decrease in mean plasma ornithine levels following vitamin B6 (pyridoxine) supplementation probably by increasing the activity of the pyridoxine-dependent OAT enzyme [18]. The dose of vitamin B6 supplementation used in studies is variable.

Dietary modifications to lower ornithine levels can also be helpful in treating cystoid macular edema. In addition, vitamin B6 supplementation, topical carbonic anhydrase inhibitors, topical NSAIDs, intravitreal or subtenon steroid injections, and intravitreal anti-VEGF agents might be effective [19, 20].

16.3 Central Areolar Choroidal Dystrophy (CACD)

Central areolar choroidal dystrophy (CACD) is a hereditary macular disorder characterized by progressive loss of photoreceptors and atrophy of RPE and choriocapillaris, resulting in paracentral or central scotoma and a decrease in visual acuity.

16.3.1 Genetics

CACD is mostly inherited as an autosomal dominant trait, although autosomal recessive cases have been reported. Autosomal dominant CACD is genetically heterogeneous, but *PRPH2* mutations have been frequently reported including p.Arg142Trp, p.Arg172Trp, p.Arg172Gln, p. Arg195Leu, and p.Leu307fsX83. GUCY2D also has been associated with CACD [21]. Hughes et al. reported a novel GUCY2D V933A mutation causing CACD [22].

Boon et al. [21] reported data of 103 patients with CACD from the Netherlands caused by *PRPH2* mutations (p.Arg142Trp and p. Arg172Gln). In this study, the mean age at onset of visual loss was 46 years and 98 patients carried a p.Arg142Trp mutation in *PRPH2*, whereas 5 affected members carried a p.Arg172Gln *PRPH2* mutation. Interestingly, nonpenetrance was seen up to the age of 64 years, in up to 21% of mutation carriers. The age at onset and phenotypic characteristics showed overlap with geographic atrophy in age-related macular degeneration. The authors concluded that CACD by a *PRPH2* p.Arg142Trp mutation caused a central cone dystrophy phenotype and in the elderly patient, CACD may be confused with AMD, especially in cases with decreased penetrance.

16.3.2 Pathogenesis

Boon et al. [21] proposed a pathophysiologic sequence of CACD caused by *PRPH2* mutation. The amino acid substitution by *PRPH2* mutation probably has a disturbing effect on peripherin/rds protein structure, resulting in dysmorphic cone and possibly rod outer segments, resulting in increased phagocytosis of the abnormal outer segments. This results in increased levels of lipofuscin and toxic byproducts in the RPE, resulting in RPE and photoreceptor cell death.

16.3.3 Ocular Features

In 1996, Hoyng and Deutman [23] described four clinical stages of CACD. In stage 1, slight parafoveal pigmentary RPE changes can be observed; In stage 2, RPE mottling encircling fovea; fundus autofluorescence (FAF) shows a speckled FAF pattern; In stage 3, atrophy of the choriocapillaris without central involvement; In stage 4, the atrophic area involves the fovea.

Paracentral scotoma may develop by the third or fourth decade, when parafoveal pigmentary changes may be visible. Over time, a depigmented macular lesion develops, which can be well-visualized on FAF. The RPE, choriocapillaris, and retina become atrophic in the affected lesions.

References

1. Rafuse EV, McCulloch C. Choroideremia. A pathological report. Can J Ophthalmol. 1968;3:347–52.
2. Rubin ML, Fishman RS, McKay RA. Choroideremia. Study of a family and literature review. Arch Ophthalmol. 1966;76:563–74.
3. van den Hurk JA, Schwartz M, van Bokhoven H, van de Pol TJ, Bogerd L, Pinckers AJ, et al. Molecular basis of choroideremia (CHM): mutations involving the Rab escort protein-1 (REP-1) gene. Hum Mutat. 1997;9:110–7.
4. Pennesi ME, Birch DG, Duncan JL, Bennett J, Girach A. CHOROIDEREMIA: retinal degeneration with an unmet need. Retina. 2019;39:2059–69.
5. Jolly JK, Xue K, Edwards TL, et al. Characterizing the natural history of visual function in choroideremia using microperimetry and multimodal retinal imaging. Invest Ophthalmol Vis Sci. 2017;58:5575–83.
6. Furgoch MJ, Mewes-Ares J, Radziwon A, Macdonald IM. Molecular genetic diagnostic techniques in choroideremia. Mol Vis. 2014;20:535–44.
7. Tolmachova T, Tolmachov OE, Barnard AR, et al. Functional expression of Rab escort protein 1 following AAV2-mediated gene delivery in the retina of choroideremia mice and human cells ex vivo. J Mol Med (Berl). 2013;91:825–37.
8. MacLaren RE, Groppe M, Barnard AR, Cottriall CL, Tolmachova T, Seymour L, et al. Retinal gene therapy in patients with choroideremia: initial findings from a phase 1/2 clinical trial. Lancet. 2014;383:1129–37.
9. Fischer MD, Ochakovski GA, Beier B, Seitz IP, Vaheb Y, Kortuem C, Reichel FFL, Kuehlewein L, Kahle NA, Peters T, Girach A, Zrenner E, Ueffing M, MacLaren RE, Bartz-Schmidt KU, Wilhelm B. Efficacy and safety of retinal gene therapy using adeno-associated virus vector for patients with choroideremia: a randomized clinical trial. JAMA Ophthalmol. 2019;137:1247–54.
10. Lam BL, Davis JL, Gregori NZ, MacLaren RE, Girach A, Verriotto JD, Rodriguez B, Rosa PR, Zhang X, Feuer WJ. Choroideremia gene therapy phase 2

clinical trial: 24-month results. Am J Ophthalmol. 2019;197:65–73.
11. Valle D, Kaiser-Kupfer MI, Del Valle LA. Gyrate atrophy of the choroid and retina: deficiency of ornithine aminotransferase in transformed lymphocytes. Proc Natl Acad Sci U S A. 1977;74:5159–61.
12. Takki KK, Milton RC. The natural history of gyrate atrophy of the choroid and retina. Ophthalmology. 1981;88:292–301.
13. Sergouniotis PI, Davidson AE, Lenassi E, Devery SR, Moore AT, Webster AR. Retinal structure, function, and molecular pathologic features in gyrate atrophy. Ophthalmology. 2012;119:596–605.
14. Wilson DJ, Weleber RG, Green WR. Ocular clinicopathologic study of gyrate atrophy. Am J Ophthalmol. 1991;111:24–33.
15. Kaiser-Kupfer MI, Caruso RC, Valle D. Gyrate atrophy of the choroid and retina. Long-term reduction of ornithine slows retinal degeneration. Arch Ophthalmol. 1991;109:1539–48.
16. Kaiser-Kupfer MI, Caruso RC, Valle D. Gyrate atrophy of the choroid and retina: further experience with long-term reduction of ornithine levels in children. Arch Ophthalmol. 2002;120:146–53.
17. Vannas-Sulonen K, Simell O, Sipilä I. Gyrate atrophy of the choroid and retina. The ocular disease progresses in juvenile patients despite normal or near normal plasma ornithine concentration. Ophthalmology. 1987;94:1428–33.
18. Michaud J, Thompson GN, Brody LC, Steel G, Obie C, Fontaine G, Schappert K, Keith CG, Valle D, Mitchell GA. Pyridoxine-responsive gyrate atrophy of the choroid and retina: clinical and biochemical correlates of the mutation A226V. Am J Hum Genet. 1995;56:616–22.
19. Heller D, Weiner C, Nasie I, Anikster Y, Landau Y, Koren T, Pokroy R, Abulafia A, Pras E. Reversal of cystoid macular edema in gyrate atrophy patients. Ophthalmic Genet. 2017;38:549–54.
20. Salvatore S, Fishman GA, Genead MA. Treatment of cystic macular lesions in hereditary retinal dystrophies. Surv Ophthalmol. 2013;58:560–84.
21. Boon CJ, Klevering BJ, Cremers FP, Zonneveld-Vrieling MN, Theelen T, Den Hollander AI, Hoyng CB. Central areolar choroidal dystrophy. Ophthalmology. 2009;116:771–82, 782.e1.
22. Hughes AE, Meng W, Lotery AJ, Bradley DT. A novel GUCY2D mutation, V933A, causes central areolar choroidal dystrophy. Invest Ophthalmol Vis Sci. 2012;53:4748–53.
23. Hoyng CB, Deutman AF. The development of central areolar choroidal dystrophy. Graefes Arch Clin Exp Ophthalmol. 1996;234:87–93.

Retinal Disorders Mimicking Inherited Retinal Diseases

17

Un Chul Park

17.1 Introduction

Various retinal conditions can mimic inherited retinal diseases, especially retinitis pigmentosa (RP). Some are phenocopies of RP, and they can be differentiated from RP based on careful fundus examination and thorough systemic review. Meanwhile, others are pseudo-RP diseases, which are not true genetic diseases but are panretinal damage caused by conditions other than heredity. A number of acquired conditions can present with diffuse chorioretinal atrophy which is very difficult to distinguish from advanced RP. Specific medical history and asymmetry of retinal degenerative change are important clues for differential diagnosis, which is critical because it can prevent the burden of genetic and prognostic counseling and some conditions may be treatable.

U. C. Park (✉)
Seoul National University College of Medicine, Jongno-gu, Seoul, Korea
e-mail: ucpark@snu.ac.kr

17.2 Phenocopies of Retinitis Pigmentosa

17.2.1 Pigmented Paravenous Chorioretinal Atrophy (PPCRA)

PPCRA is a rare form of chorioretinal atrophy which was first described as retinochoroiditis radiata in 1937 [1]. It is characterized by aggregations of pigment clumps and radial zones of retinal pigment epithelial atrophy that are distributed along the retinal veins [2]. It is usually bilateral and symmetric, but the proportion of patients with a markedly asymmetric pattern was 40% in a recent study. Patients are usually asymptomatic, but one-third of patients may have nyctalopia [3]. The diagnosis is primarily based on its characteristic fundus findings, but detailed multimodal retinal imaging and electrophysiology are helpful to confirm the diagnosis of PPCRA. When chorioretinal atrophy with bony spicule is extensively combined, it is likely to be mistaken for RP (Fig. 17.1).

The etiology of PPCRA is unknown, and inflammatory, genetic, and infectious causes have been suggested. Most cases develop sporadically, but there have been several cases of familial occurrence. One study reported a heterozygous *CRB1* mutation identified in a family with dominantly inherited PPCRA with variable expressivity [4]. Although there have been various speculations on the mode of inheritance, but there

H.-G. Yu (ed.), *Inherited Retinal Disease*, https://doi.org/10.1007/978-981-16-7337-5_17

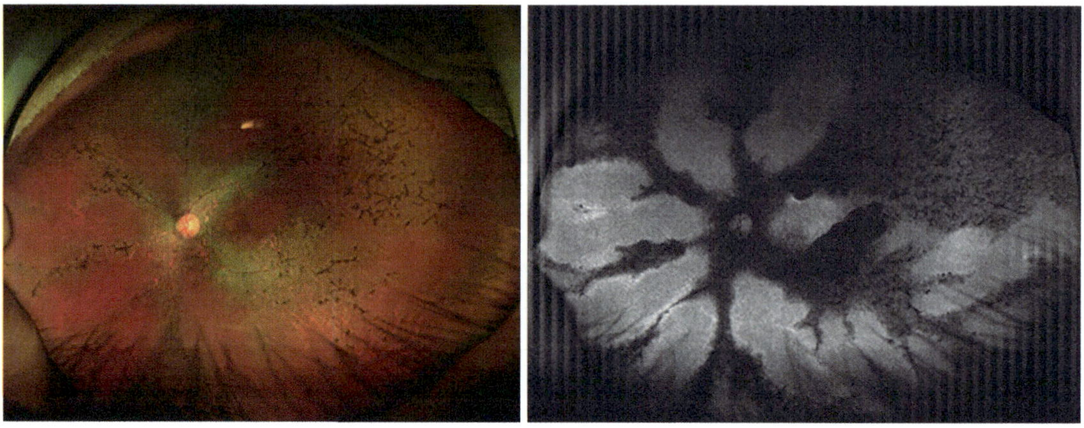

Fig. 17.1 Ultra-widefield fundus image and autofluorescence image of a 45-year-old female with pigmented paravenous chorioretinal atrophy

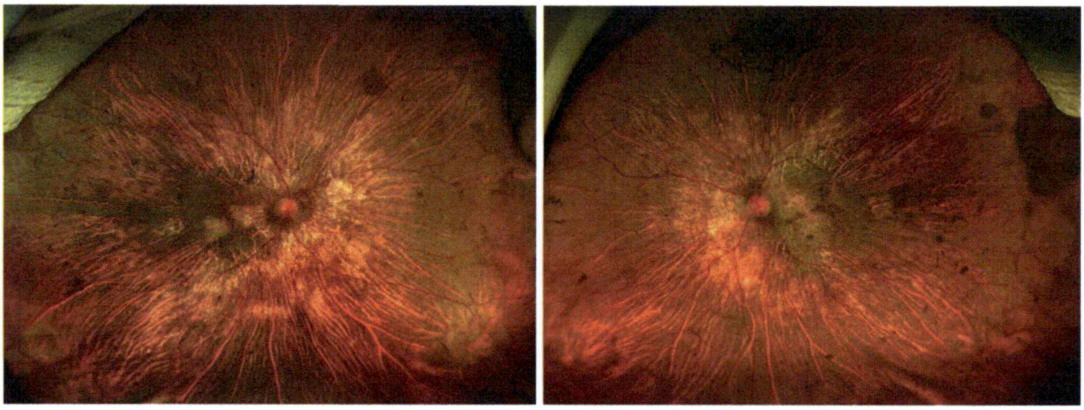

Fig. 17.2 Ultra-widefield fundus image of a 37-year-old male with choroideremia. He had pathogenic variants of *CHM* gene (c.315_318del, p.Ser105Argfs*20)

remains no convincing evidence. Meanwhile, early studies described PPCRA that developed after an inflammatory disease, including Behçet disease [5], measles [6], and uveitis [7]. Some studies have suggested that choroidal thinning or hypoperfusion is associated with the development of PPCRA [8].

17.2.2 Choroideremia

Choroideremia is rare chorioretinal dystrophy with an estimated prevalence of 1 in 50,000. This disease is inherited as an X-linked recessive trait and is caused by mutations in the *CHM* gene that encodes Rab Escort Protein 1 (REP1) [9]. As a result of loss of REP1 function, normal intracellular trafficking posttranscriptional lipid modification of Rab protein is disrupted leading to progressive degeneration of choroid, retinal pigment epithelium (RPE), and photoreceptors [10]. Clinically, male patients report nyctalopia in their first or second decade of life as the first symptom. In the fundus, fine pepper-like retinal pigment mottling at the mid-peripheral retina and posterior pole is observed. At a later stage, focal distinct regions of chorioretinal atrophy develop showing the exposure of bare sclera and eventual loss of overlying choroid and RPE (Fig. 17.2). Peripheral visual field loss progresses but central vision is substantially reduced later in their fifth or sixth decade of life.

Female carriers have considerable milder fundus changes compared to affected males [11]. Pigment mottling described as "moth-eaten appearance" is observed in the mid-peripheral retina, but the degree of pigmentary change is not associated with the age of carrier. They are usually asymptomatic but may show subtle changes in electroretinogram and dark adaptation.

17.2.3 Gyrate Atrophy of the Choroid and Retina

Gyrate atrophy of the choroid and retina is a rare choroidal disease with a prevalence of 1 in 50,000 in Finland. It was first described as an example of atypical retinitis pigmentosa in 1888 but was recognized as a distinct clinical entity later by Cutler and Fuchs. This disease is inherited as an autosomal recessive trait and caused by the absence of marked reduction in the enzyme ornithine-delta-aminotransferase, gene of which is located on chromosome 10. In patients with gyrate atrophy, plasma level of ornithine is increased up to 10–15 times of normal level. Patients experience poor night vision and constriction of peripheral vision which begin during the second or third decades. Fundus changes begin in the mid-peripheral retina as an RPE atrophic region with a scalloped border. Separate lesions become confluent as they progress both centrifugally and centripetally, eventually showing annular ring of choroidal atrophy sparing the macula. At an advanced stage, total choroidal atrophy leads to exposure of white sclera. Visual function depends on the extent of choroid involvement. A full-field electroretinogram may show mild abnormality during the early stage, but as the disease progresses, the responses may eventually become undetectable.

17.3 Pseudo-inherited Retinal Disease

17.3.1 Traumatic Retinopathy

Trauma is one of the most common etiologies of monocular blindness, especially in young people in their 20s and 30s. After blunt trauma, fundus may show retinal cloudiness and a creamy discoloration of the RPE which has been described as RPE edema or RPE contusion [12]. It may eventually result in depigmentation and pigment clumping at the affected region. Incidence of this RPE sequela in patients with history of blunt trauma was 20% in a recent multicenter study [13]. The RPE sequelae typically present as hyperpigmentation within the well-demarcated hypopigmented region, and optical coherence tomography shows loss of photoreceptors over abnormal RPE at the corresponding region. Although photoreceptors within the commotio retinae without RPE sequelae usually recover over time, permanent loss of photoreceptor and persistent visual field defect can occur in eyes with RPE sequelae. The presence of subretinal fluid was associated with the development of RPE sequelae during follow-up [13], and this may suggest that impaired barrier function of RPE due to mechanical damage to the RPE. When diffuse area of retina is affected by RPE sequelae, fundus finding may mimic inherited retinal disease, and thus, history of blunt trauma should be checked.

17.3.2 Autoimmune Retinopathy

Autoimmune retinopathy represents pathologic condition of retina caused by inflammation reaction to circulating autoantibodies against retinal antigens. It is characterized by otherwise unexplained vision loss accompanied by visual field defect and photoreceptor dysfunction. In autoimmune retinopathy, fundus often looks normal, though some may show diffuse retinal atrophy, waxy disc pallor, and attenuated retinal vessel. When pigmentary changes are also present, fundus with diffuse atrophic change may resemble advanced RP. Autoimmune retinopathy is almost bilateral, although involvement can be asymmetric. There is a female predominance. Diffuse retinal atrophy is observed in the majority of patients, while pigmentary deposits are observed in less than half of cases [14–16]. Patients manifest with subacute or acute vision loss, color vision change, constricted visual field, photopsia, and nyctalopia.

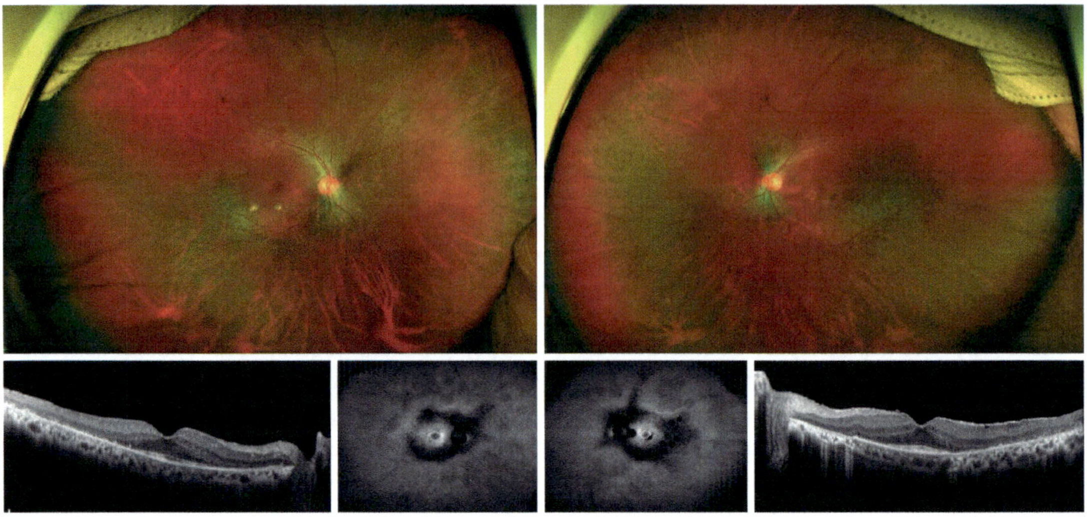

Fig. 17.3 Ultra-widefield fundus image, autofluorescence image, and optical coherence tomography (OCT) horizontal section image of a 62-year-old male with autoimmune retinopathy associated with multiple myeloma. Note the preserved foveal structure and outer retinal loss in the parafoveal area in OCT images, which resemble retinitis pigmentosa. His vision was 20/25 in both eyes

Autoimmune retinopathy can be categorized into two forms; paraneoplastic retinopathy which is associated with cancer or other malignancies and non-paraneoplastic retinopathy without any evidence of malignancy (Fig. 17.3). Cancers can produce remote effects on tissue without direct spread of tumor, and primary carcinoma of the lung is the most common cause [17]. Ophthalmologists should be aware of this condition so that they can prompt ancillary testing for cancers.

17.3.3 Retinal Infections

Some ocular manifestations of infectious diseases may be occasionally confused with RP, including rubella, syphilis, and toxoplasmosis, or herpes infection.

Rubella retinopathy is one of the most characteristic ocular manifestations of congenital rubella and can resemble fundus appearance of RP [18]. Pigmentary changes may be diffusely observed to the peripheral retina, while some patients only reveal speckling of pigment granules in the macula [19]. In particular, this confusion is more likely in children with congenital deafness due to rubella, because these can raise the suspicion for Usher syndrome. Correct differential diagnosis can be established based on clinical features and electroretinography, which is only mildly decreased in rubella retinopathy while patients with Usher syndrome may reveal severely decreased amplitude.

Congenital or acquired syphilis may also manifest as a pigmentary retinopathy that resemble the fundus appearance of advanced RP [20]. Interstitial keratitis is commonly observed in patients with congenital syphilis. Unlike typical bony spicule in RP, pigment deposits are clumps or large patches of black pigment in syphilis. Toxoplasmosis and herpes infection are rare causes of pigmentary retinopathy, but patches of retinal degeneration tend to be randomly distributed compared to typical RP.

17.3.4 Chronic Uveitis

As the term "retinitis pigmentosa" coined in nineteenth century implies, inflammation of the retina was initially believed to be the main pathogenesis of the disease. Although some features commonly observed in uveitic eyes, such as cystoid macular edema and increased aqueous flare, are also observed in patients with RP, these are secondary changes due to retinal degeneration. On the other hand, long-standing intraocular inflammation can result in a variety of posterior segment sequele, such as severe chorioretinal atrophy, extensive pigmentary changes, retinal vessel attenuation, disc pallor, and pigment clumping, which can mimic the fundus appearance of inherited retinal diseases such as RP [21]. Although early presentation of inherited retinal diseases and ocular inflammatory diseases are different, some patients with chronic intraocular inflammation, particularly when the disease has not been treated at its active phase, can present with fundus that could be confused with inherited retinal diseases (Fig. 17.4). Differentiation between the intraocular inflammatory disease and inherited retinal diseases is more challenging at an end-stage of uveitis because inflammatory activity has sometimes subsided or minimal. Therapeutic options are very different between inherited retinal diseases and uveitis, and precise diagnosis is important to provide optimal management to a patient. In particular, proper intervention can prevent further destruction of ocular tissue in patients with fundal change attributed to long-standing intraocular inflammation.

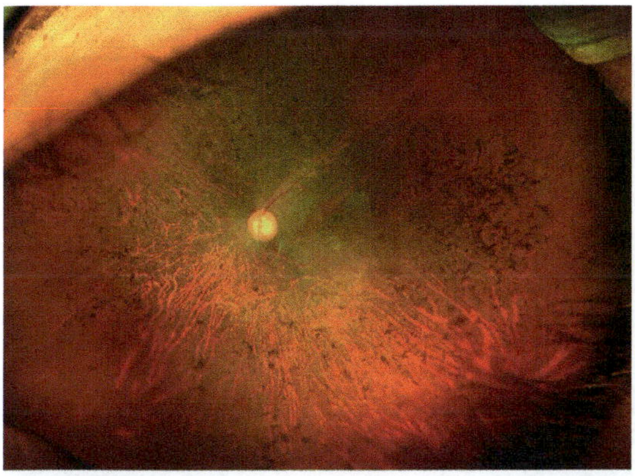

Fig. 17.4 Ultra-widefield fundus image of a 59-year-old male with Behçet disease. Note the diffuse pigmentary change and retinal vessel attenuation resembling retinitis pigmentosa

Because prognoses of uveitis and inherited retinal diseases differ very much, making precise and timely diagnosis is of great importance to prevent further chorioretinal destruction. It is important to maintain a high index of suspicion for the probability of chronic uveitis when a patient presents with extensive retinal atrophic or pigmentary changes. A careful review of past medical history, a detailed examination of signs for the previous intraocular inflammation, and ancillary testing are necessary to make a precise diagnosis. Some clues can be used to distinguish intraocular inflammatory disorder from the primary inherited retinal diseases. First, patients with uveitis show responses to treatment with corticosteroid or immunomodulatory agents, which are not generally expected in patients with inherited retinal diseases. Second, significant retinal vascular leakage or deep multifocal leakage on fluorescein angiography is more suggestive of uveitis than inherited retinal diseases [22], though the prevalence of retinal vascular or peripheral leakage was reported to range 17–60% [22, 23]. In addition, pigmentary change due to inflammation may be localized to a region where severe inflammation was present, and the localized pigmentation, especially for the extensively observed perivascular pigmentary and atrophic changes, may support a diagnosis of intraocular inflammation rather than inherited retinal diseases [22]. Peripheral visual field loss and dark adaptation abnormalities may suggest inherited retinal diseases rather than uveitis [24].

17.3.5 Drug Toxicity

A variety of systemic medications can result in fundus change with retinal toxicity. Progressive and permanent retinopathy retinal change associated with vision loss can occur even after cessation of causative drug in some instances. Various patterns of retinal toxicity have been described, and medications that can result in the disruption of the retina and RPE, such as chloroquine derivatives, thioridazine, and chlorpromazine, may mimic fundus appearance of inherited retinal diseases.

Chloroquine is used for the treatment of amebiasis, rheumatoid arthritis, and systemic lupus erythematosus. As a result of long-term use, usually, a total cumulative dose between 100 and 300 g, retinal toxicity with degeneration of the RPE and neurosensory retina can occur [25]. It binds to melanin and concentrates in the RPE and uveal tissues [26]. A paracentral scotoma may be the first manifestation of retinal toxicity and followed by ophthalmoscopic or electroretinographic abnormalities. Typical appearance of advanced chloroquine toxicity is a bull's eye maculopathy, and pigmentary changes with bony spicule may be observed in the mid-peripheral retina [27]. With the availability of hydroxychloroquine, which is less toxic, use of chloroquine has decreased.

Hydroxychloroquine can also result in identical retinal toxicity to chloroquine when used long-term, although its occurrence is much less common (Fig. 17.5) [28]. Currently, annual ophthalmologic examination including static perimetric visual field and at least one objective test among the spectral domain optical coherence tomography, multifocal electroretinogram, and fundus autofluorescence are recommended when the duration of use is longer than 5 years [29], particularly when daily dose is greater than 6.5 kg/mg/day [30]. Asian patients are more likely to have perifoveal retinopathy rather than central involvement. Coexisting kidney diseases and concurrent use of tamoxifen may increase the risk of hydroxychloroquine toxicity [31]. In most cases, the use of hydroxychloroquine should be stopped and alternative treatment options can be discussed with the prescribing physician.

Thioridazine binds to melanin and concentrates in the uveal tract and RPE and can cause pigmentary retinopathy that resembles fundus appearance of RP. Toxicity depends more on the daily dose rather than on the cumulative dose used, and a higher daily dose of thioridazine can result in rapid progression of toxicity even within several weeks [32]. Toxicity at daily dose of less than 800 mg is rare. At early stage, only mild granular pigment stippling or nummular area of RPE loss at posterior pole or mid-peripheral retina is observed [33]. At later stage, hyperpigmented plaques are seen within the widespread area of depigmentation and chorioretinal atrophy [34].

17.3.6 Unilateral Pigmentary Retinopathy

Although inherited retinal disease is usually bilateral and relatively symmetrical, there have been reports of unilateral RP in the literature [35]. A long-standing concept is that unilateral RP is a diagnosis of exclusion, and most reported cases were not genetically confirmed and had no evidence of inheritance. Several acquired retinal disorders such as inflammation or trauma can

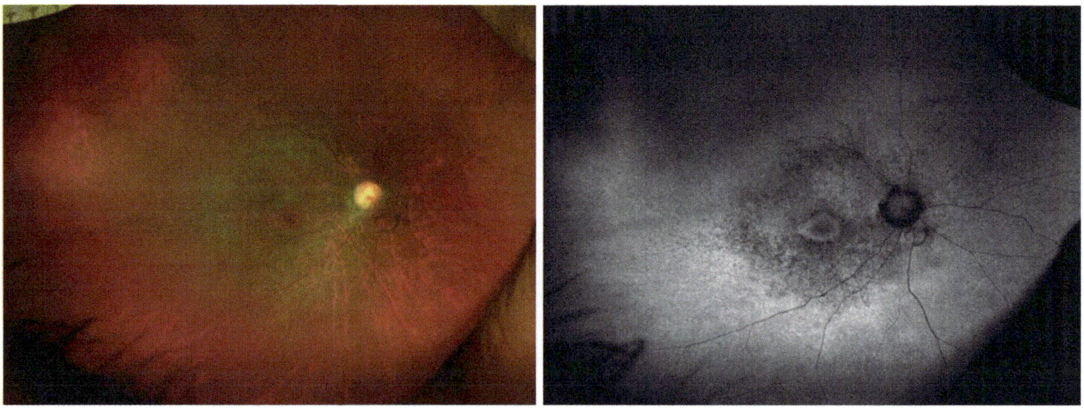

Fig. 17.5 Ultra-widefield fundus image and autofluorescence image of a 63-year-old female who had been on hydroxychloroquine for more than 10 years for the treatment of systemic lupus erythematosus

have fundoscopic features that resemble RP only in one eye, and other etiology includes birth trauma, choroidal melanoma [36], drug toxicity, ocular toxoplasmosis, and diffuse unilateral subacute neuroretinitis (DUSN) [37]. Although it is unclear, the mechanism of characteristic bony spicule appearance observed in RP, which is presumed to be inner migration of RPE triggered by direct contract between retinal vessels and RPE after photoreceptor loss and outer retinal degeneration, may also occur in pigmentary retinopathy secondary to other etiologies such as inflammation and trauma [38].

In a retrospective cohort study of 42 patients with unilateral pigmentary retinopathy, 36% of patients had relevant history or diagnosis that can explain the unilateral funduscopic finding, including acute zonal occult outer retinopathy, trauma, paraneoplastic syndrome, systemic autoimmune disease, retinal vasculitis, and choroidal ischemia during pregnancy [39]. Only two (4.8%) were identified as true RP depending on genetic tests showing mutation in *RP1* and *RPGR* genes. One possible cause of true unilateral RP may be mosaicism, in which a somatic mutation occurs only for precursor cells for unilateral retina during embryonic development [40]. In the remaining patients, electroretinography did not adhere to the typical RP pattern of more prominent impairment of rod function compared to cone, suggesting that hereditary pathogenesis is unlikely in those patients (Fig. 17.6).

Comprehensive electrophysiologic and clinical examinations are important to determine the etiology for this clinical situation, although most cases may remain idiopathic rather than hereditary.

17.3.7 Diffuse Unilateral Subacute Neuroretinitis (DUSN)

DUSN is a pan-retinal degeneration caused by the presence of a nematode in the subretinal space. This disease affects mostly young adults and causes severe unilateral vision loss, mimicking unilateral involvement of RP. At acute stage, the disease presents with subacute retini-

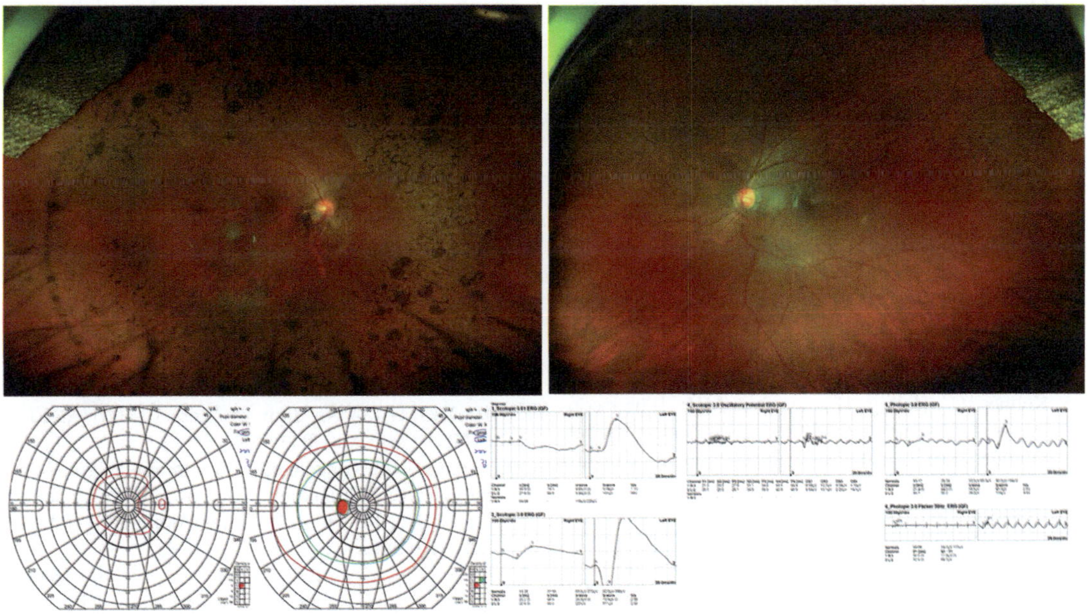

Fig. 17.6 Ultra-widefield fundus image, Goldmann perimetry, and full-field electroretinogram of a 58-year-old female with unilateral pigmentary retinopathy in her right eye. Visual acuity was 20/32 in the right eye and 20/20 in the left eye. Visual field in the right eye is constricted, and rod and cone responses were both decreased in the right eye. She denied any systemic disease or family history of retinal dystrophy

tis, optic disc swelling, mild to moderate vitritis, and retinal vessel narrowing. Main symptoms are floaters, central or paracentral scotoma, and ocular discomfort [41]. If the nematode is not recognized and the infection is not treated, this disease evolves to later stage. Diffuse pigmentary clumping, marked degenerative change of RPE, and progressive optic disc atrophy resembling the advanced RP development. Pigmentary change of DUSN is in the form of accumulation of medium to coarse clumping of pigment rather than bony spicule. Elevated gliotic mass in the mid-peripheral retina that represents the encased worm may be observed occasionally. Treatment of DUSN includes laser photocoagulation of the identified nematode during fundus examination [42] and systemic anti-helminthic drugs such as thiabendazole or ivermectin [43].

References

1. Brown TH. Retino-choroiditis radiata. Br J Ophthalmol. 1937;21(12):645–8. https://doi.org/10.1136/BJO.21.12.645.
2. Limaye SR, Mahmood MA. Retinal microangiopathy in pigmented paravenous chorioretinal atrophy. Br J Ophthalmol. 1987;71(10):757–61. https://doi.org/10.1136/BJO.71.10.757.
3. Lee EK, Lee SY, Oh BL, Yoon CK, Park UC, Yu HG. Pigmented paravenous chorioretinal atrophy: clinical spectrum and multimodal imaging characteristics. Am J Ophthalmol. 2021;224:120–32. https://doi.org/10.1016/J.AJO.2020.12.010.
4. McKay GJ, Clarke S, Davis JA, Simpson DAC, Silvestri G. Pigmented paravenous chorioretinal atrophy is associated with a mutation within the crumbs homolog 1 (CRB1) gene. Invest Ophthalmol Vis Sci. 2005;46(1):322–8. https://doi.org/10.1167/IOVS.04-0734.
5. Kellner U, Helbig H, Foerster MH. [Phenocopies of hereditary retinal degenerations]. Ophthalmologe. 1996;93(6):680–7. https://doi.org/10.1007/S003470050058
6. Peduzzi M, Guerrieri F, Torlai F, Prampolini ML. Bilateral pigmented paravenous retinochoroidal degeneration following measles. Int Ophthalmol. 1984;7(1):11–4. https://doi.org/10.1007/BF00138263.
7. Yamaguchi K, Hara S, Tanifuji Y, Tamai M. Inflammatory pigmented paravenous retinochoroidal atrophy. Br J Ophthalmol. 1989;73(6):463–7. https://doi.org/10.1136/BJO.73.6.463.
8. Cicinelli MV, Giuffrè C, Rabiolo A, Parodi MB, Bandello F. Optical coherence tomography angiography of pigmented paravenous retinochoroidal atrophy. Ophthalmic Surg Lasers Imaging Retina. 2018;49(5):381–3. https://doi.org/10.3928/23258160-20180501-14.
9. Kalatzis V, Hamel CP, Macdonald IM. Choroideremia: towards a therapy. Am J Ophthalmol. 2013;156(3):433–7.e3. https://doi.org/10.1016/J.AJO.2013.05.009
10. Preising M, Ayuso C. Rab escort protein 1 (REP1) in intracellular traffic: a functional and pathophysiological overview. Ophthalmic Genet. 2004;25(2):101–10. https://doi.org/10.1080/13816810490514333.
11. Sanchez-Alcudia R, Garcia-Hoyos M, Lopez-Martinez MA, et al. A comprehensive analysis of choroideremia: from genetic characterization to clinical practice. PLoS One. 2016;11(4):e0151943. https://doi.org/10.1371/JOURNAL.PONE.0151943.
12. Friberg TR. Traumatic retinal pigment epithelial edema. Am J Ophthalmol. 1979;88(1):18–21. https://doi.org/10.1016/0002-9394(79)90745-1.
13. Ahn SJ, Woo SJ, Park KH, Lee BR. Retinal pigment epithelium sequelae caused by blunt ocular trauma: incidence, visual outcome, and associated factors. Sci Rep. 2017;7(1):1–8. https://doi.org/10.1038/s41598-017-14659-4
14. Adamus G, Ren G, Weleber RG. Autoantibodies against retinal proteins in paraneoplastic and autoimmune retinopathy. BMC Ophthalmol. 2004;4:1–9. https://doi.org/10.1186/1471-2415-4-5.
15. Mantel I, Ramchand KV, Holder GE, et al. Macular and retinal dysfunction of unknown origin in adults with normal fundi: evidence for an autoimmune pathophysiology. Exp Mol Pathol. 2008;84(2):90–101. https://doi.org/10.1016/J.YEXMP.2007.10.006.
16. Weleber RG, Watzke RC, Shults WT, et al. Clinical and electrophysiologic characterization of paraneoplastic and autoimmune retinopathies associated with antienolase antibodies. Am J Ophthalmol. 2005;139(5):780–94. https://doi.org/10.1016/J.AJO.2004.12.104.
17. Chan JW. Paraneoplastic retinopathies and optic neuropathies. Surv Ophthalmol. 2003;48(1):12–38. https://doi.org/10.1016/S0039-6257(02)00416-2.
18. Cooper LZ, Krugman S. Clinical manifestations of postnatal and congenital rubella. Arch Ophthalmol. 1967;77(4):434–9. https://doi.org/10.1001/ARCHOPHT.1967.00980020436004.
19. Menne K. Kongenitale Rötelnretinopathie—eine progressive Erkrankung. Klin Monbl Augenheilkd. 2008;189(10):326–9. https://doi.org/10.1055/S--2008-1050812.
20. Cristiani R. [Sectorial pigmented retinopathy secondary to acquired syphilis]. Ann Ottalmol Clin Ocul. 1967;93(10):1099–108. https://pubmed.ncbi.nlm.nih.gov/5605815/. Accessed July 12, 2021.
21. Hamel C. Retinitis pigmentosa. Orphanet J Rare Dis. 2006;1(1):1–12. https://doi.org/10.1186/1750-1172-1-40

22. Sevgi DD, Davoudi S, Comander J, Sobrin L. Retinal pigmentary changes in chronic uveitis mimicking retinitis pigmentosa. Graefes Arch Clin Exp Ophthalmol. 2017;255(9):1801–10. https://doi.org/10.1007/S00417-017-3689-7.
23. Newsome DA. Retinal fluorescein leakage in retinitis pigmentosa. Am J Ophthalmol. 1986;101(3):354–60. https://doi.org/10.1016/0002-9394(86)90831-7.
24. Consugar MB, Navarro-Gomez D, Place EM, et al. Panel-based genetic diagnostic testing for inherited eye diseases is highly accurate and reproducible, and more sensitive for variant detection, than exome sequencing. Genet Med. 2014;17(4):253–61. https://doi.org/10.1038/gim.2014.172.
25. Tobin DR, Krohel GB, Rynes RI. Hydroxychloroquine: seven-year experience. Arch Ophthalmol. 1982;100(1):81–3. https://doi.org/10.1001/ARCHOPHT.1982.01030030083006.
26. Kellner U, Kellner S, Weinitz S. Chloroquine retinopathy: lipofuscin- and melanin-related fundus autofluorescence, optical coherence tomography and multifocal electroretinography. Doc Ophthalmol. 2007;116(2):119–27. https://doi.org/10.1007/S10633-007-9105-6.
27. Farag TI, Teebi AS. Bardet-Biedl and Laurence-Moon syndromes in a mixed Arab population. Clin Genet. 1988;33(2):78–82. https://doi.org/10.1111/J.1399-0004.1988.TB03414.X.
28. Levy GD, Munz SJ, Paschal J, Cohen HB, Pince KJ, Peterson T. Incidence of hydroxychloroquine retinopathy in 1,207 patients in a large multicenter outpatient practice. Arthritis Rheum. 1997;40(8):1482–6. https://doi.org/10.1002/ART.1780400817.
29. Mavrikakis I, Sfikakis PP, Mavrikakis E, et al. The incidence of irreversible retinal toxicity in patients treated with hydroxychloroquine: a reappraisal. Ophthalmology. 2003;110(7):1321–6. https://doi.org/10.1016/S0161-6420(03)00409-3.
30. Marmor MF, Carr RE, Easterbrook M, Farjo AA, Mieler WF. Recommendations on screening for chloroquine and hydroxychloroquine retinopathy: a report by the American Academy of Ophthalmology. Ophthalmology. 2002;109(7):1377–82. https://doi.org/10.1016/S0161-6420(02)01168-5.
31. Marmor MF, Kellner U, Lai TYY, Melles RB, Mieler WF, Lum F. Recommendations on screening for chloroquine and hydroxychloroquine retinopathy (2016 revision). Ophthalmology. 2016;123(6):1386–94. https://doi.org/10.1016/J.OPHTHA.2016.01.058.
32. Hagopian V, Stratton DB, Busiek RD. Five cases of pigmentary retinopathy associated with thioridazine administration. Am J Psychiatry. 1996;123(1):97–100. https://doi.org/10.1176/AJP.123.1.97.
33. Meredith TA, Aaberg TM, Willerson WD. Progressive chorioretinopathy after receiving thioridazine. Arch Ophthalmol. 1978;96(7):1172–6. https://doi.org/10.1001/ARCHOPHT.1978.03910060006002.
34. Miller FS, Bunt-Milam AH, Kalina RE. Clinical-ultrastructural study of thioridazine retinopathy. Ophthalmology. 1982;89(12):1478–88. https://doi.org/10.1016/S0161-6420(82)34613-8.
35. Farrell DF. Unilateral retinitis pigmentosa and cone-rod dystrophy. Clin Ophthalmol. 2009;3(1):263–70. https://doi.org/10.2147/OPTH.S5130.
36. Lommatzsch PK, Jensen OA, Prause JU, Bauke G. [Pseudoneuritis pigmentosa in malignant melanoma of the choroid]. Klin Monbl Augenheilkd. 1988;193(1):69–74. https://doi.org/10.1055/S--2008-1050226
37. Silveira C, Belfort R Jr, Nussenblatt R, et al. Unilateral pigmentary retinopathy associated with ocular toxoplasmosis. Am J Ophthalmol. 1989;107(6):682–4. https://doi.org/10.1016/0002-9394(89)90274-2.
38. Jaissle GB, May CA, van de Pavert SA, et al. Bone spicule pigment formation in retinitis pigmentosa: insights from a mouse model. Graefes Arch Clin Exp Ophthalmol. 2010;248(8):1063–70. https://doi.org/10.1007/S00417-009-1253-9.
39. Errera M-H, Robson AG, Wong T, et al. Unilateral pigmentary retinopathy: a retrospective case series. Acta Ophthalmol. 2019;97(4):e601–17. https://doi.org/10.1111/AOS.13981.
40. Poduri A, Evrony GD, Cai X, Walsh CA. Somatic mutation, genomic variation, and neurological disease. Science. 2013;341(6141). https://doi.org/10.1126/SCIENCE.1237758
41. Gass JDM, Gilbert WR, Guerry RK, Scelfo R. Diffuse unilateral subacute neuroretinitis. Ophthalmology. 1978;85(5):521–45. https://doi.org/10.1016/S0161-6420(78)35645-1.
42. Gass JDM, Braunstein RA. Further observations concerning the diffuse unilateral subacute neuroretinitis syndrome. Arch Ophthalmol. 1983;101(11):1689–97. https://doi.org/10.1001/ARCHOPHT.1983.01040020691004.
43. Gass JDM, Callanan DG, Bowman CB. Oral therapy in diffuse unilateral subacute neuroretinitis. Arch Ophthalmol. 1992;110(5):675–80. https://doi.org/10.1001/ARCHOPHT.1992.01080170097031.

Correction to: Other Macular Dystrophies 2

Correction to: Chapter 14 in: H.-G. Yu (ed.), Inherited Retinal Disease, https://doi.org/10.1007/978-981-16-7337-5_14

This chapter was inadvertently published with missing references in figures 14.1 and 14.2 which has now been corrected as below:

1) “Courtesy of Prof. Eun Kyoung Lee, Seoul National University, Seoul, Korea" has been added at the end of legends for figures 14.1 and 14.2.
2) New reference no. 36 "Song JS, BL Oh, UC Park, HG Yu, EK Lee. Autosomal Dominant Drusen Confirmed by Molecular Genetics. Journal of the Korean Ophthalmological Society 2021;62(1):120-126 has been added in pages 200, 201 and 206.
3) The references 36–54 were re-numbered sequentially due to addition of new reference 36 as mentioned in point 2.

The updated version of the book can be found at
https://doi.org/10.1007/978-981-16-7337-5_14

H.-G. Yu (ed.), *Inherited Retinal Disease*, https://doi.org/10.1007/978-981-16-7337-5_18

GPSR Compliance

The European Union's (EU) General Product Safety Regulation (GPSR) is a set of rules that requires consumer products to be safe and our obligations to ensure this.

If you have any concerns about our products, you can contact us on ProductSafety@springernature.com

In case Publisher is established outside the EU, the EU authorized representative is:

Springer Nature Customer Service Center GmbH
Europaplatz 3
69115 Heidelberg, Germany

Batch number: 10732801

Printed by Printforce, the Netherlands